Atlas of PET/CT in Pediatric Patients

Angelina Cistaro
Editor

Atlas of PET/CT in Pediatric Patients

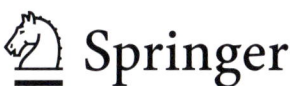 Springer

Editor
Angelina Cistaro
Department of Nuclear Medicine
Positron Emission Tomography Center
IRMET S.p.A.
Euromedic Inc.
Turin
Italy

Institute of Cognitive Sciences
and Technologies
National Research Council
Rome
Italy

Angelina Cistaro is Coordinator of the PET-Pediatric Study Intergroup of the Italian Association of Nuclear Medicine

ISBN 978-88-470-5357-1   ISBN 978-88-470-5358-8 (eBook)
DOI 10.1007/978-88-470-5358-8
Springer Milan Heidelberg New York Dordrecht London

Library of Congress Control Number: 2013947598

© Springer-Verlag Italia 2014
This work is subject to copyright. All rights are reserved by the Publisher, whether the whole or part of the material is concerned, specifically the rights of translation, reprinting, reuse of illustrations, recitation, broadcasting, reproduction on microfilms or in any other physical way, and transmission or information storage and retrieval, electronic adaptation, computer software, or by similar or dissimilar methodology now known or hereafter developed. Exempted from this legal reservation are brief excerpts in connection with reviews or scholarly analysis or material supplied specifically for the purpose of being entered and executed on a computer system, for exclusive use by the purchaser of the work. Duplication of this publication or parts thereof is permitted only under the provisions of the Copyright Law of the Publisher's location, in its current version, and permission for use must always be obtained from Springer. Permissions for use may be obtained through RightsLink at the Copyright Clearance Center. Violations are liable to prosecution under the respective Copyright Law.
The use of general descriptive names, registered names, trademarks, service marks, etc. in this publication does not imply, even in the absence of a specific statement, that such names are exempt from the relevant protective laws and regulations and therefore free for general use.
While the advice and information in this book are believed to be true and accurate at the date of publication, neither the authors nor the editors nor the publisher can accept any legal responsibility for any errors or omissions that may be made. The publisher makes no warranty, express or implied, with respect to the material contained herein.

Printed on acid-free paper

Springer is part of Springer Science+Business Media (www.springer.com)

To my children Simone Amedeo and Sylvia Teresa, for giving meaning to my life.
To the memory of my father, Domenico, who taught me what is important in life.
To my mother, Teresa, who helped me to become what I am and gave me the courage to embrace life.
For my brother and sisters, who preciously enriched my existence.
To the memory of a lost love.
To the love found again, who gives me strength each day.
For all of my young patients and their parents, for their trust, love, and generosity.
And finally, to my friends and colleagues, who patiently supported me throughout this project.
"Life is a sequence of breaths and beats to which we give our own interpretation."

Angelina Cistaro

Contents

Part I Basic Science and Practical Issues

1. The ^{18}F–FDG–Positron Emission Tomography/Computed Tomography Examination 3
   Andrea Skanjeti and Angelina Cistaro

2. Method and Patient Preparation 5
   Andrea Skanjeti and Angelina Cistaro

3. ^{18}F-FDG Administration and Dosimetry 13
   Andrea Skanjeti and Angelina Cistaro

4. Physiological Patterns and Pitfalls of ^{18}F-FDG Biodistribution 17
   Andrea Skanjeti and Angelina Cistaro

Part II Oncology

5. Malignant Lymphoma in Children 31
   Francesco Cicone and Stefania Uccini

6. ^{18}F-FDG–PET/CT in Pediatric Lymphoma 39
   Andrea Skanjeti, Luca Guerra, and Angelina Cistaro

7. Other Hematological Diseases (Leukemia) 61
   Angelina Cistaro

8. Primary Bone Tumors 67
   Natale Quartuccio and Angelina Cistaro

9. Utility of ^{18}F-FDG–PET/CT in Soft Tissue Sarcomas 87
   Somali Gavane, Angelina Cistaro, and Heiko Schoder

10. Primary Hepatic Tumors 93
    Natale Quartuccio and Angelina Cistaro

11. Neuroendocrine Tumors 103
    Egesta Lopci and Angelina Cistaro

12. Neuroblastoma 113
    Egesta Lopci, Umberto Ficola, and Angelina Cistaro

Part III Other Tumors

13 Pediatric Nasopharyngeal Carcinoma 131
Silvia Morbelli

14 Poorly Differentiated Thyroid Carcinoma 137
Somali Gavane and Heiko Schoder

15 Phylloid Tumor of the Breast 141
Mariapaola Cucinotta and Angelina Cistaro

16 Wilms' Tumor 143
Natale Quartuccio

17 Adrenal Gland Cancers 147
Natale Quartuccio and Angelina Cistaro

18 Ovarian Teratomas 151
Angelina Cistaro

Part IV Neurology

**19 Role of Amino Acid PET Tracers
in Pediatric Brain Tumors** 157
Arnoldo Piccardo and Giovanni Morana

**20 ^{18}F-FDG in the Imaging
of Brain Tumors** 165
Angelina Cistaro, Piercarlo Fania, and
Maria Consuelo Valentini

**21 PET/CT in the Clinical Evaluation
of Pediatric Epilepsy** 181
Valentina Garibotto, Maria Isabel Vargas,
Margitta Seeck, and Fabienne Picard

22 Epilepsia Partialis Continua 187
Silvia Morbelli

**23 Brain ^{18}F-FDG–PET/CT Imaging
in Hemolytic Uremic Syndrome During
and After the Acute Phase** 189
Riccardo Benti and Angelina Cistaro

Part V Infection and Inflammation

24 Inflammatory Bowel Diseases 199
Giorgio Treglia and Pierpaolo Alongi

25 Appendicitis 201
Mariapaola Cucinotta and Angelina Cistaro

26	**Spondylodiscitis**.. Mariapaola Cucinotta and Angelina Cistaro	205
27	**Other Bone Lesions**.................................... Angelina Cistaro	209
28	**Pulmonary Aspergillosis**.............................. Mariapaola Cucinotta and Angelina Cistaro	213
29	**Mycobacteriosis**....................................... Giorgio Treglia and Angelina Cistaro	217

Part VI Other Applications

30	**Sarcoidosis**... Giorgio Treglia and Angelina Cistaro	223
31	**Neurofibromatosis**.................................... Giorgio Treglia and Angelina Cistaro	229
32	**Autoimmune Lymphoproliferative Syndrome**.............. Angelina Cistaro	233
33	**Castleman's Disease**.................................. Mariapaola Cucinotta and Angelina Cistaro	241
34	**Fever of Unknown Origin**.............................. Alireza Mojtahedi, Daniele Penna, and Angelina Cistaro	245
35	**Congenital Hyperinsulinism**.......................... Vittoria Rufini and Milena Pizzoferro	249
36	**Myocardial Perfusion Imaging with ^{82}Rb Cardiac PET/CT**........................... Emmanuel Deshayes, Stefano Di Bernardo, and John O. Prior	253

Index... 259

Contributors

Pierpaolo Alongi Nuclear Medicine Unit, IRCCS Scientific Institute San Raffaele, Milan, Italy

Riccardo Benti Department of Nuclear Medicine, Fondazione IRCCS, Maggiore-Policlinico Mangiagalli Hospital, Regina Elena, Milan, Italy

Francesco Cicone Nuclear Medicine Department, Sant'Andrea Hospital, Faculty of Medicine and Psychology, "Sapienza" University of Rome, Rome, Italy

Angelina Cistaro Department of Nuclear Medicine, Positron Emission Tomography Center IRMET S.p.A., Euromedic Inc., Turin, Italy

Institute of Cognitive Sciences and Technologies, National Research Council, Rome, Italy

Mariapaola Cucinotta Nuclear Medicine Unit, Department of Radiological Sciences, Policlinico Gaetano Martino Hospital, University of Messina, Messina, Italy

Emmanuel Deshayes Department of Nuclear Medicine, Lausanne University Hospital, Lausanne, Switzerland

Stefano Di Bernardo Pediatric Catheterization Laboratory, Department of Pediatrics, Lausanne University Hospital, Lausanne, Switzerland

Piercarlo Fania Brain Tumors Project, San Paolo IMI Foundation for Neuroradiology Department, CTO Hospital, Turin, Italy

Umberto Ficola Nuclear Medicine Unit, La Maddalena Hospital, Palermo, Italy

Valentina Garibotto Nuclear Medicine Division, Department of Medical Imaging, Geneva University and Geneva University Hospitals, Geneva, Switzerland

Somali Gavane Nuclear Medicine Department, Memorial Sloan-Kettering Cancer Center, New York, NY, USA

Luca Guerra Nuclear Medicine Department, Azienda Ospedaliera San Gerardo di Monza, Monza (MI), Italy

Egesta Lopci Nuclear Medicine Unit, Humanitas Cancer Center, IRCCS Humanitas, Rozzano (MI), Italy

Alireza Mojtahedi Nuclear Medicine Department, Memorial Sloan-Kettering Cancer Center, New York, NY, USA

Giovanni Morana Unit of Pediatric Neuroradiology, Department of Radiology, G. Gaslini Children's Research Hospital, Genoa, Italy

Silvia Morbelli Nuclear Medicine Unit, IRCCS AOU San Martino – IST, Genoa, Italy

Daniele Penna Department of Nuclear Medicine, Positron Emission Tomography Center IRMET S.p.A., Euromedic Inc., Turin, Italy

Fabienne Picard EEG and Epilepsy Unit, Neurology Division, Department of Clinical Neurosciences, Geneva University and Geneva University Hospitals, Geneva, Switzerland

Arnoldo Piccardo Nuclear Medicine Department, E.O. Ospedali Galliera, Genoa, Italy

Milena Pizzoferro Unit of Nuclear Medicine, Department of Radiology, Bambino Gesù Children's Hospital, Rome, Italy

John O. Prior Department of Nuclear Medicine, Lausanne University Hospital, Lausanne, Switzerland

Natale Quartuccio Nuclear Medicine Unit, Department of Biomedical Sciences and Morphological and Functional Images, University of Messina, Messina, Italy

Vittoria Rufini Unit of Nuclear Medicine, Department of Radiological Sciences, Agostino Gemelli Hospital, Università Cattolica del Sacro Cuore, Rome, Italy

Heiko Schoder Nuclear Medicine Department, Memorial Sloan-Kettering Cancer Center, New York, NY, USA

Andrea Skanjeti Nuclear Medicine Division, San Luigi Gonzaga Hospital, University of Turin, Turin, Italy

Medical Science Department, University A. Avogadro, Novara, Italy

Margitta Seeck EEG and Epilepsy Unit, Neurology Division, Department of Clinical Neurosciences, Geneva University and Geneva University Hospitals, Geneva, Switzerland

Giorgio Treglia Department of Nuclear Medicine, Oncology Institute of Southern Switzerland, Bellinzona, Switzerland

Stefania Uccini Pathology Department, Sant'Andrea Hospital, Faculty of Medicine and Psychology, "Sapienza" University of Rome, Rome, Italy

Maria Consuelo Valentini Neuroradiology InterDepartment, CTO – M.Adelaide-OIRM – S.Anna Hospitals and San Giovanni Battista Hospital, Turin, Italy

Maria Isabel Vargas Neuroradiology Division, Department of Medical Imaging, Geneva University and Geneva University Hospitals, Geneva, Switzerland

Part I
Basic Science and Practical Issues

The ^{18}F-FDG–Positron Emission Tomography/Computed Tomography Examination

Andrea Skanjeti and Angelina Cistaro

Although the ^{18}F-FDG–PET/CT scan is a recently introduced imaging technique, it has rapidly become well established, particularly in patients with malignant disease. A CT scan concomitantly performed with ^{18}F-FDG–PET has two purposes: to correct the attenuation associated with PET and to provide a map of ^{18}F-FDG uptake. Both the sensitivity and the specificity of the imaging study are increased by this "happy marriage". ^{18}F-fluorodeoxyglucose (^{18}F- FDG) is a radio-labeled structural analogue of 2-deoxyglucose and therefore serves as a tracer of glucose metabolism. Three mechanisms of transport are responsible for the uptake of glucose, and thus of ^{18}F-FDG, into mammalian cells: (1) passive diffusion, (2) active transport in kidney epithelial cells and in the intestinal tract by a Na+-dependent glucose transporter (GLUT), and (3) a facultative GLUT mediated mechanism involving GLUT-1-13 enzymes [1]. Once ^{18}F-FDG has entered the cell, it is subsequently phosphorylated to FDG-6 phosphate by the enzyme hexokinase. In contrast to glucose-6-phosphate, FDG-6 phosphate is not a substrate for enzymes of either the glycolytic pathway or the pentose–phosphate shunt. Most tumors express only low levels of glucose-6-phosphatase, capable of reversing the phosphorylation of ^{18}F-FDG. In the absence of this enzyme, FDG-6 phosphate is trapped in the cell because it cannot be metabolized nor can it diffuse back into the extracellular space. In organs and cells with high concentrations of glucose-6-phosphatase, such as the liver, and in leukocytes, FDG-6 phosphate uptake decreases after a rapid initial accumulation.

Following its intravenous administration, 18F-FDG is preferably taken up in tissues with high glucose consumption. The tracer is filtered in the kidney glomeruli, with only a small amount reabsorbed by renal tubular cells. Rapid clearance of ^{18}F-FDG from the intravascular compartment results in a high target-to-background ratio within a short time (Fig. 1.1). High concentrations of ^{18}F-FDG accumulate in the brain, especially in the cortex and basal ganglia, whereas cardiac uptake is minimal and typically patchy. The accumulation of ^{18}F-FDG activity in urine interferes with the visualization of pelvic and, potentially, abdominal abnormalities. Circumscribed or diffuse gastrointestinal uptake may result from smooth muscle peristalsis. Uptake of ^{18}F-FDG in the reticuloendothelial system, especially in the bone marrow, varies [2]. Glucose is also strongly taken up by inflammatory cells, especially in response to inflammatory stimuli [3].

A. Skanjeti, MD
Nuclear Medicine Division, San Luigi Gonzaga Hospital, University of Turin, Regione Gonzole 10, 10043 Orbassano, Turin 10100, Italy

Medical Science Department,
University A. Avogadro, Novara, Italy
e-mail: askanjeti@yahoo.it

A. Cistaro, MD (✉)
Department of Nuclear Medicine, Positron Emission Tomography Center IRMET S.p.A., Euromedic Inc., Via Onorato Vigliani 89, Turin 10100, Italy

Institute of Cognitive Sciences and Technologies, National Research Council, Rome, Italy
e-mail: a.cistaro@irmet.com

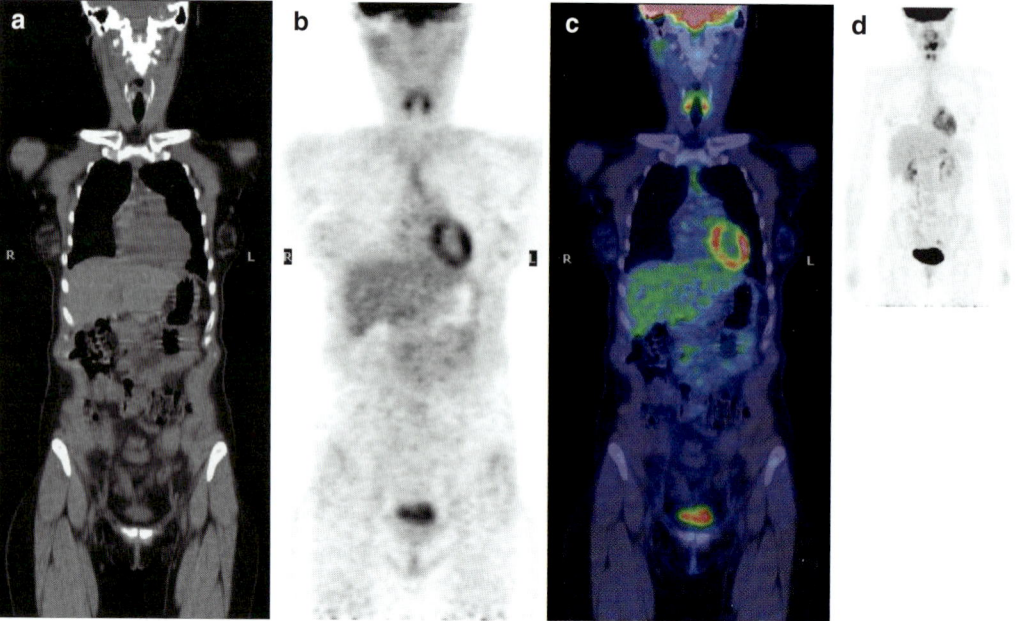

Fig. 1.1 Coronal CT (**a**), PET (**b**), and PET/CT fusion (**c**) images and (**d**) maximal intensity projection (MIP) show the physiological biodistribution of ^{18}F-FDG (Discovery ST-E PET/CT system, General Electric Healthcare, Milwaukee, WI. Images collected 60 min after intravenous injection of ^{18}F-FDG. At the time of the tracer injection, the patient had fasted for over 6 h, and his glucose blood level was 94 mg/dl. The data was acquired in 3D mode, with attenuation correction calculated by coregistered CT images)

In 1930, O. Warburg described what came to be known as the "Warburg effect", in which glucose uptake is enhanced in malignant cells due to their overexpression of glucose transporters and hexokinases [4]. Moreover, the tumoral stroma, made up of fibroblasts, glial cells, lymphocytes, macrophages, and dendritic cells, also accumulates glucose [5]. These observations underlie the use of the ^{18}F-FDG–PET/CT exam for the staging and restaging of a wide range of adult neoplasms, such as lymphoma, head and neck carcinoma, colon cancer, and lung cancer. However, this imaging modality is also able to localize other pathologies, among them, abdominal or pelvic abscesses and bone, joint, and soft tissue infections, including infected joint prostheses, as well as vasculitis, and tuberculosis. While most of these conditions are not common in the pediatric population, others, such as sarcomas, blastomas, lymphomas, post-transplantation lymphoproliferative diseases, cerebral tumors, spondylodiscitis, and aspergillosis, have been studied in children by mean of ^{18}F-FDG–PET/CT.

References

1. Shepherd PR, Kahn BB (1999) Glucose transporters and insulin action: implications for insulin resistance and diabetes mellitus. N Engl J Med 341:248–257
2. Meller J, Sahlmann CO, Scheel AK (2007) 18F-FDG-PET and PET/CT in fever of unknown origin. J Nucl Med 48:35–45
3. Jacobs DB, Lee TP, Jung CY, Mookerjee BK (1989) Mechanism of mitogen-induced stimulation of glucose transport in human peripheral blood mononuclear cells. J Clin Invest 83:437–443
4. Pauwels EK, Sturm EJ, Bombardieri E, Cleton FJ, Stokkel MP (2000) Positron-emission tomography with fluorodeoxyglucose. Part I. Biochemical uptake mechanism and its implication for clinical studies. J Cancer Res Clin Oncol 126:549–559
5. Kubota R, Yamada S, Kubota K, Ishiwata K, Tamahashi N, Ido T (1992) Intratumoral distribution of fluorine-18-fluorodeoxyglucose in vivo: high accumulation in macrophages and granulocytes studied by microautoradiography. J Nucl Med 33:1972–1980

Method and Patient Preparation

Andrea Skanjeti and Angelina Cistaro

Bilateral communication between the nuclear medicine physician and the child and his/her parents is essential to achieve good patient compliance as well as an accurate ^{18}F-FDG–PET/CT report. A detailed history, similar to that obtained from adult patients and including symptoms and complaints as well as a list of medications, is carefully acquired from the child and family. Additional clinical information, contained in the patient's medical record, includes the type of suspected or known primary tumor, the dates and results of previous imaging studies and therapies (surgery, chemotherapy, radiotherapy), the detection of morphological and/or functional abnormalities involving other organs, and potential drug interferences [1]. Instead of a conventional brain or total body scan (Fig. 2.1), in some cases, a more specific protocol will improve the study of a tumor confined to a single area of the body, for example, the oral cavity (Fig. 2.2) [2], or it may help to alleviate pain or discomfort, e.g., related to the presence of catheters or surgical instruments.

Since the patient must be in a fasting state beginning 4–6 h before the exam and for approximately 2 h during the exam and thereafter, the PET study should be scheduled early in the morning, shortly before breakfast, since, especially in children, a hungry patient is less likely to be compliant with the demands of the imaging study. A serum glucose level of 170 mg/dL in adults and 140 mg/dL in the pediatric patient is generally acceptable.

In case of hyperglycemia, PET has a lower sensitivity in revealing disease because ^{18}F-FDG competes with circulating glucose (Fig. 2.3) [1]. Thus, in children, once the typical diseases have been ruled out, if neoplasms involving the muscles (sarcomas) or other organs (e.g., hepatoblastoma) are suspected, an ^{18}F-FDG–PET/CT study is warranted but with aggressive control of serum glucose levels in order to optimize the accuracy of the study. In diabetic patients, this can be achieved with fast-acting insulin. If a good glycemic level proves to be challenging, we recommend the protocol used in our center: 250 mL of saline solution (NaCl 0.9 %) containing 100 IU fast-acting insulin/L is infused at a maximum rate of 50 mL/h until the serum glucose is reduced to a correct level. Thirty minutes later, the radiotracer is injected. For nursing infants, the injection should be administered before the next milk feed [3] which should be 20–30 min later.

A. Skanjeti, MD
Nuclear Medicine Division,
San Luigi Gonzaga Hospital, University of Turin,
Regione Gonzole 10, Orbassano 10043,
Turin 10100, Italy

Medical Science Department,
University A. Avogadro, Novara, Italy
e-mail: askanjeti@yahoo.it

A. Cistaro, MD (✉)
Department of Nuclear Medicine, Positron Emission Tomography Center IRMET S.p.A., Euromedic Inc.,
Via Onorato Vigliani 89, Turin 10100, Italy

Institute of Cognitive Sciences and Technologies,
National Research Council, Rome, Italy
e-mail: a.cistaro@irmet.com

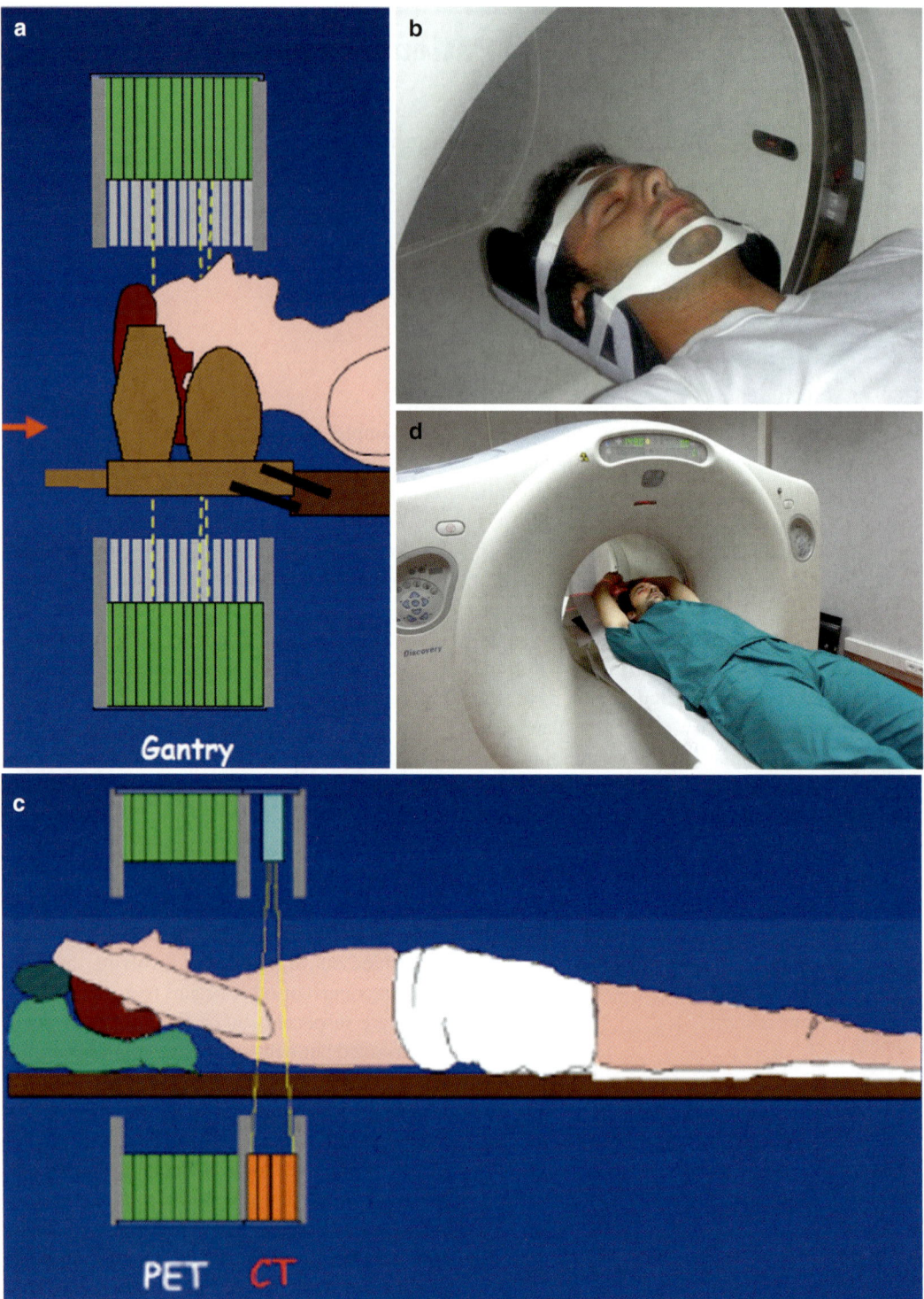

Fig. 2.1 Position of the patient during a brain study (**a**, **b**) and total body acquisition (**c**, **d**) (Discovery ST-E PET/CT system, General Electric Healthcare, Milwaukee, WI)

2 Method and Patient Preparation 7

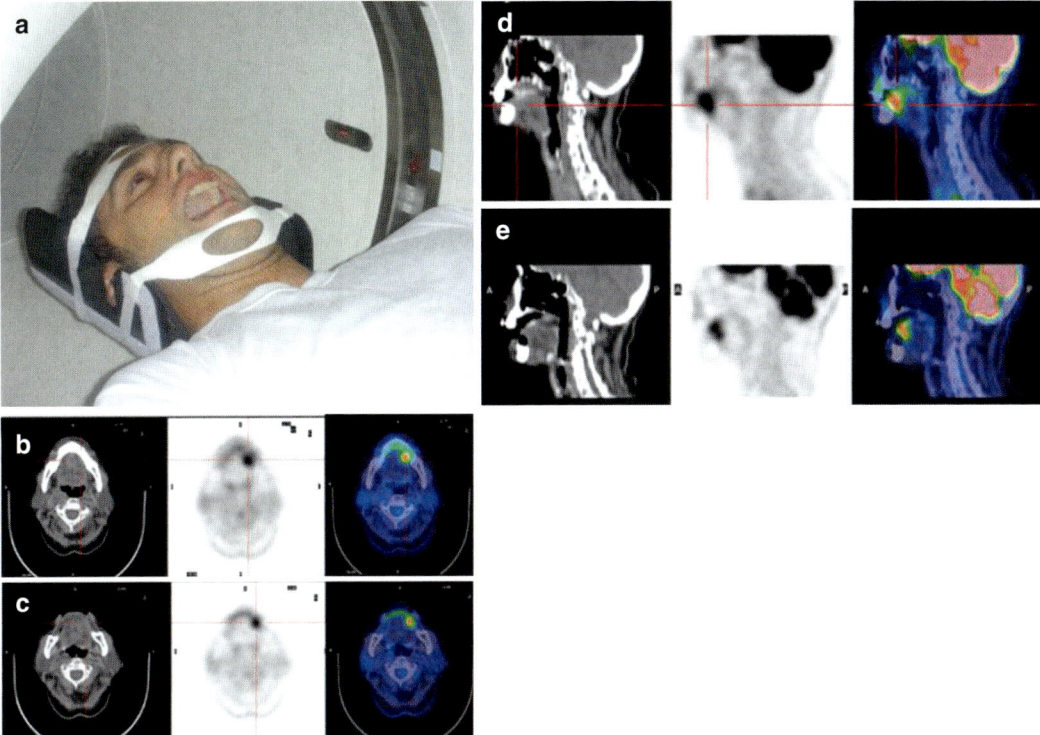

Fig. 2.2 (**a**) Open-mouth acquisition (Discovery ST-E PET/CT system, General Electric Healthcare, Milwaukee, WI). A 19-year-old male treated 10 years earlier for osteosarcoma of the tibia and now diagnosed with squamous carcinoma of the left border of the tongue. (**b**, **c**) Axial and sagittal projections of a conventional closed-mouth acquisition show pathological uptake in the left anterior mouth. Involvement of the mandibular bone or floor of the mouth is difficult to evaluate. (**d**, **e**) Axial and sagittal projections obtained in an open-mouth acquisition clearly show that the tumor is confined to the tongue

Both the child and his/her parents should be fully informed of the details of the imaging study, including the potential role of ^{18}F-FDG–PET/CT in disease management and the absolute and relative (vs. a common exam such as X-ray or CT scan) radiation doses. Given the complexity of the procedure for the patient and family, it is important to ensure that they fully understand the procedure as this will greatly facilitate compliance. Similarly, it is essential to establish a good relationship with the child before and after tracer injection. This relationship should be tailored to the child's developmental stage. A child who cries during the uptake phase will activate the diaphragm and intercostal muscles; continuous movement of the facial muscles, such as by chewing, during the uptake phase will activate the salivary glands and buccal cavity muscles (Fig. 2.4); in a child distracted by video games, the extraocular muscles and those of the upper limbs will be activated (Fig. 2.5). Also, the activation of brown adipose tissue, as will occur in a child who waits in a cold room during the uptake phase, must be avoided (Figs. 2.6 and 2.7). Brown adipose tissue is mostly present in the laterocervical regions of the neck, paravertebral thoracic regions, mediastinum, and epiphrenic area as well as around the kidneys and adrenal glands. Its activation can be mistakenly attributed to disease, leading to upstaging during the cancer staging phase and underestimation of the efficacy of therapy during treatment evaluation.

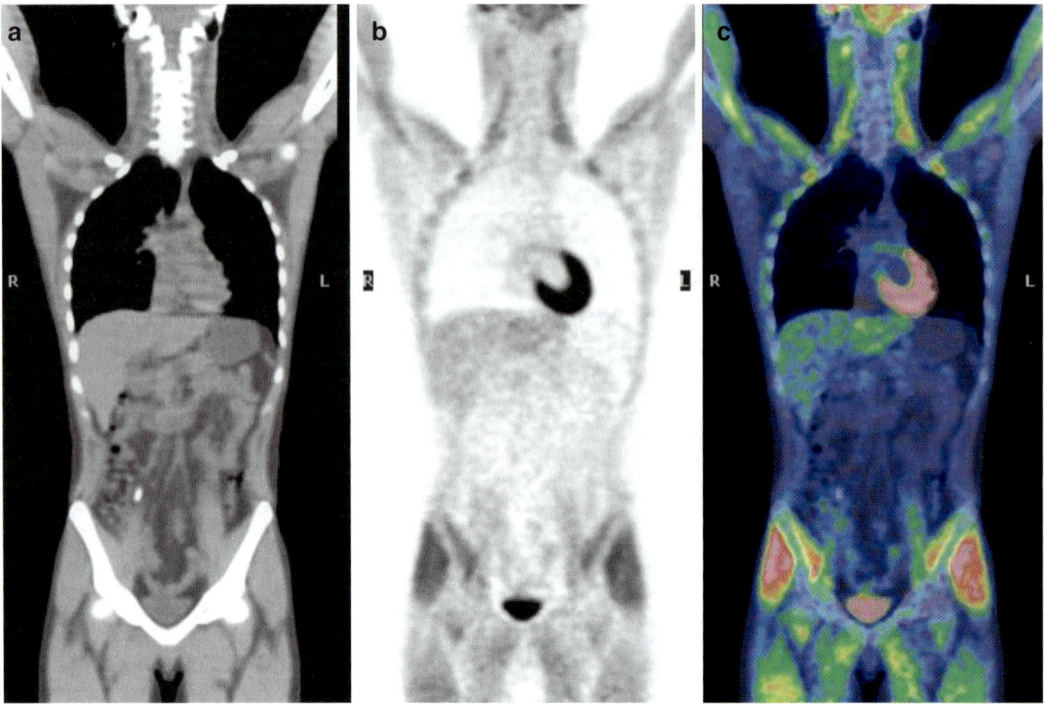

Fig. 2.3 A 17-year-old male treated for Ewing's sarcoma. The patient did not comply with the fasting requirement. Coronal CT (**a**), PET (**b**), and PET/CT (**c**) fusion images accordingly show diffuse ^{18}F-FDG uptake by the skeletal muscles

It is therefore crucial that during the uptake phase, the child minimizes his or her movements. This is best achieved by having a technician or parent distract and reassure the child, who should be seated in a comfortable chair inside a warm, quiet room. Anesthesia, sedation, and the use of benzodiazepines have been described in noncompliant children but this requires the relevant medications, equipment, and personnel to manage potential pediatric emergency situations. Recently, hypnosis has been shown to be effective in calming young patients.

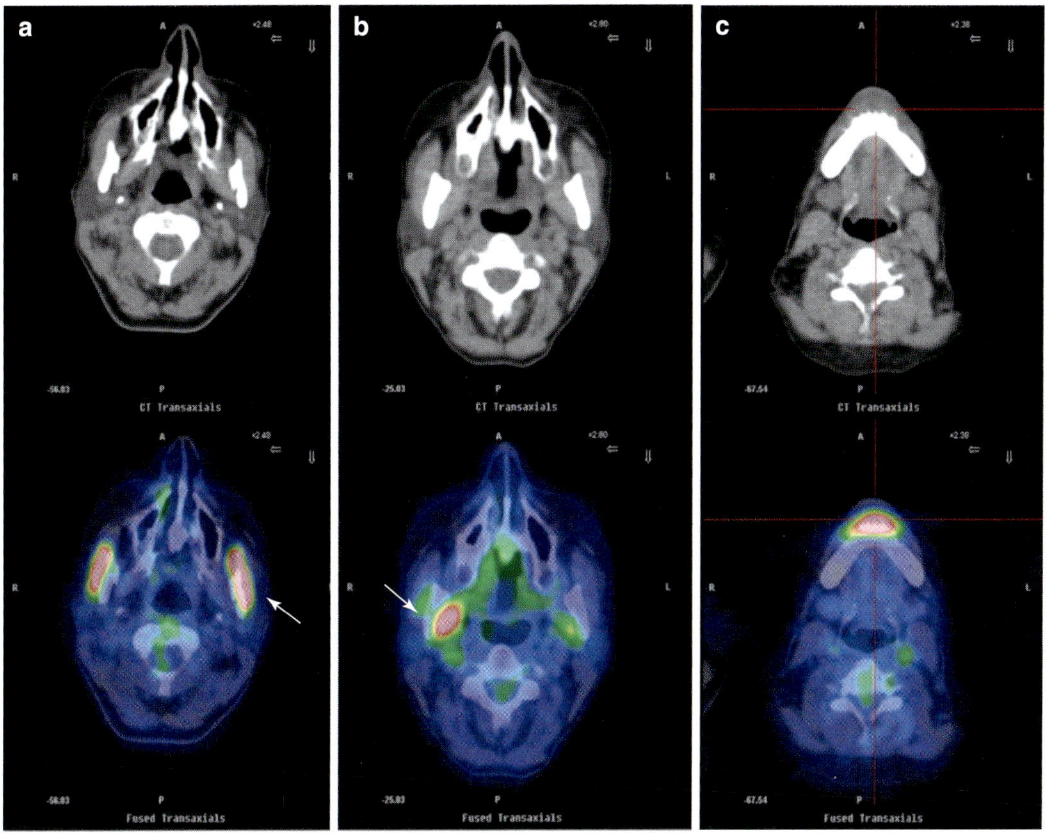

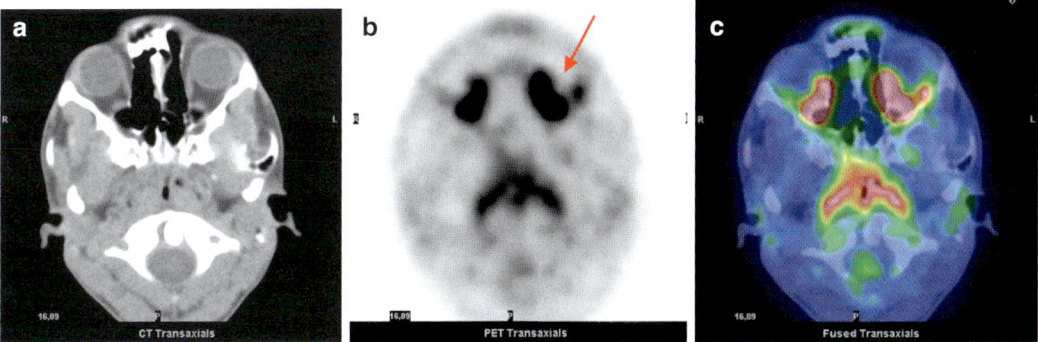

Fig. 2.4 Axial CT and PET/CT fusion images show uptake by the masseter (**a**), *by the* lateral pterygoid muscles (**b**), and (**c**) by the orbicular muscles of the mouth

Fig. 2.5 Axial CT (**a**), PET (**b**), and PET/CT fusion (**c**) images showing uptake by the extraocular muscles, especially the medial and lateral rectus muscles (*red arrow* in **b**). The patient had played a video game during the waiting time after the FDG injection

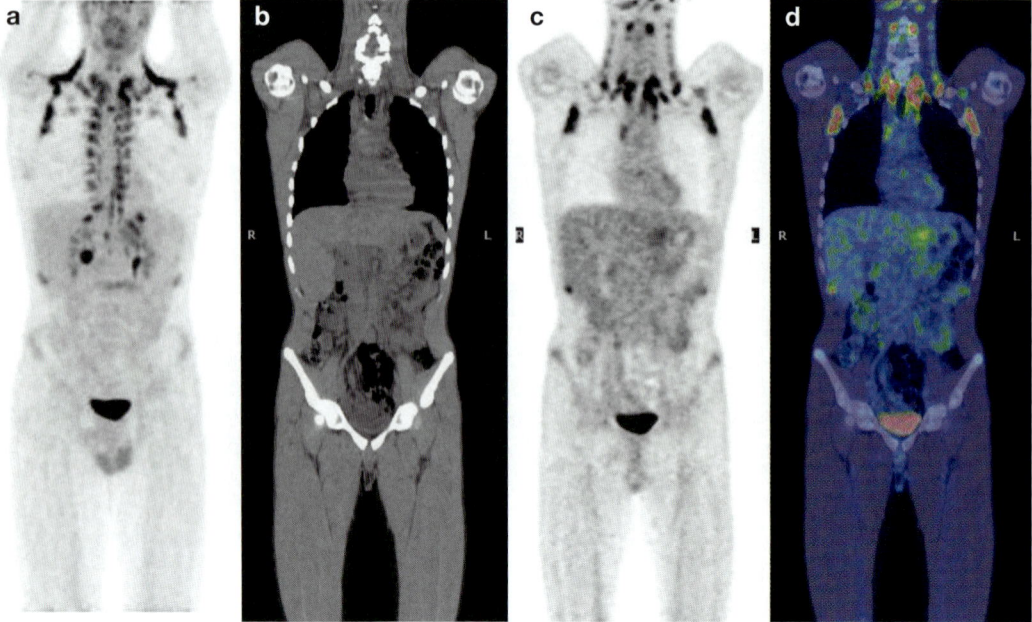

Fig. 2.6 Maximal intensity projection bilaterally showing laterocervical, supraclavicular, and axillary ^{18}F-FDG uptake (**a**). Coronal CT (**b**), PET (**c**), and PET/CT fusion (**d**) images show brown fat uptake in the laterocervical and supraclavicular regions

2 Method and Patient Preparation

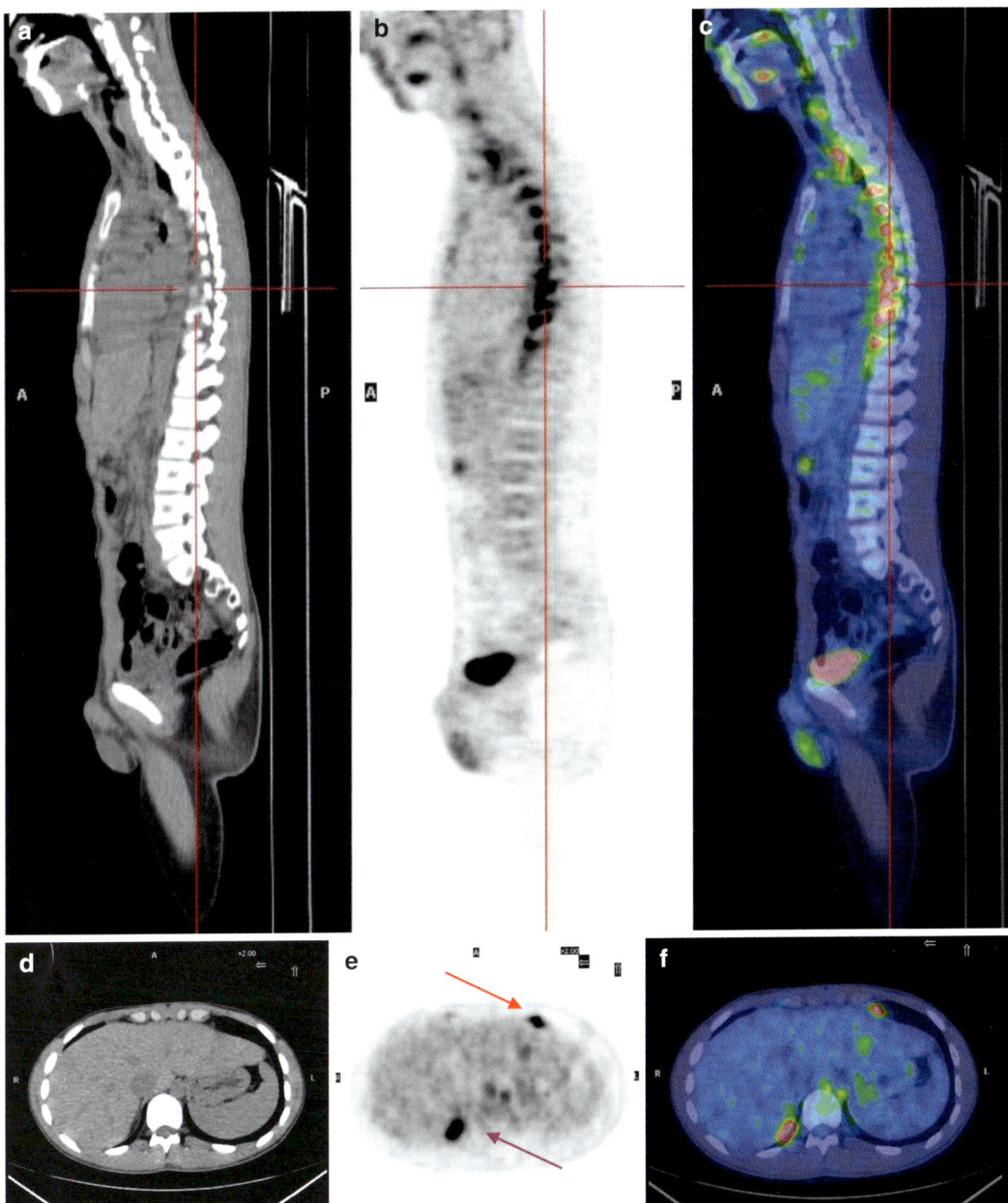

Fig. 2.7 The same patient as in Fig. 2.6. Sagittal CT (**a**), PET (**b**), and PET/CT fusion (**c**) images show brown fat uptake in the paravertebral regions. The axial CT (**d**), PET (**e**), and PET/CT fusion (**f**) images show focal FDG uptake in the anterior left (*red arrow* in **e**) and posterior right (*violet arrow* in **e**) epiphrenic region

References

1. Stauss J, Franzius C, Pfluger T, Juergens KU, Biassoni L, Begent J, Kluge R, Amthauer H, Voelker T, Højgaard L, Barrington S, Hain S, Lynch T, Hahn K, European Association of Nuclear Medicine (2008) Guidelines for 18F-FDG PET and PET-CT imaging in paediatric oncology. Eur J Nucl Med Mol Imaging 35:1581–1588
2. Cistaro A, Palandri S, Balsamo V, Migliaretti G, Pentenero M, Testa C, Cusmà S, Ceraudo F, Gandolfo S, Ficola U (2011) Assessment of a new 18F-FDG PET/CT protocol in the staging of oral cavity carcinomas. J Nucl Med Technol 39:7–13
3. Franzius C, Juergens KU (2009) PET/CT in paediatric oncology: indications and pitfalls. Pediatr Radiol 39(Suppl 3):446–449

^{18}F-FDG Administration and Dosimetry

3

Andrea Skanjeti and Angelina Cistaro

The dose to be administered to a child is dependent on his/her weight. While several institutions have their own dose recommendation [1], in our practice, we commonly use the dose suggested by the pediatric and dosimetry committees of the EANM [2], performing a 3D scan according to the same guidelines. Since the dosage must be adjusted to the time needed to acquire the scan, in some cases, a low dose of tracer can be compensated by increasing the acquisition time (taking into account the child's compliance). The pre- and postinjection levels of the tracer should be noted as well as the injection time as this will ensure accurate dosimetry in addition to allowing the synchronization of the dose calibrator and the PET scanner. Since intravenous access can be a serious problem in very young pediatric patients, nor do parents tolerate multiple access attempts [3], the most experienced staff should administer the injections. A better option is to establish a peripheral intravenous line before radiotracer injection as this will also avoid dose extravasation. Alternatively, a central venous line may be advantageous, in which case we advise abundant flushing with saline solution to avoid significant residual activity. In fact, the line should be thoroughly rinsed with saline before tracer injection and the tracer should be "pushed" with saline after the injection to avoid artifacts arising from a bolus of tracer in the line wall (Figs. 3.1 and 3.2). In addition, the line should be heparinized.

Pediatric radiation dosimetry recommendations are contained in the ICRP guidelines, which identified the bladder wall as the critical organ for the effective dose received (range: 25.6–50.5 mGy varying on the basis of the body weight with a maximum administered FDG activity of 370 MBq for large-size children weighting ≥70 kg). In ^{18}F-FDG–PET/CT, due to the high energy of photons emitted after tracer disintegration, radiation exposure to individuals accompanying the child must be considered. A good compromise is, for example, the presence of only one parent and not the child's siblings during the uptake phase. The acquisition parameters of the CT scan should be tailored to the patient's size. Those used in our center are 60–80 mA, 80–140 kV, and a helical pitch of 3.75:1. A 30–50 % reduction in exposure of the child patient relative to that of an adult will not

A. Skanjeti, MD
Nuclear Medicine Division,
San Luigi Gonzaga Hospital, University of Turin,
Regione Gonzole 10, Orbassano 10043,
Turin 10100, Italy

Medical Science Department,
University A. Avogadro, Novara, Italy
e-mail: askanjeti@yahoo.it

A. Cistaro, MD (✉)
Department of Nuclear Medicine,
Positron Emission Tomography Center
IRMET S.p.A., Euromedic Inc.,
Via Onorato Vigliani 89, Turin 10100, Italy

Institute of Cognitive Sciences and Technologies,
National Research Council, Rome, Italy
e-mail: a.cistaro@irmet.com

cause an important loss of information. After the scan is completed, a fast review of the exam is recommended before the child leaves the scanning bed in order to avoid movements during the acquisition that can provoke the necessity to repeat it.

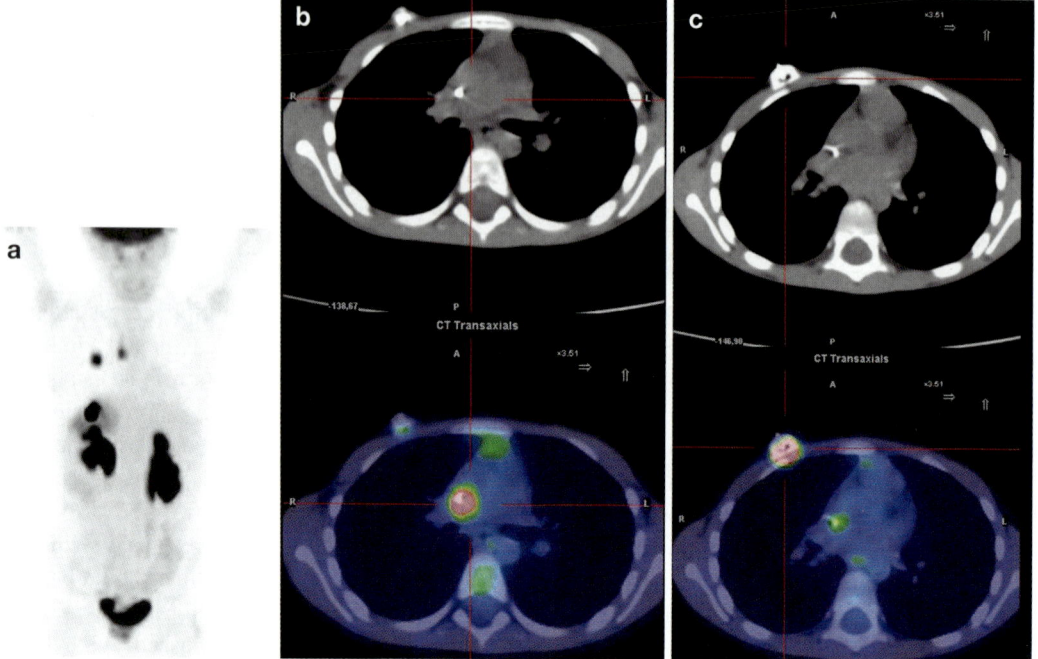

Fig. 3.1 (**a**) Maximal intensity projection showing focal ^{18}F-FDG uptake in the mediastinum and right lung. (**b**, **c**) Axial CT and PET/CT fusion images show mediastinal uptake at the summit of the central venous line (**b**) and tracer stasis in the catheter reservoir (**c**)

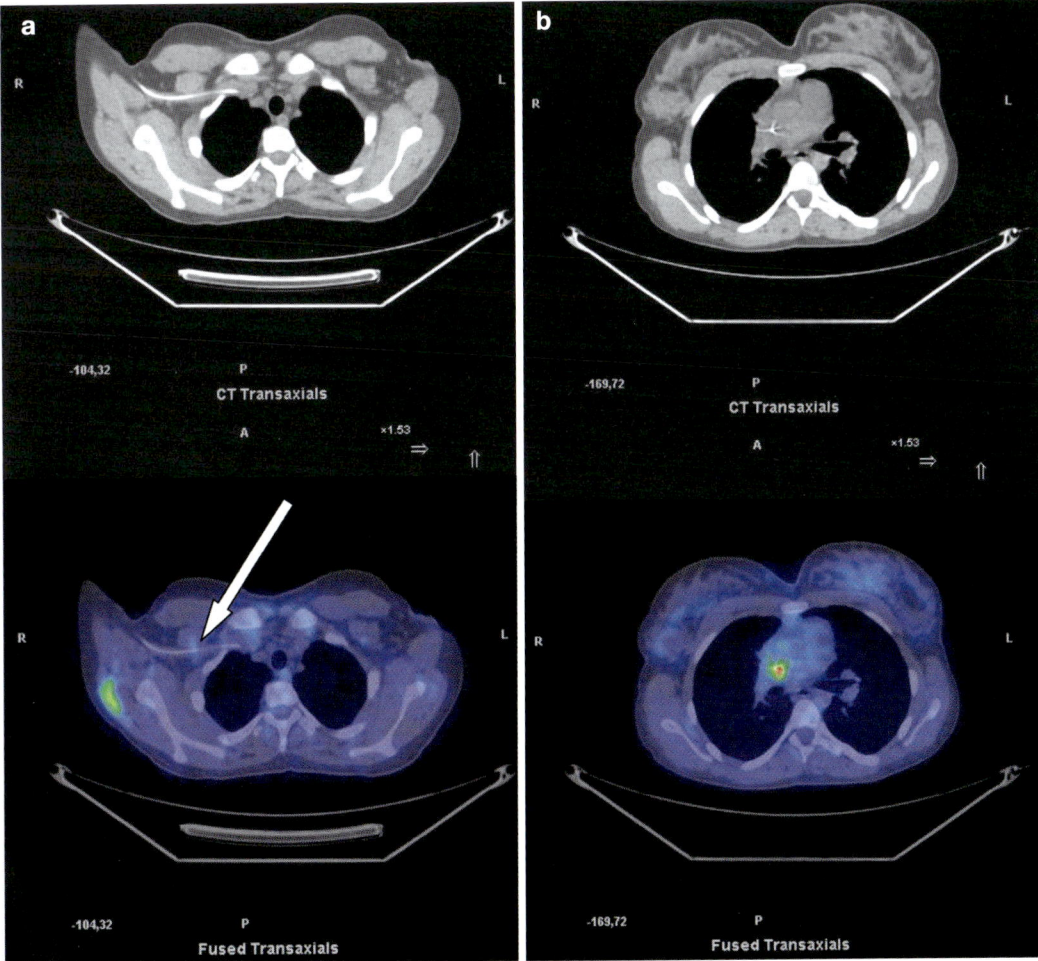

Fig. 3.2 (**a**) Axial CT and PET/CT fusion images show the axillary venous line (*white arrow*) and (**b**) focal mediastinal uptake at the terminus of the central venous line due to tracer stasis

References

1. McQuattie S (2008) Pediatric PET/CT imaging: tips and techniques. J Nucl Med Technol 36:171–180
2. Jacobs F, Thierens H, Piepsz A, Bacher K, Van de Wiele C, Ham H, Dierckx RA, European Association of Nuclear Medicine (2005) Optimised tracer-dependent dosage cards to obtain weight-independent effective doses. Eur J Nucl Med Mol Imaging 32:581–588
3. Jadvar H, Connolly LP, Fahey FH, Shulkin BL (2007) PET and PET/CT in pediatric oncology. Semin Nucl Med 37:316–331

Physiological Patterns and Pitfalls of ^{18}F-FDG Biodistribution

Angelina Cistaro

^{18}F-FDG is normally accumulated in very high concentrations in the cerebral cortex, basal ganglia, and, in some cases, in cardiac muscle. Due to its renal excretion, ^{18}F-FDG also accumulates in the entire urinary system, from the renal parenchyma to the bladder. The liver is highly involved in glucose metabolism, but as hepatic cells reversibly dephosphorylate ^{18}F-FDG by the action of phosphatases, the initial uptake of 18F-FDG in the liver is followed by a significant washout [1]. Moderate uptake of ^{18}F-FDG occurs also in breast, particularly in dense tissues. In women, there is increased uptake by the ovaries during the ovulatory or secretory phases of the menstrual cycle (Fig. 4.1), while in men, accumulation may be seen in the testes [2].

In young patients, the thymus is frequently seen on PET as an inverted-V-shaped structure (Fig. 4.2), or as a unilateral structure with right or left extensions (Fig. 4.3), with homogeneous or patchy tracer uptake (Fig. 4.4). In children and in young adults who have undergone chemotherapy, the thymus is an important site of ^{18}F-FDG uptake as this organ uptake may persist for as long as 2 years after the end of therapy. Jerushalmi and coworkers studied a population of 160 patients (age 3–40 years) and found that 28 % exhibited thymic ^{18}F-FDG uptake. Within this subgroup, 80 % were younger than 10 years, 17 % showed uptake only at the baseline study, 6 % during treatment, 8 % at the end of treatment, and 27–40 % during follow-up [3]. It is also important to be aware of normal anatomic variants and variants in FDG uptake patterns. For example, there is a normal variant in which the thymus extends superiorly to the left brachiocephalic vein and anteriorly to the brachiocephalic artery or left common carotid artery (Fig. 4.5). This superior extension of the thymus should not be mistaken for a mediastinal mass or lymphadenopathy [4].

In addition to the thymus, significant uptake is frequently seen in the bone marrow and spleen, probably due to normal growth. After chemotherapy or granulocyte colony-stimulating factor therapy, this activation is significantly increased such that homogeneity is an important criterion for the diagnosis of non-tumoral disease (Fig. 4.6) [5].

In children, it is possible to observe the metaphysis in long bones such as the femur or tibiae, because during growth, the interface between the epiphysis and diaphysis is ^{18}F-FDG avid (Fig. 4.7).

The palatine and nasopharyngeal tonsils and Waldeyer's ring are lymphoepithelial tissues located near the oropharynx and nasopharynx (Figs. 4.8 and 4.9). These immunocompetent tissues are the immune system's first line of defense

A. Cistaro, MD
Department of Nuclear Medicine, Positron Emission Tomography Center IRMET S.p.A., Euromedic Inc., Via Onorato Vigliani 89, Turin 10100, Italy

Institute of Cognitive Sciences and Technologies, National Research Council, Rome, Italy
e-mail: a.cistaro@irmet.com

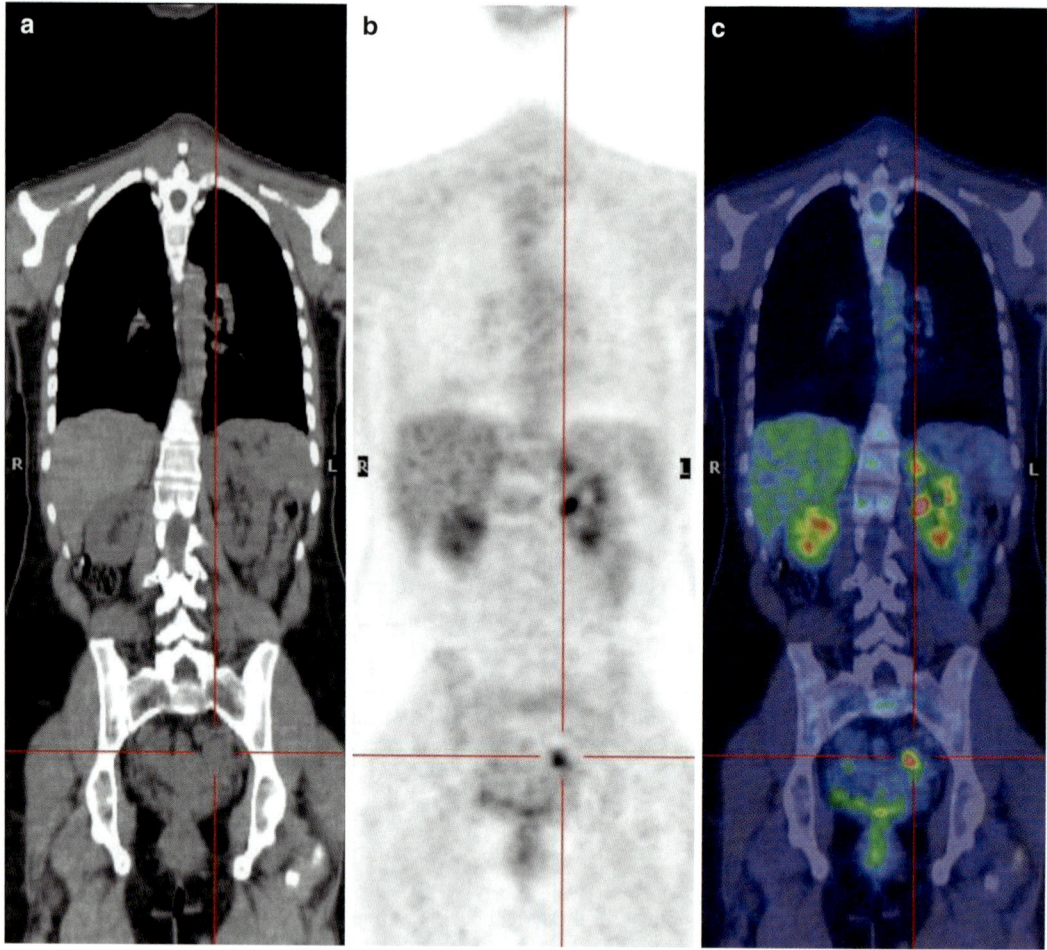

Fig. 4.1 Coronal CT (**a**), PET (**b**), and PET/CT fusion (**c**) images show focal ^{18}F-FDG uptake in the left pelvis, corresponding to the ovarian follicle

against ingested or inhaled foreign pathogens. In children, the PET study frequently shows enhanced and symmetric uptake, which helps to distinguish neoplasms from inflammatory pathologies.

^{18}F-FDG–PET/CT imaging of the pediatric intestine does not follow the same rules as in adults. In the latter, there may be modest to intense uptake in the intestine whereas this is generally not the case in the healthy intestine of children. Therefore, intestinal uptake in young patients, especially in those who have undergone stem cell or organ transplantation, warrants attention as it may indicate posttransplantation lymphoproliferative disease (PTLD) (Fig. 4.10).

However, benign causes of inflammation in young patients, such as appendicitis, must be ruled out (Figs. 4.11 and 4.12).

The acne vulgaris is another benign condition in young patients that is better to keep in mind, particularly during the staging of cutaneous malignant diseases. Acne is a common skin disease that affects an estimated 80 % of teens and young adults during their lives. It is characterized by noninflammatory open or closed comedones and by inflammatory papules, pustules, and nodules. Acne typically affects the areas of skin with the densest population of sebaceous follicles including the face, the upper part of the chest, and the back (Fig 4.13).

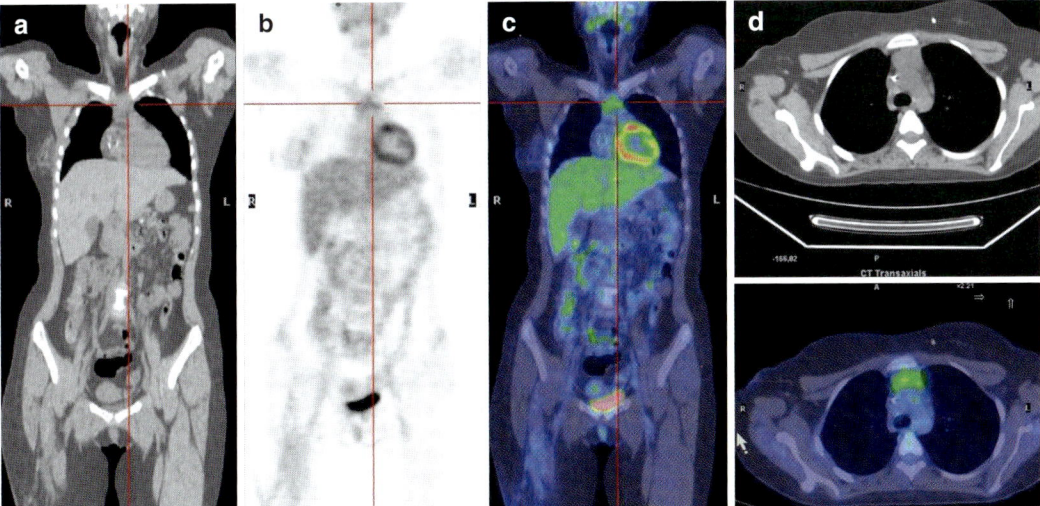

Fig. 4.2 A 14-year-old girl administered chemotherapy for osteoblastic osteosarcoma of the right femur. Coronal CT (**a**), PET (**b**), and PET/CT fusion (**c**) images show soft tissue ^{18}F-FDG uptake by the inverted-V-shaped thymus in the anterior mediastinum. (**d**) Axial CT and PET/CT fusion images show the thickened thymus in the anterior mediastinum, in front of the aortic arch

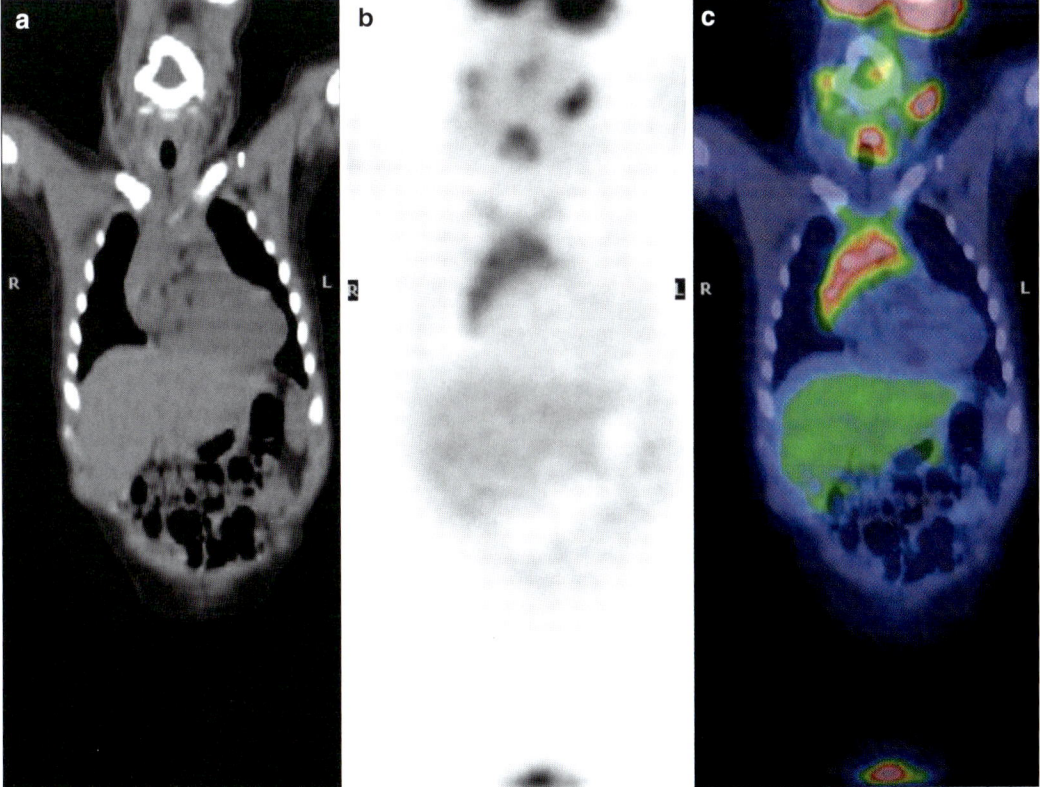

Fig. 4.3 A 5-year-old boy 4 months after the end of chemotherapy for non-Hodgkin's lymphoma. Coronal CT (**a**), PET (**b**), and PET/CT fusion (**c**) images show intense ^{18}F-FDG uptake by the thymus, which has a unilateral right extension

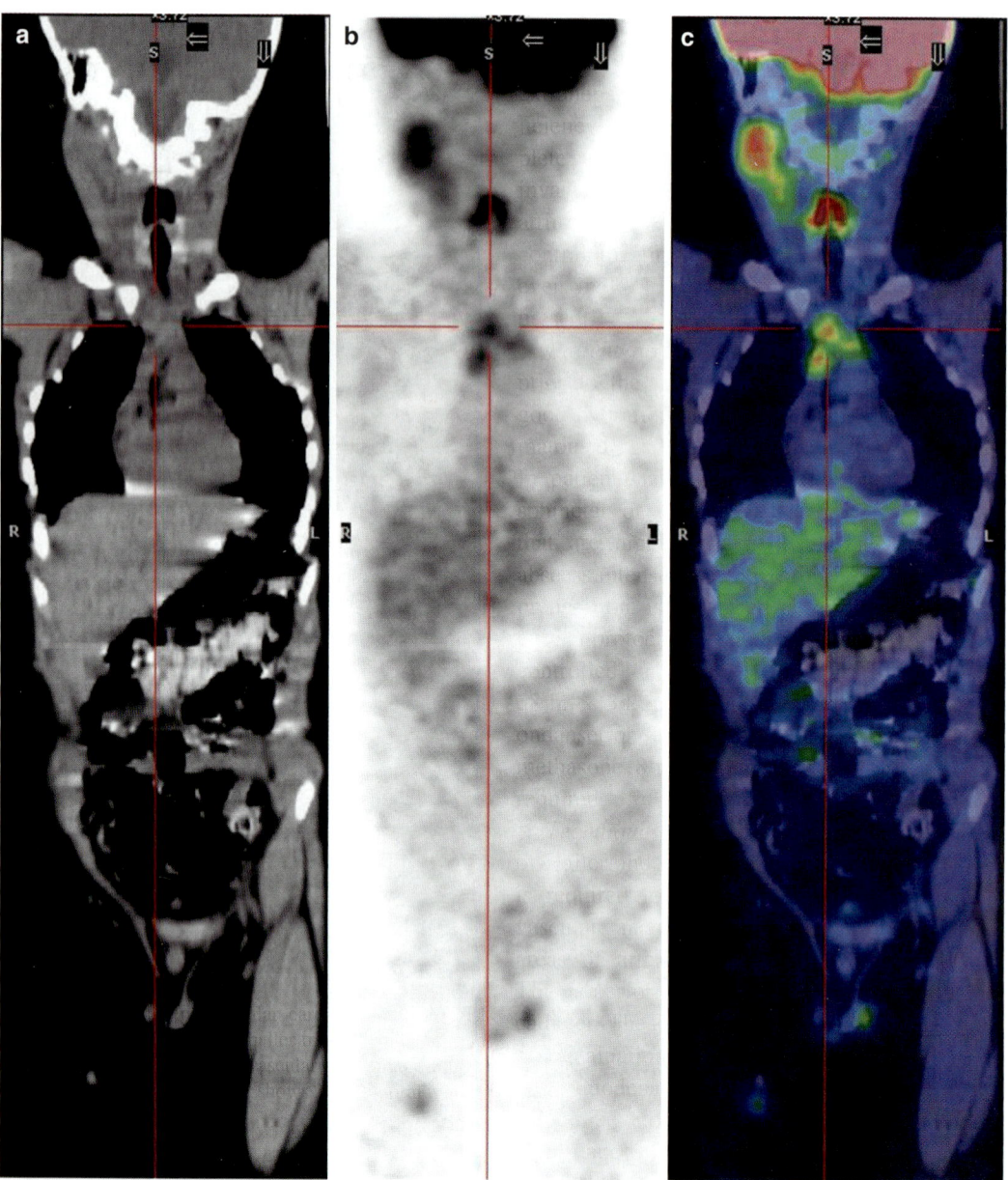

Fig. 4.4 A 6-year-old boy with autoimmune lymphoproliferative syndrome (ALPS). Coronal CT (**a**), PET (**b**), and PET/CT fusion (**c**) images show patchy ^{18}F-FDG by the inverted-V-shaped thymus

4 Physiological Patterns and Pitfalls of ¹⁸F-FDG Biodistribution

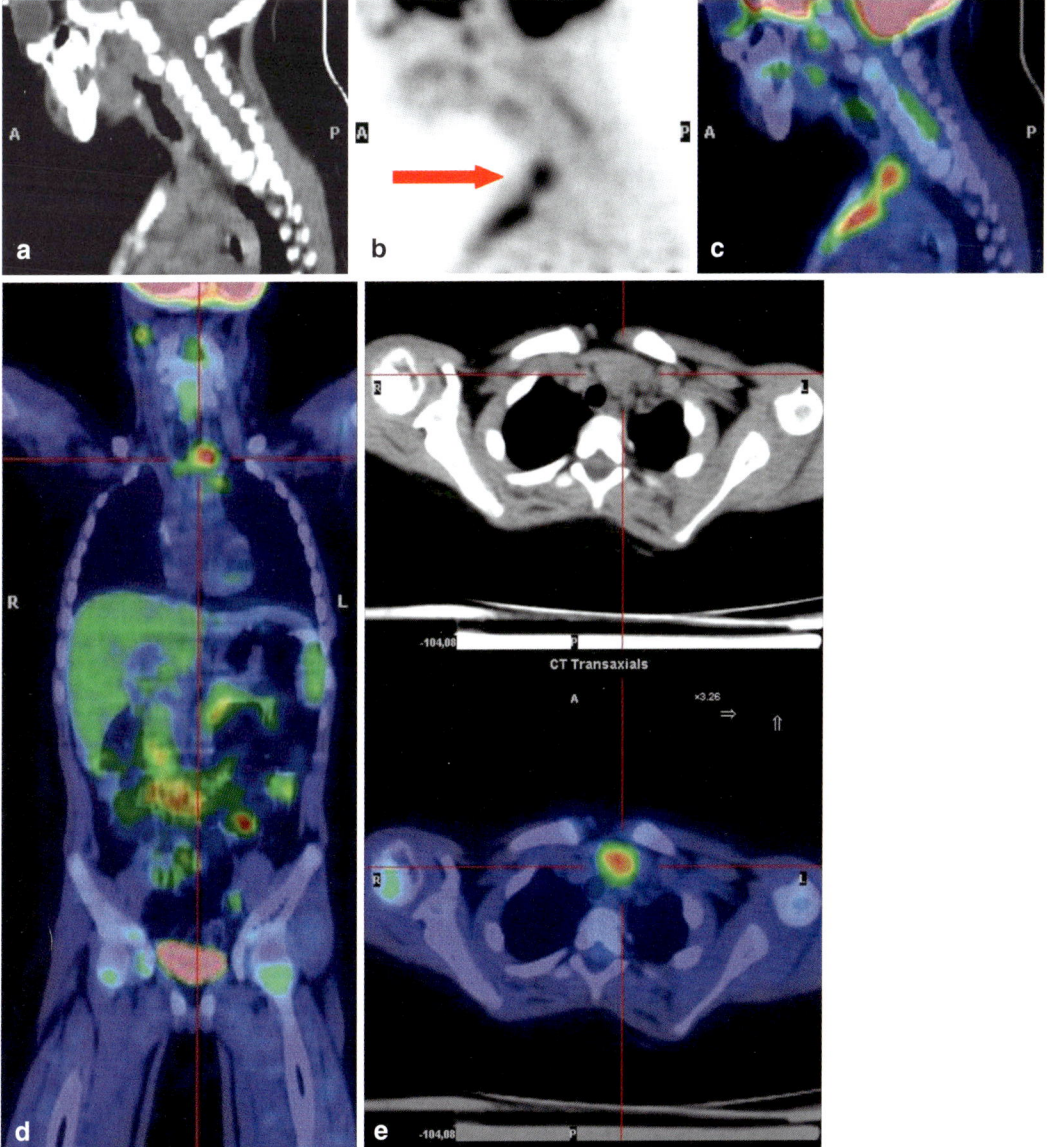

Fig. 4.5 A 4-year-old boy treated for acute lymphoblastic leukemia (ALL). Sagittal CT (**a**), PET (**b**), and PET/CT fusion (**c**) images show an extension of the thymus to the superior mediastinum (*red arrow* in **b**). Coronal PET/CT fusion image (**d**) and axial CT and PET/CT fusion images (**e**) show the extension of the thymus superiorly to the left brachiocephalic vein and anteriorly to the left common carotid artery

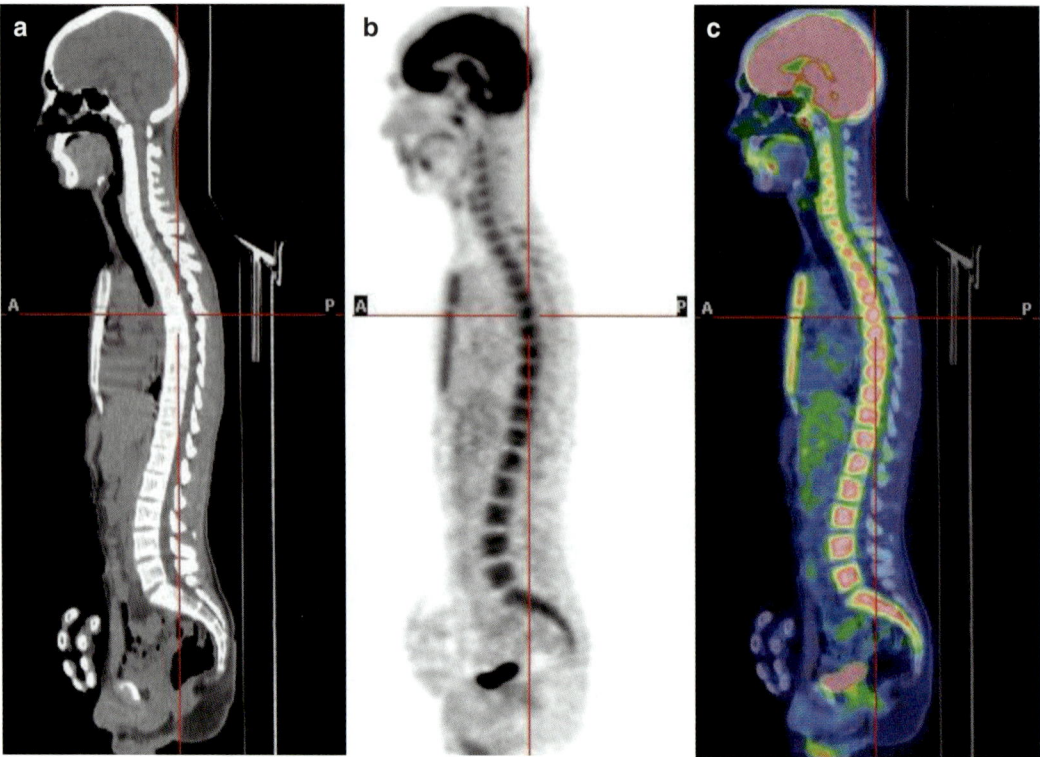

Fig. 4.6 Coronal CT (**a**), PET (**b**), and PET/CT fusion (**c**) images in a patient undergoing chemotherapy for Hodgkin's lymphoma. Note the intense accumulation of ^{18}F-FDG in the sternum and in the spine

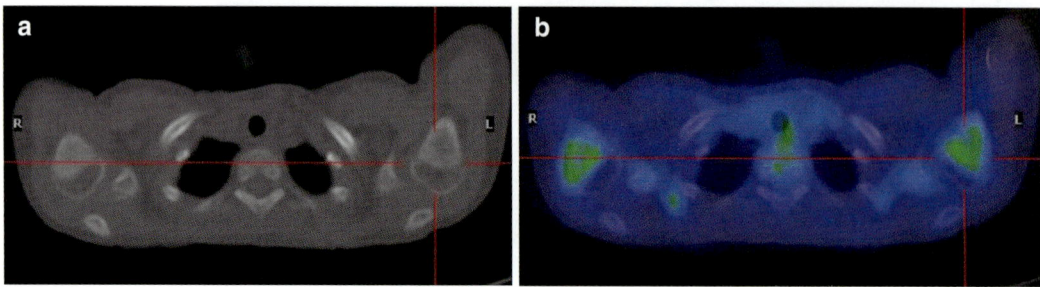

Fig. 4.7 A 6-year-old girl who underwent surgery for adrenal gland carcinoma. Axial CT (**a**) and PET/CT fusion (**b**) images show physiologically symmetric ^{18}F-FDG uptake by the epiphyseal growth cartilage of the humerus

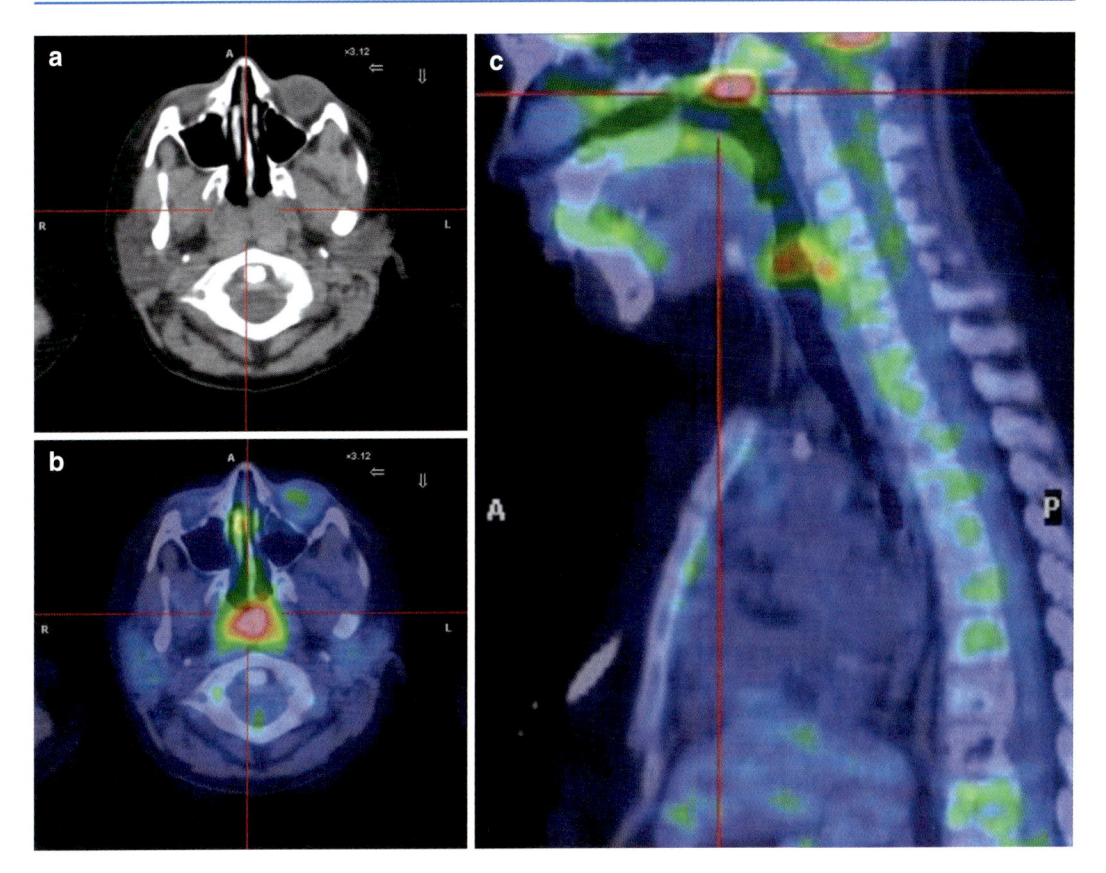

4 Physiological Patterns and Pitfalls of ^{18}F-FDG Biodistribution

Fig. 4.8 Axial CT (**a**) and PET/CT fusion (**b**) images show ^{18}F-FDG nasopharyngeal uptake, also evident in the sagittal PET/CT fusion image (**c**)

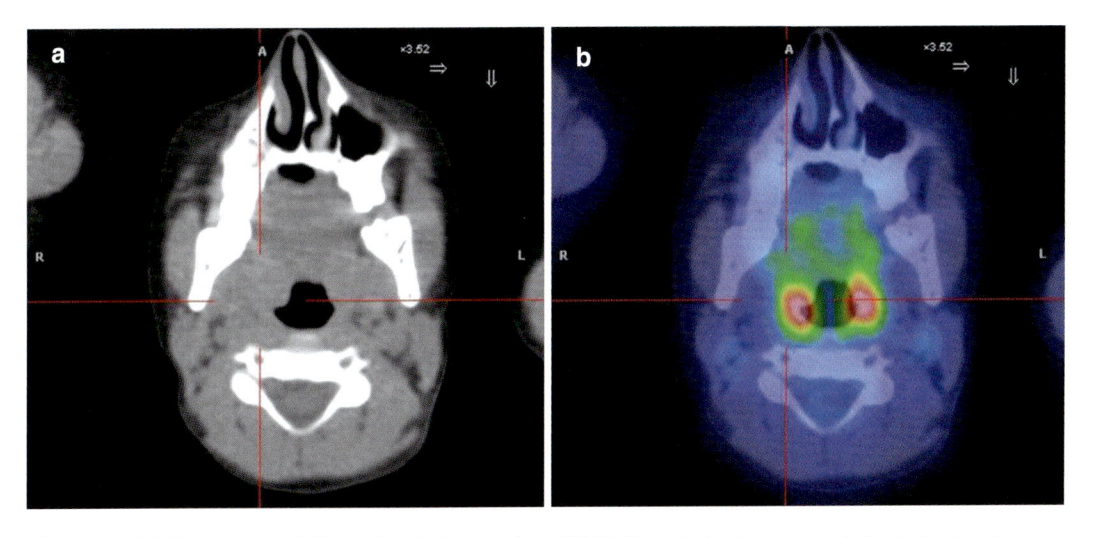

Fig. 4.9 Axial CT (**a**) and PET/CT fusion (**b**) images show ^{18}F-FDG uptake by the symmetrical palatine tonsils

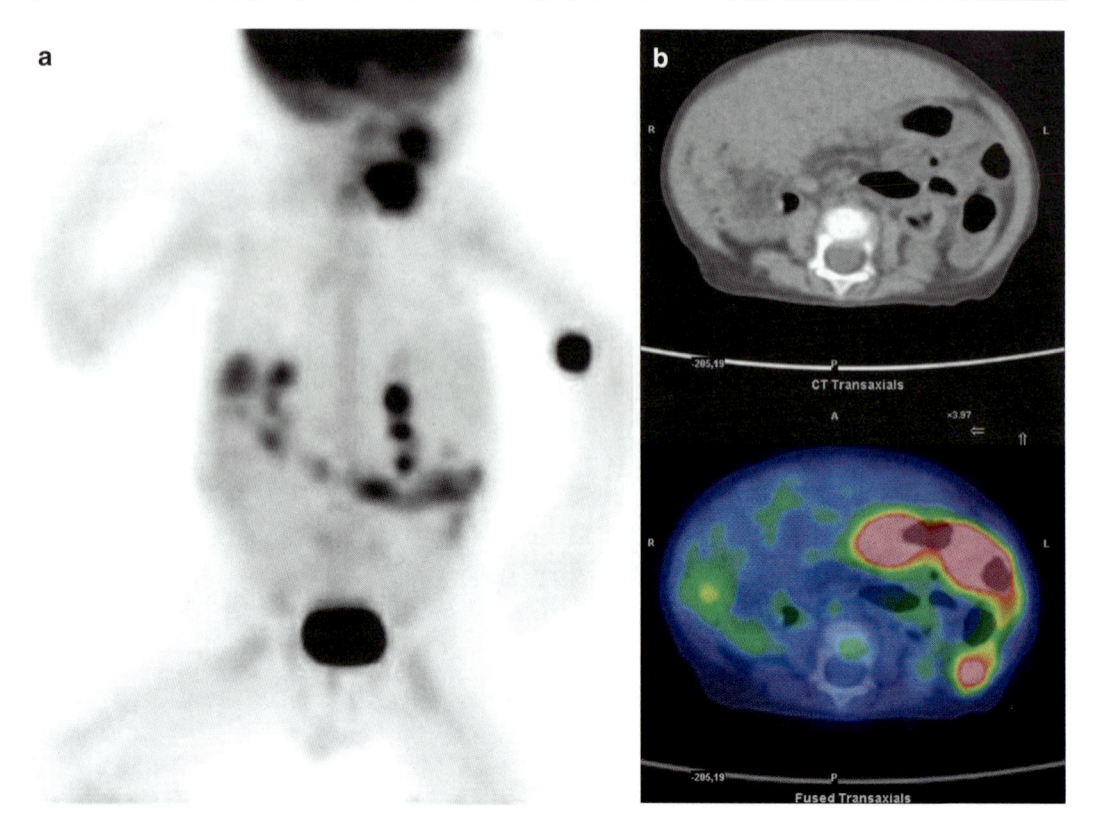

Fig. 4.10 A 1-year-old boy underwent liver transplantation for congenital biliary atresia, the most common lethal liver disease in children, for whom surgery offers the only chance of cure. The patient was treated with tacrolimus, an immunosuppressive drug that is mainly used after allogeneic organ transplantation to reduce the risk of organ rejection. However, the patient subsequently developed Epstein–Barr virus (EBV)-associated PTLD, correlated with large bowel involvement. (**a**) The maximal intensity projection and (**b**) axial CT and PET/CT fusion images show pathological ^{18}F-FDG uptake in the transverse colon

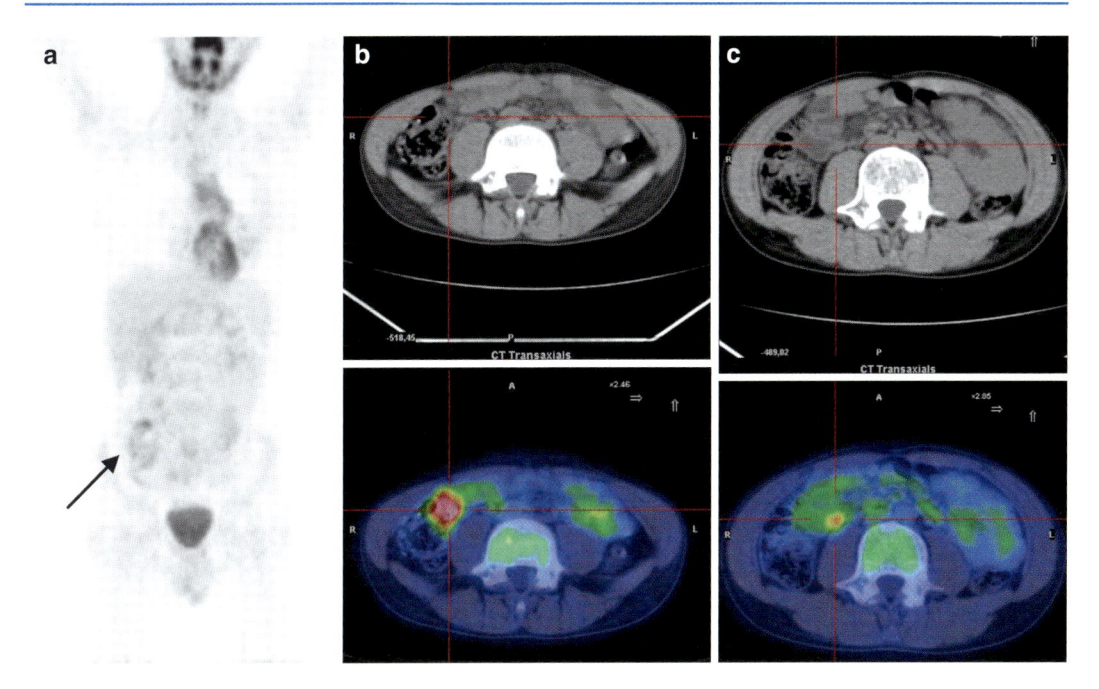

Fig. 4.11 A 13-year-old boy received chemotherapy and radiotherapy for primitive neuroectodermal tumor (PNET) of the chest. (**a**) Maximal intensity projection shows nonhomogeneous and mild FDG uptake of the large right bowel (*black arrow*). (**b**, **c**) Axial CT and PET/CT fusion images show FDG accumulation at the level of the terminal ileum (**b**) and pericolic lymph node (**c**) due to an inflammation process

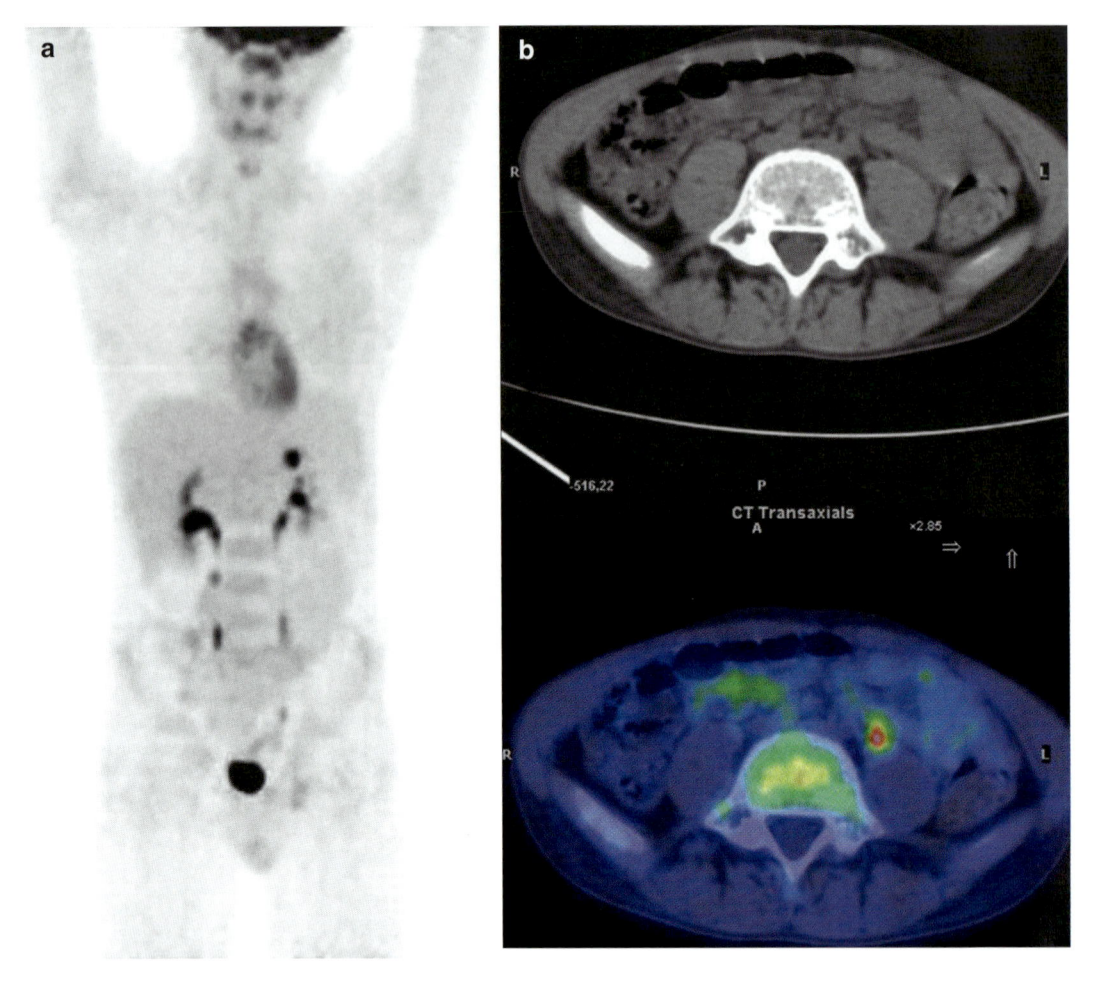

Fig. 4.12 (**a**, **b**) The same patient as in Fig. 4.11 underwent antibiotic treatment before the last PET/CT study, which showed the disappearance of abdominal FDG uptake

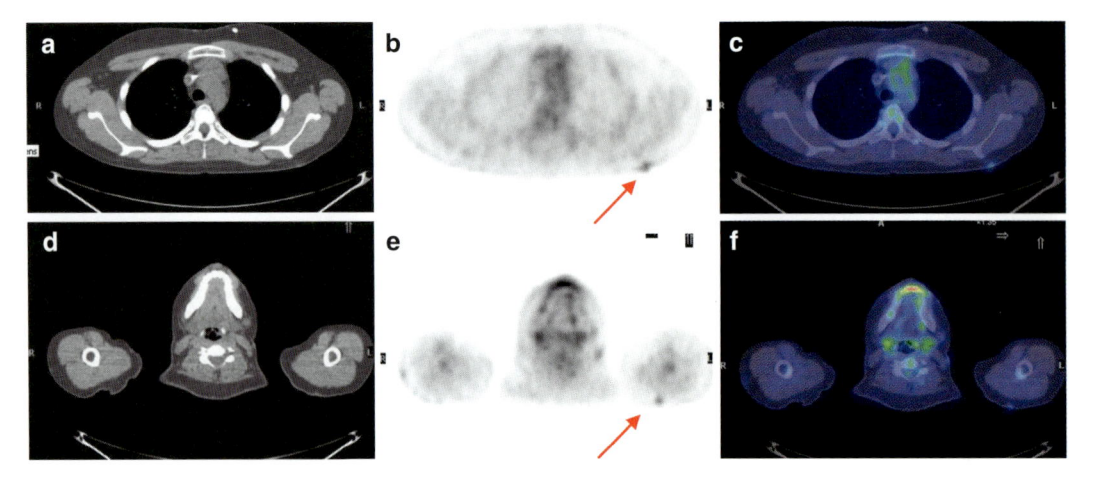

Fig. 4.13 A 13-year-old boy who underwent chemotherapy for large cell non-Hodgkin's lymphoma. Axial CT (**a**, **d**), PET (**b**, **e**), and PET/CT fusion (**c**, **f**) images show slight cutaneous FDG uptake in the left back (*red arrow* in **b**) and homolaterally in the arm (*red arrow* in **e**). The clinical examination revealed inflammatory acne

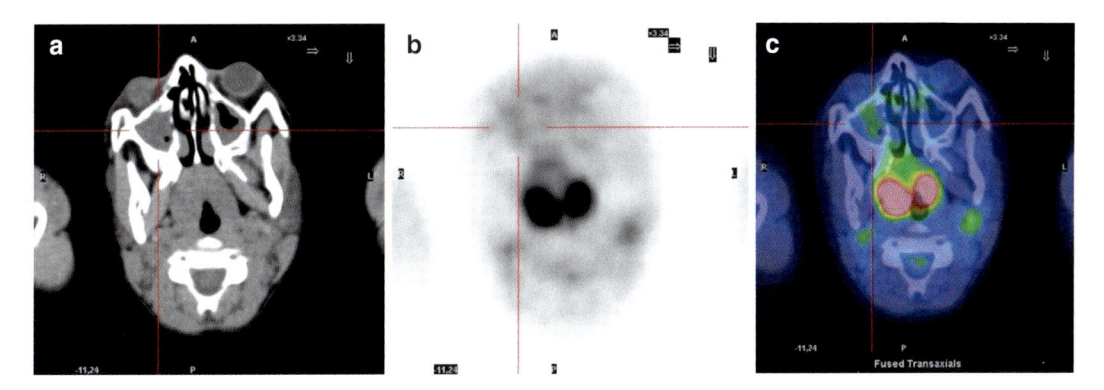

Fig. 4.14 Axial CT (**a**), PET (**b**), and PET/CT fusion (**c**) images show slight FDG uptake in a patient with right maxillary sinusitis

The same reasoning is valid for sinusitis, a common condition caused by acute or chronic inflammation of the paranasal sinuses. Maxillary sinusitis is the most common type of sinusitis. The ethmoid, frontal, and sphenoid sinuses are less frequently affected (Fig 4.14).

References

1. Pauwels EK, Sturm EJ, Bombardieri E, Cleton FJ, Stokkel MP (2000) Positron-emission tomography with fluorodeoxyglucose. Part I. Biochemical uptake mechanism and its implication for clinical studies. J Cancer Res Clin Oncol 126:549–559
2. Shammas A, Lim R, Charron M (2009) Pediatric FDG PET/CT: physiologic uptake, normal variants, and benign conditions. Radiographics 29:1467–1486
3. Jerushalmi J, Frenkel A, Bar-Shalom R, Khoury J, Israel O (2009) Physiologic thymic uptake of 18- in children and young adults: a PET/CT evaluation of incidence, patterns, and the relationship to treatment. J Nucl Med 50:849–853
4. Smith CS, Schöder H, Yeung HW (2007) Thymic extension in the superior mediastinum in patients with thymic hyperplasia: potential cause of false-positive findings on 18F-FDG PET/CT. AJR Am J Roentgenol 188:1716–1721
5. Sugawara Y, Zasadny KR, Kison PV, Baker LH, Wahl RL (1999) Splenic fluorodeoxyglucose uptake increased by granulocyte colony-stimulating factor therapy: PET imaging results. J Nucl Med 40:1456–1462

Part II
Oncology

Malignant Lymphoma in Children

Francesco Cicone and Stefania Uccini

5.1 Introduction

Lymphomas are among the most common malignancies in childhood (0–14 years of age) and the third most frequent pediatric cancer after leukemia and brain tumors [1]. In adolescence (15–19 years of age), lymphoma is the most prevalent malignancy, accounting for >25 % of newly diagnosed cancers [2].

The focus of this chapter is Hodgkin's lymphoma (HL) and non-Hodgkin's lymphoma (NHL), which are two separate entities with different pathological and clinical characteristics. In addition, there are several differences between young and adult HL and NHL in terms of histological subtype, patterns of presentation, treatment, and outcome, and they should be kept in mind by the nuclear medicine specialist evaluating the pediatric PET/CT exam.

F. Cicone (✉)
Nuclear Medicine Department,
Sant'Andrea Hospital, Faculty of Medicine
and Psychology, "Sapienza" University of Rome,
Via di Grottarossa 1035-1039, Rome 00189, Italy
e-mail: f.cicone@iol.it

S. Uccini, MD
Pathology Department,
Sant'Andrea Hospital, Faculty of Medicine
and Psychology, "Sapienza" University of Rome,
Via di Grottarossa 1035-1039, Rome 00189, Italy
e-mail: stefania.uccini@uniroma1.it

5.2 Hodgkin's Lymphoma

5.2.1 Background

Hodgkin's lymphomas comprise two disease entities, nodular lymphocyte predominant Hodgkin's lymphoma (NLPHL) and classical Hodgkin's lymphoma (cHL), which differ in their clinical features, behavior, morphology, immunophenotype, and cellular background. Classical HL accounts for nearly 45 % of all lymphomas in children and typically presents in one of two distinct geographical incidence patterns. In Asia and tropical regions, up to 100 % of cHL cases are Epstein–Barr virus (EBV)-positive, whereas in western countries, only 30–50 % of the cHL are EBV associated. Moreover, in developing countries, the peak incidence of cHL is in children 3–14 years of age, in contrast to the peak occurrence in adolescents in western countries, with a sharp increase after 10 years of age. Diagnosis of HL requires the presence of the hallmark "Reed–Sternberg" (RS) cells, although they make up only 0.1–2 % of the total cellular population. RS cells are characterized by multiple polymorphic nuclei with prominent acidophilic nucleoli (Fig. 5.1a). They nearly always express CD30 and usually CD15 while a minority also express the B-cell-associated antigens CD20 and CD79a. Based on the characteristics of the surrounding inflammatory infiltrate, four subtypes of cHL are distinguished: nodular sclerosis, mixed cellularity, lymphocyte rich, and lymphocyte depleted. Classical HL most often involves lymph nodes of

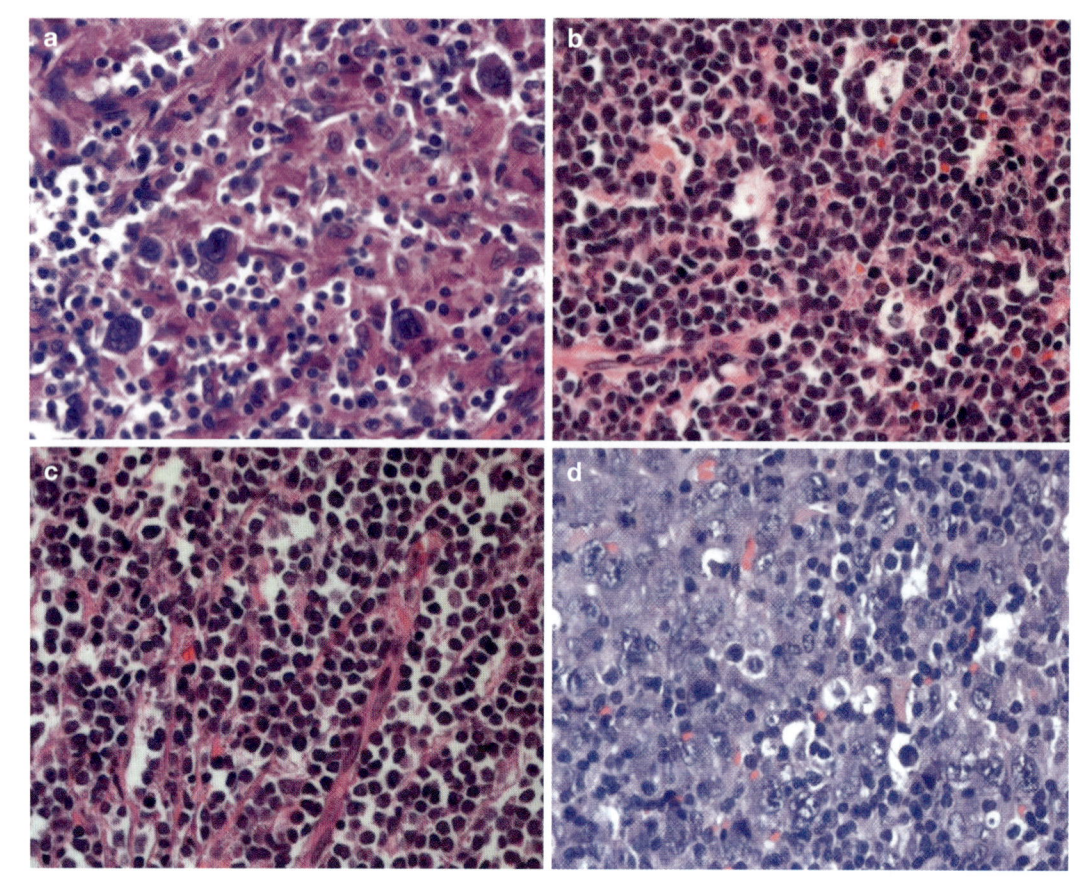

Fig. 5.1 (**a**) Hodgkin's lymphoma, mixed cellularity subtype. The hallmark "Reed–Sternberg" cells are scattered and surrounded by an inflammatory infiltrate composed of histiocytes and mature lymphocytes (H&E ×400). (**b**) Burkitt's lymphoma. A proliferation of intermediate-sized neoplastic cells is associated with scattered macrophages containing cellular debris, resulting in the typical "starry sky" appearance (H&E ×400). (**c**) Lymphoblastic lymphoma. There is diffuse tissue involvement by small, round, blue, monomorphic tumor cells with dense chromatin and scant cytoplasm (H&E ×400). (**d**) Anaplastic large B-cell lymphoma. The neoplastic cells have bizarre, lobulated, or wreath-like nuclei and abundant cytoplasm (H&E ×400)

the cervical region; primary extranodal involvement is rare.

NLPHL represents less than 5 % of all HLs and has a peak incidence around the age of 40. It is a monoclonal B-cell neoplasm, mainly characterized by a nodular infiltrate consisting of B lymphocytes, histiocytes, and intermingled lymphocyte predominant (LP) variants of RS cells, also termed "popcorn" cells. LP cells are positive for the B-cell markers CD20 and CD79a and consistently lack CD15 and CD30. The natural history of the disease is relatively indolent, with most patients cured with local radiotherapy or surgery alone.

5.2.2 Staging System and Treatment Strategies

HL prognostic score relies on the Ann Arbor staging system [3], modified during the Cotswolds meeting [4] (Table 5.1). Radiotherapy alone was the standard treatment for HL until the 1960s, when the first chemotherapeutic regimen, MOPP (mechlorethamine, vincristine, procarbazine, and prednisone), was introduced. Concerns about late toxicities prompted reductions in both the dose delivered by radiotherapy and the number and intensity of chemotherapy cycles [5]. To minimize the use of alkylating agents, in order

Table 5.1 Ann Arbor staging system, with Cotswolds modifications [3, 4]

Stage I
Involvement of a single lymph node region or lymphoid structure such as spleen, thymus, or Waldeyer's ring

Stage II
Involvement of two or more lymph node regions or lymphoid structures on the same side of the diaphragm. The number of anatomic regions involved should be indicated by a subscript (e.g., II$_3$)

Stage III
Involvement of two or more lymph node regions or lymphoid structures on both sides of the diaphragm. This may be subdivided into stage III1 or stage III2, stage III1 for patients with spleen or splenic, hilar, celiac, or portal node involvement and stage III2 for those with para-aortic, iliac, or mesenteric node involvement

Stage IV
Extensive extranodal disease, beyond the definition of bulky and extranodal disease [4]

to avoid male infertility and secondary leukemia, the ABVD protocol was introduced, consisting of six cycles of doxorubicin, bleomycin, vinblastine, and dacarbazine [6]. Today, ABVD is given to most patients with or without additional radiotherapy. Higher-risk patients are treated with more intensive chemotherapies, such as BEACOPP (bleomycin, etoposide, doxorubicin, cyclophosphamide, vincristine, procarbazine, and prednisone).

Five-year overall survival (OS) is ≥95 in low-risk patients and about 85 % in those at high risk [7]. However, according to some studies, the outcomes are less encouraging, with the 20-year OS as low as 68 %. Event-free survival (EFS) rates are even lower. Younger age at onset seems to be associated with better survival [8].

5.3 Non-Hodgkin's Lymphoma

5.3.1 Background

NHL accounts for 55 % of childhood lymphomas. The incidence increases dramatically in children between 1 and 3 years of age (from about two cases/million to nine cases/million) and reaches a plateau thereafter, such that in adolescence, NHLs represent about one-third of all diagnosed lymphomas.

The majority of pediatric NHL cases fall into one of four categories: Burkitt's lymphoma (BL), lymphoblastic lymphoma (LBL), anaplastic large cell lymphoma (ALCL), and diffuse large B-cell lymphoma (DLBCL). Indolent lymphomas composed of small lymphocytes (e.g., small lymphocytic lymphoma, marginal zone lymphoma, mantle cell lymphoma, follicle center cell lymphoma) are extremely rare in children and should be diagnosed with caution.

5.3.2 Staging System and Treatment Strategies

The Ann Arbor staging system does not apply to pediatric NHLs. Indeed, unlike HLs, NHLs spread non-contiguously, with a high frequency of extranodal disease. This pattern prompted researchers to develop a different staging approach, resulting in the St Jude/Murphy's system [9, 10], in which mediastinal and abdominal localizations are distinct from tumors arising in the remainder of the body and differ in their prognostic significance. Moreover, the classification also considers the extent of surgical excision of abdominal masses (Table 5.2).

Classically, the treatment modality was chosen based on the histological subtype, with treatment intensity modulated according to disease stage and other parameters [11].

At least two major treatment strategies are identifiable for treatment of different NHL subtypes: the first strategy was initially developed for leukaemia and is based on the continuous exposure to cytostatics over a long period of time. It is represented by ten drugs LSA$_2$-L$_2$ (cyclophosfamide, vincristine, methotrexate, daunorubicin, prednisone, cytarabine, thioguanine, asparaginase, carmustine, hydroxyurea) or LSA$_2$-L$_2$ –type protocols. The second strategy consists of shortly repeated, dose-intense combinations of cytotoxic drugs and is represented by the COMP (cyclophosphamide, vincristine, methotrexate, prednisone) or COMP-like regimens. The former has proved to be mostly effective

Table 5.2 St Jude/Murphy's pediatric NHL staging system [8, 9]

Stage I
A single tumor (extranodal) or single anatomic area (nodal), with the exclusion of the mediastinum and abdomen

Stage II
A single tumor (extranodal) with regional lymph node involvement
Two or more nodal areas on the same side of the diaphragm
Two single (extranodal) tumors with or without regional lymph node involvement on the same side of the diaphragm
A resectable primary tumor of the gastrointestinal tract, usually in the ileocecal area, with or without involvement of associated mesenteric nodes only

Stage III
Two single tumors (extranodal) on opposite sides of the diaphragm
Two or more nodal areas above and below the diaphragm
All primary intrathoracic tumors (mediastinal, pleural, thymic)
All extensive primary unresectable intra-abdominal disease
All paraspinal or epidural tumors, regardless of other tumor sites

Stage IV
Any of the above with initial involvement of the central nervous system, bone marrow, or both

for treatment of precursor NHL (T- and B-LBL), the latter shows the best results in treatment of mature B-NHL (BL, DLCBL) [12]. A summary of treatment modalities for each NHL subtype is provided in specific paragraphs.

5.3.3 Burkitt's Lymphoma

As the most common NHL subtype in children, BL accounts for up to 40 % of all cases. Three epidemiological variants have been described: endemic, sporadic, and immunodeficiency related [13, 14]. Endemic BL is most commonly seen in male children in equatorial Africa and New Guinea and is strongly associated with EBV infection, which probably leads to the genetic hallmark of endemic BL, the t(8;14)(q24;q32) translocation. This alteration, present in 70–80 % of cases, causes constitutive expression of the *MYC* oncogene in immunoglobulin-codifying DNA [15]. Sporadic BL is less commonly related to EBV infection and affects both children and adults, with a bimodal age distribution. Immunodeficiency-related BL occurs in the setting of congenital immunodeficiency, HIV infection, and posttransplantation.

The typical presentation of endemic BL is jaw and periorbital swelling, due to the unexplained predilection of EBV for the sockets around the deciduous teeth of young children. The abdomen, and particularly the small bowel, is the most common site of presentation in sporadic and immunodeficiency-associated BL, with symptoms related to obstruction or perforation. Bone marrow infiltration is more common in sporadic BL (~20 % of all cases) than in endemic BL.

Histologically, BL is diagnosed based on the detection of a monomorphic proliferation of intermediate-sized cells with a proliferative index >95 %. Evenly distributed macrophages containing cellular debris result in a mottled "starry sky" appearance at low magnification (Fig. 5.1b). The immunophenotype is that of a mature surface Ig+ B cell, and both CD20 and CD79a antigens are expressed. The cells are also CD10-positive while terminal deoxynucleotidyl transferase (TdT) expression is lacking.

Localized stages are successfully treated with complete surgical excision followed by two cycles of chemotherapy (cyclophosphamide, doxorubicin, vincristine, and prednisolone). Advanced stages warrant between four and eight cycles of chemotherapy, augmented by varying combinations of high-dose methotrexate, cytarabine, and etoposide. Prophylactic intrathecal therapy is also administered to high-risk patients in order to prevent central nervous system (CNS) recurrence.

In developed countries, OS is excellent (>90 %, with differences according to stage at presentation) whereas, regretfully, it is much worse in endemic sub-Saharan countries. The incidence of relapse is highest within 6 months after the completion of treatment and the prognosis of patients who suffer a relapse after optimized treatment is dismal.

5.3.4 T-Cell and B-Cell Lymphoblastic Lymphoma

LBL is the second most common NHL of childhood after BL, comprising 20–30 % of all pediatric NHLs. About 80–90 % of LBLs are of T-cell lineage and present as a bulky mediastinal mass and diffuse systemic disease. LBL of B-cell origin (B-LBL) is less frequent and often limited to the skin, bone, or lymph nodes.

The differential diagnosis of LBL vs. precursor T-cell and B-cell acute lymphoblastic leukemia (ALL) depends on the percentage of blasts in the bone marrow biopsy specimen: LBL is defined as <25 % blasts, while ALL is diagnosed when blasts are >25 % [16]. Tissue involvement is characterized by the diffuse proliferation of small and intermediate cells with dense chromatin and scant cytoplasm; the mitotic rate is frequently elevated (Fig. 5.1c). The immunophenotype of TdT-positive cells with variable expression of the immature T-cell antigens CD1a, CD4, and CD5, together with cytoplasmic CD3 positivity and (usually) surface CD3 negativity, is indicative of T-LBL. By contrast, a phenotype comprising TdT+, CD79+, CD10+, and CD20− is indicative of B-LBL.

The backbone of LBL therapy is the LSA_2-L_2 regimen and its variants [17–20], which are administered over a period of 18–24 months and divided into induction, consolidation, reintensification, and maintenance phases. Prophylactic intrathecal methotrexate is often sufficient for preventing CNS recurrences such that prophylactic cranial irradiation is progressively disappearing from standard treatments. The OS of patients with limited-stage disease is 85–90 %, while trials of advanced stages have reported 3- to 6-year EFS rates of 70–90 % [16]. The majority of relapses occur within 12–24 months after diagnosis. These patients have poor prognosis, with a 5-year OS of 10 % [11]. Re-induction treatments include platinum-based protocols. Patients with chemosensitive relapses benefit from stem cell transplantation procedures (auto or allo) [21–23].

5.3.5 Anaplastic Large Cell Lymphoma

Between 10 and 15 % of childhood NHLs are ALCL. In children, the most frequent presentation is systemic, with nodal and extranodal involved sites including skin, bone, soft tissues, lung, and liver. Mediastinal localization is uncommon and bone marrow and CNS invasions are rare.

Although T-cell antigens are not necessarily expressed, ALCLs are classified as lymphomas of mature T-cell origin because T-cell receptor (TCR) gene rearrangements are nearly always present [16]. Two different clinical entities are defined according to the presence or absence of a gene translocation involving anaplastic lymphoma kinase (*ALK*), the t(2;5) (p23;q35)/NPM-ALK translocation [24]. Unlike adult ALCLs, >90 % of pediatric ALCLs are *ALK*+, which have a better prognosis. The hallmark neoplastic cells have bizarre, lobulated, or wreath-like nuclei with abundant cytoplasm. CD30 positivity is required for the diagnosis (Fig. 5.1d). Epithelial membrane antigen (EMA) and CD45 are usually but not always positive [25].

Optimal primary treatment for ALCL has not been clearly established. Localized ALCL is almost always cured after a few cycles of short-course chemotherapy. For advanced-stage ALCL, EFS rates of 65–75 % have been reported with either LSA_2-L_2-like regimens or mature B-NHL-like chemotherapies [26, 27]. Poor prognostic features include ALK negativity or visceral, mediastinal, or diffuse skin involvement. Unlike other NHL subtypes, relapsed ALCL is commonly chemosensitive, with satisfying EFS rates achieved after chemotherapy with or without transplantation procedures. Trials of specific treatments targeting ALK proteins, CD30 antigen, or other signaling pathway components are underway.

5.3.6 Diffuse Large B-Cell Lymphoma

DLBCL is rare in childhood, but its incidence increases in adolescence. However, in patients with congenital, iatrogenic (posttransplantation lymphoproliferative disorders, PTLD), or acquired immunodeficiency, DLBCL is the most common lymphoma subtype and has an extremely poor prognosis. Patients may present with nodal or extranodal disease, but a solely gastrointestinal extranodal presentation is not uncommon. A rare primary mediastinal DLBCL has also been described in children. In DLBCL, the typical cells are large, with round nuclei and prominent central nucleoli. Immunophenotypically, they express pan B-cell markers such as CD20 and CD79a [28, 29].

Most treatment protocols aimed at advanced stages of the disease employ a combination of cyclophosphamide, high-dose methotrexate, cytarabine, and intrathecal prophylaxis, resulting in EFS rates >90 %. Lower-risk patients are treated with chemotherapies of reduced duration and intensity and survival is excellent [30].

References

1. Horner MJ, Ries LAG, Krapcho M (2008) Cancer in children (ages 0–14 and ages 0–19). SEER Cancer Statistics Review, 1975–2006. National Cancer Institute, Bethesda
2. Hochberg J, Waxman IM, Kelly KM et al (2009) Adolescent non-Hodgkin lymphoma and Hodgkin lymphoma: state of the science. Br J Haematol 144:24–40
3. Carbone PP, Kaplan HS, Musshoff K et al (1971) Report of the committee on Hodgkin's disease staging classification. Cancer Res 31:1860–1861
4. Lister TA, Crowther D, Sutcliffe SB et al (1989) Report of a committee convened to discuss the evaluation and staging of patients with Hodgkin's disease: Cotswolds meeting. J Clin Oncol 7:1630–1636
5. Donaldson SS (2002) Pediatric Hodgkin's disease – up, up, and beyond. Int J Radiat Oncol Biol Phys 54:1–8
6. Bonadonna G, Zucali R, Monfardini S et al (1975) Combination chemotherapy of Hodgkin's disease with adriamycin, bleomycin, vinblastine, and imidazole carboxamide versus MOPP. Cancer 36:252–259
7. Nachman JB, Sposto R, Herzog P et al (2002) Randomized comparison of low-dose involved-field radiotherapy and no radiotherapy for children with Hodgkin's disease who achieve a complete response to chemotherapy. J Clin Oncol 20:3765–3771
8. Yung L, Smith P, Hancock BW et al (2004) Long term outcome in adolescents with Hodgkin's lymphoma: poor results using regimens designed for adults. Leuk Lymphoma 45:1579–1585
9. Murphy SB (1978) Childhood non-Hodgkin's lymphoma. N Engl J Med 299:1446–1448
10. Murphy SB (1980) Classification, staging and end results of treatment of childhood non-Hodgkin's lymphomas: dissimilarities from lymphomas in adults. Semin Oncol 7:332–339
11. Reiter A (2007) Diagnosis and treatment of childhood non-hodgkin lymphoma. Hematology Am Soc Hematol Educ Program 2007(1):285–296. doi: 10.1182/asheducation-2007.1.285
12. Anderson JR, Jenkin RD, Wilson JF et al (1993) Long-term follow-up of patients treated with COMP or LSA2L2 therapy for childhood non-Hodgkin's lymphoma: a report of CCG-551 from the Childrens Cancer Group. J Clin Oncol 11:1024–1032
13. de-Thé G (1985) The Epstein-Barr virus (EBV): a Rosetta Stone for understanding the role of viruses in immunopathological disorders and in human carcinogenesis. Biomed Pharmacother 39:49–51
14. Molyneux EM, Rochford R, Griffin B et al (2012) Burkitt's lymphoma. Lancet 379:1234–1244
15. Bellan C, Lazzi S, Hummel M et al (2005) Immunoglobulin gene analysis reveals 2 distinct cells of origin for EBV-positive and EBV-negative Burkitt lymphomas. Blood 106:1031–1036
16. El-Mallawany NK, Frazer JK, Van Vlierberghe P et al (2012) Pediatric T- and NK-cell lymphomas: new biologic insights and treatment strategies. Blood Cancer J 2:e65
17. Schrappe M, Reiter A, Ludwig WD et al (2000) Improved outcome in childhood acute lymphoblastic leukemia despite reduced use of anthracyclines and cranial radiotherapy: results of trial ALL-BFM 90. German-Austrian-Swiss ALL-BFM Study Group. Blood 95:3310–3322
18. Pillon M, Piglione M, Garaventa A et al (2009) Long-term results of AIEOP LNH-92 protocol for the treatment of pediatric lymphoblastic lymphoma: a report of the Italian Association of Pediatric Hematology and Oncology. Pediatr Blood Cancer 53:953–959
19. Burkhardt B, Woessmann W, Zimmermann M et al (2006) Impact of cranial radiotherapy on central nervous system prophylaxis in children and adolescents with central nervous system-negative stage III or IV lymphoblastic lymphoma. J Clin Oncol 24:491–499
20. Abromowitch M, Sposto R, Perkins S et al (2008) Shortened intensified multi-agent chemotherapy and non-cross resistant maintenance therapy for advanced lymphoblastic lymphoma in children and adolescents: report from the Children's Oncology Group. Br J Haematol 143:261–267
21. Bureo E, Ortega JJ, Muñoz A et al (1995) Bone marrow transplantation in 46 pediatric patients with non-Hodgkin's lymphoma. Spanish Working Party for Bone Marrow Transplantation in Children. Bone Marrow Transplant 15:353–359
22. Kleiner S, Kirsch A, Schwaner I et al (1997) High-dose chemotherapy with carboplatin, etoposide and ifosfamide followed by autologous stem cell rescue in patients with relapsed or refractory malignant lymphomas: a phase I/II study. Bone Marrow Transplant 20:953–959

23. Kobrinsky NL, Sposto R, Shah NR et al (2001) Outcomes of treatment of children and adolescents with recurrent non-Hodgkin's lymphoma and Hodgkin's disease with dexamethasone, etoposide, cisplatin, cytarabine, and l-asparaginase, maintenance chemotherapy, and transplantation: Children's Cancer Group Study CCG-5912. J Clin Oncol 19:2390–2396
24. Duyster J, Bai RY, Morris SW (2001) Translocations involving anaplastic lymphoma kinase (ALK). Oncogene 20:5623–5637
25. Benharroch D, Meguerian-Bedoyan Z, Lamant L et al (1998) ALK-positive lymphoma: a single disease with a broad spectrum of morphology. Blood 91:2076–2084
26. Seidemann K, Tiemann M, Schrappe M et al (2001) Short-pulse B-non-Hodgkin lymphoma-type chemotherapy is efficacious treatment for pediatric anaplastic large cell lymphoma: a report of the Berlin-Frankfurt-Münster Group Trial NHL-BFM 90. Blood 97:3699–3706
27. Rosolen A, Pillon M, Garaventa A et al (2005) Anaplastic large cell lymphoma treated with a leukemia-like therapy: report of the Italian Association of Pediatric Hematology and Oncology (AIEOP) LNH-92 protocol. Cancer 104:2133–2140
28. Alizadeh AA, Eisen MB, Davis RE et al (2000) Distinct types of diffuse large B-cell lymphoma identified by gene expression profiling. Nature 403:503–511
29. Oschlies I, Klapper W, Zimmermann M et al (2006) Diffuse large B-cell lymphoma in pediatric patients belongs predominantly to the germinal-center type B-cell lymphomas: a clinicopathologic analysis of cases included in the German BFM (Berlin-Frankfurt-Munster) Multicenter Trial. Blood 107:4047–4052
30. Patte C, Auperin A, Gerrard M et al (2007) Results of the randomized international FAB/LMB96 trial for intermediate risk B-cell non-Hodgkin lymphoma in children and adolescents: it is possible to reduce treatment for the early responding patients. Blood 109:2773–2780

6. ^{18}F-FDG–PET/CT in Pediatric Lymphoma

Andrea Skanjeti, Luca Guerra, and Angelina Cistaro

6.1 Background

In pediatric lymphoma, effective therapeutic regimens are now widely available and further innovations are likely. However, the efficacy of treatment still relies on accurate staging, early evaluation of the disease, post-therapeutic monitoring, and continued surveillance. Moreover, in children, high cure rates are only one of the beginnings, as the long-term potential consequences of radio- and chemotherapy, i.e., pulmonary, cardiovascular, reproductive, and thyroid complications, recurrent infections, and neurocognitive deficits, must be considered as well. Thus, a sensitive exam is not only crucial diagnostically but it also avoids overtreatment.

^{18}F-FDG–PET/CT has been studied for decades in adult lymphomas, and while its role in this setting is well defined, in childhood lymphomas, it is so far unclear. According to several authors, the usefulness of ^{18}F-FDG–PET/CT in all phases of disease management is debatable; however, it should be noted that the vast majority of these studies were retrospective, unicentric, and lacked reproducible timing of the PET scan during therapy evaluation. In fact, in addition to being a noninvasive examination, ^{18}F-FDG–PET/CT offers several other advantages. First, as a functional imaging technique, ^{18}F-FDG–PET is essential to accurately study pediatric lymphoma as morphological data alone are insufficiently informative [1, 2]. Second, ^{18}F-FDG–PET is a highly sensitive functional exam, because its high spatial resolution is higher than that of nuclear imaging techniques such as gallium scintigraphy and bone scan [3–5]. Third, it exploits the intrinsic capability of tumor cells to take up FDG. Lastly, a whole-body exam extending from the orbitomeatal line to the proximal femur can be performed both in adults and children [6].

In lymphoma, ^{18}F-FDG–PET/CT can define disease stage as well as bone involvement, and in some cases, it is better than bone marrow biopsy, as it avoids sample errors or misdiagnoses due to the absence of iliac disease [7].

During therapy, interim PET establishes treatment efficacy. ^{18}F-FDG–PET/CT results were shown to correlate with progression-free survival and had a higher specificity than the findings obtained with conventional imaging

A. Skanjeti, MD
Nuclear Medicine Division, San Luigi Hospital,
University of Turin, Regione Gonzole 10,
10043 Orbassano, Turin 10100, Italy

Medical Science Department,
University A. Avogadro, Turin, Italy
e-mail: askanjeti@yahoo.it

L. Guerra, MD
Nuclear Medicine Department, Azienda Ospedaliera San Gerardo di Monza, Via Pergolesi 33,
Monza (MI) 20900, Italy
e-mail: l.guerra@hsgerardo.org

A. Cistaro, MD (✉)
Department of Nuclear Medicine, Positron Emission Tomography Center IRMET S.p.A., Euromedic Inc.,
Via Onorato Vigliani 89, Turin 10100, Italy

Institute of Cognitive Sciences and Technologies,
National Research Council, Rome, Italy
e-mail: a.cistaro@irmet.com

[8, 9]. The relevance of functional imaging is that the first response of malignant tissues to therapy is functional and only later morphological. Furthermore, functional but not morphological imaging can easily distinguish fibrotic from tumoral tissues. However, the optimal timing of the ^{18}F-FDG–PET/CT exam has yet to be established and remains a matter of debate. According to current knowledge, a repeat ^{18}F-FDG–PET/CT should be performed after two cycles of chemotherapy.

At the end of chemotherapy, the clinical objective is to define whether the young patient will require salvage therapy or should follow a program of disease surveillance. This decision relies on the specificity and sensitivity of ^{18}F-FDG–PET/CT to stratify the disease and to avoid overtreatment in good responders. ^{18}F-FDG–PET/CT is more accurate than conventional imaging to exclude disease after treatment [9]. An open issue, at least for adults, is the minimal residual disease evaluation. To the best of our knowledge, there are no appropriate data for children with malignant lymphoma. A role for ^{18}F-FDG–PET/CT in defining the target volume prior to radiotherapy has been established in several studies [10–12].

^{18}F-FDG–PET/CT may also be beneficial during surveillance, even in the absence of suspected relapse, as it allows the earliest possible detection of recurrence. Nonetheless, the high number of false-positives, especially in Burkitt's lymphoma involving the gastrointestinal tract and abdominal lymph nodes, has discouraged its use in this setting [13–15].

In conclusion, the utility of ^{18}F-FDG–PET/CT in children with malignant lymphoma needs to be further evaluated in prospective and multicenter studies. Thus far, there is extensive evidence that the most promising applications in pediatric lymphoma will be in disease staging and stratification, early therapeutic evaluation of therapy, and in case of suspected relapse.

Case 1

In the case presented in Figs. 6.1, 6.2, and 6.3, radiography of the tibias revealed findings consistent with nonossifying fibroma. This benign condition, which is commonly encountered in radiology, is a well-circumscribed solitary proliferation of fibrous tissue usually located in the metaphysis or diametaphyseal junction of the femur or tibia. It appears as an eccentric radiolucent lesion with thinned cortex, which can have a multilocular appearance and often a sclerotic margin [1]. During the involutional phase, osteoblastic activity increases as the lesion is replaced by new bone. The mechanism for ^{18}F-FDG uptake by nonossifying fibroma and acute fractures may be similar, as the two shares increased blood flow as well as osteoblastic and metabolic activity [2]. In general, nonossifying fibroma regresses spontaneously.

Teaching Point
The PET appearance of nonossifying fibroma can mimic bone metastasis [16, 17]. When PET reveals metabolically active osseous abnormalities in children at risk for bone metastases, benign fibro-osseous lesions should be considered in the differential diagnosis.

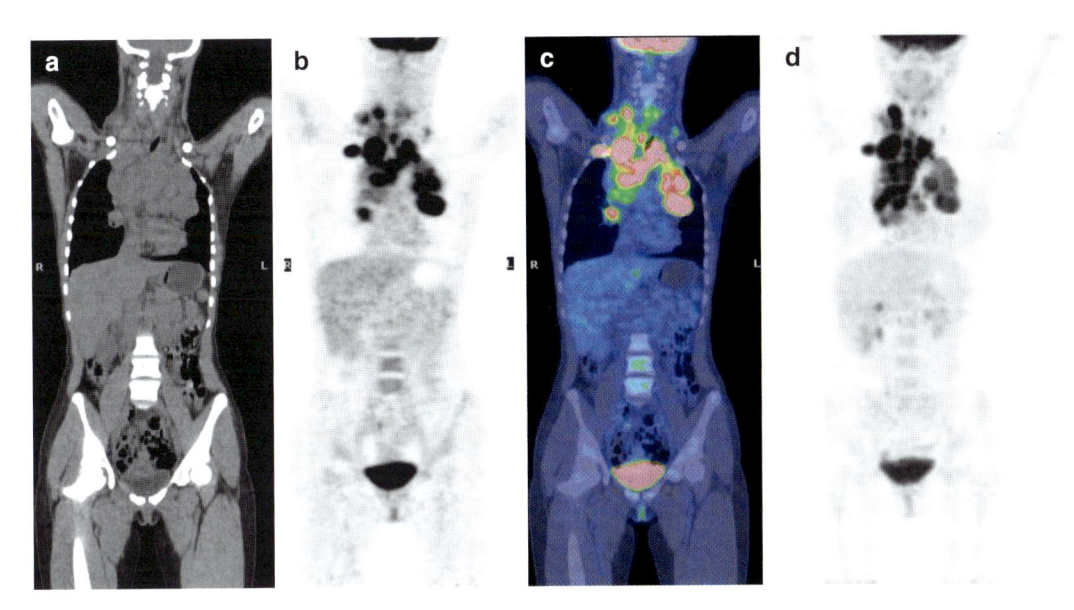

Fig. 6.1 A 15-year-old girl with Hodgkin's disease. Coronal CT (**a**), PET (**b**), PET/CT fusion (**c**), and maximum intensity projection (**d**) staging images show multiple sites of uptake in the supradiaphragmatic lymph nodes, indicative of stage II disease

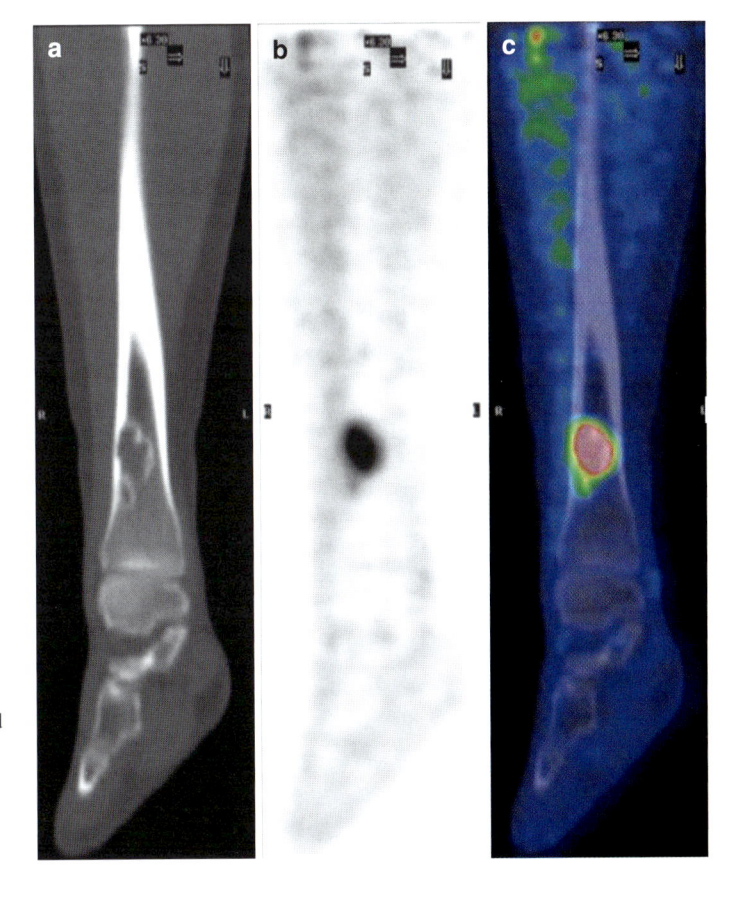

Fig. 6.2 Same patient as in Fig. 6.1. Coronal CT, PET, and PET/CT fusion images of the right tibia. The coronally reformatted CT (**a**) shows a lucent lesion in the distal right tibia, corresponding to increased uptake on coronal ^{18}F-FDG-PET (**b**) and ^{18}F-FDG-PET/CT fusion images (**c**). The disease stage has changed from stage II to stage IV based on osseous involvement

Case 1 (continued)

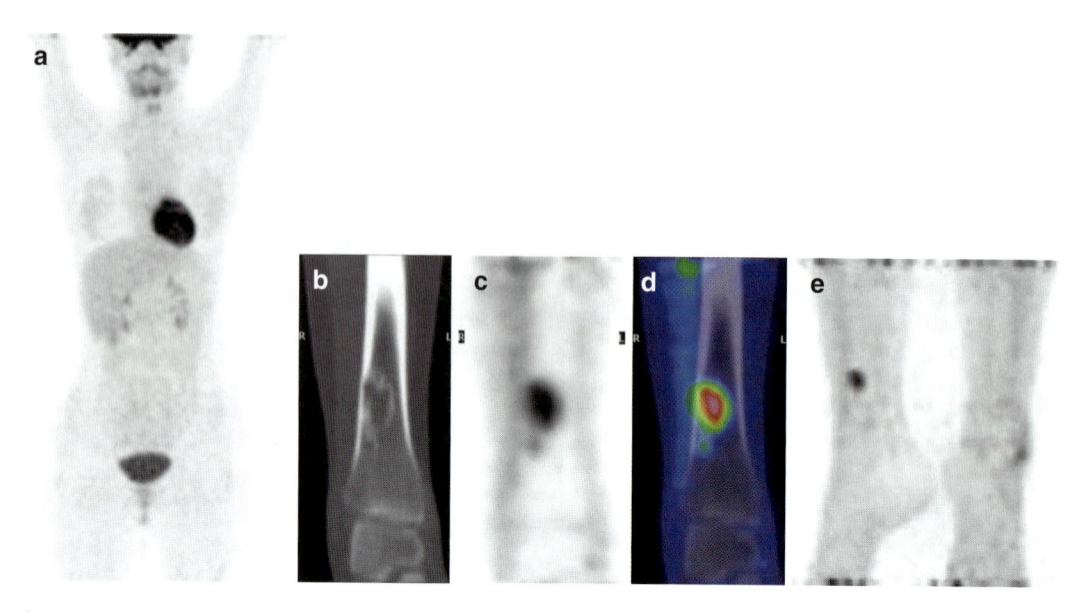

Fig. 6.3 Same patient as above. The PET study during chemotherapy showed complete resolution of the lymph node uptake, as seen on MIP (**a**). Coronal CT shows unchanged lucent tibial lesion (**b**) while persistent uptake of ^{18}F-FDG in the tibia is seen on PET (**c**) and PET/CT fusion (**d**). The evaluation at the end of treatment indicated complete lymphoma remission. Tibial uptake was unchanged on emission PET (**e**)

Case 2

Fig. 6.4 An 11-year-old boy with Hodgkin's disease. (**a**) Maximum intensity projection ^{18}F-FDG–PET image shows multiple uptake sites in the supradiaphragmatic lymph nodes. (**b**) Axial CT and PET/CT fusion images show involvement of the spleen. The final stage of the tumor was IIIs

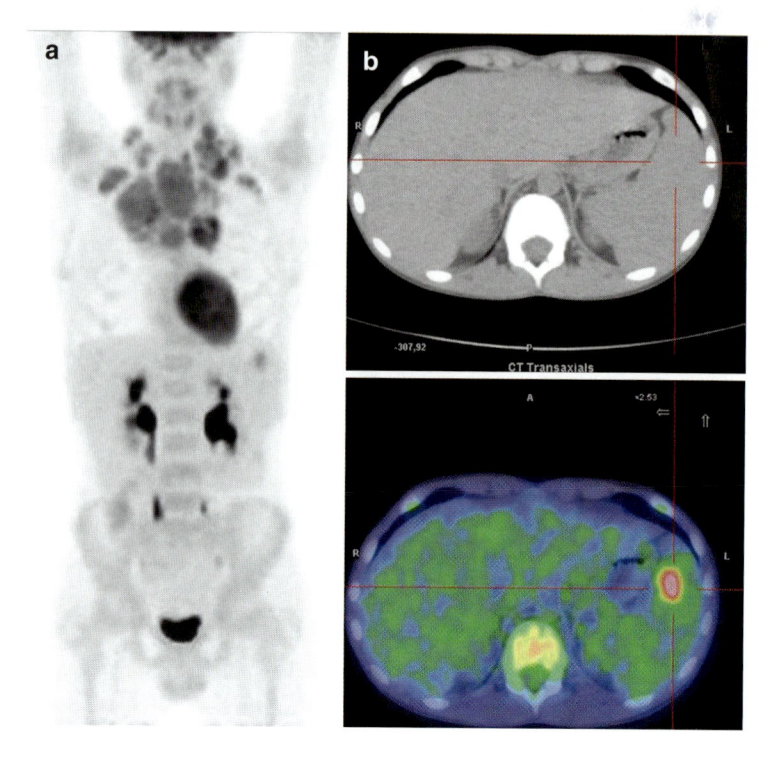

Case 3

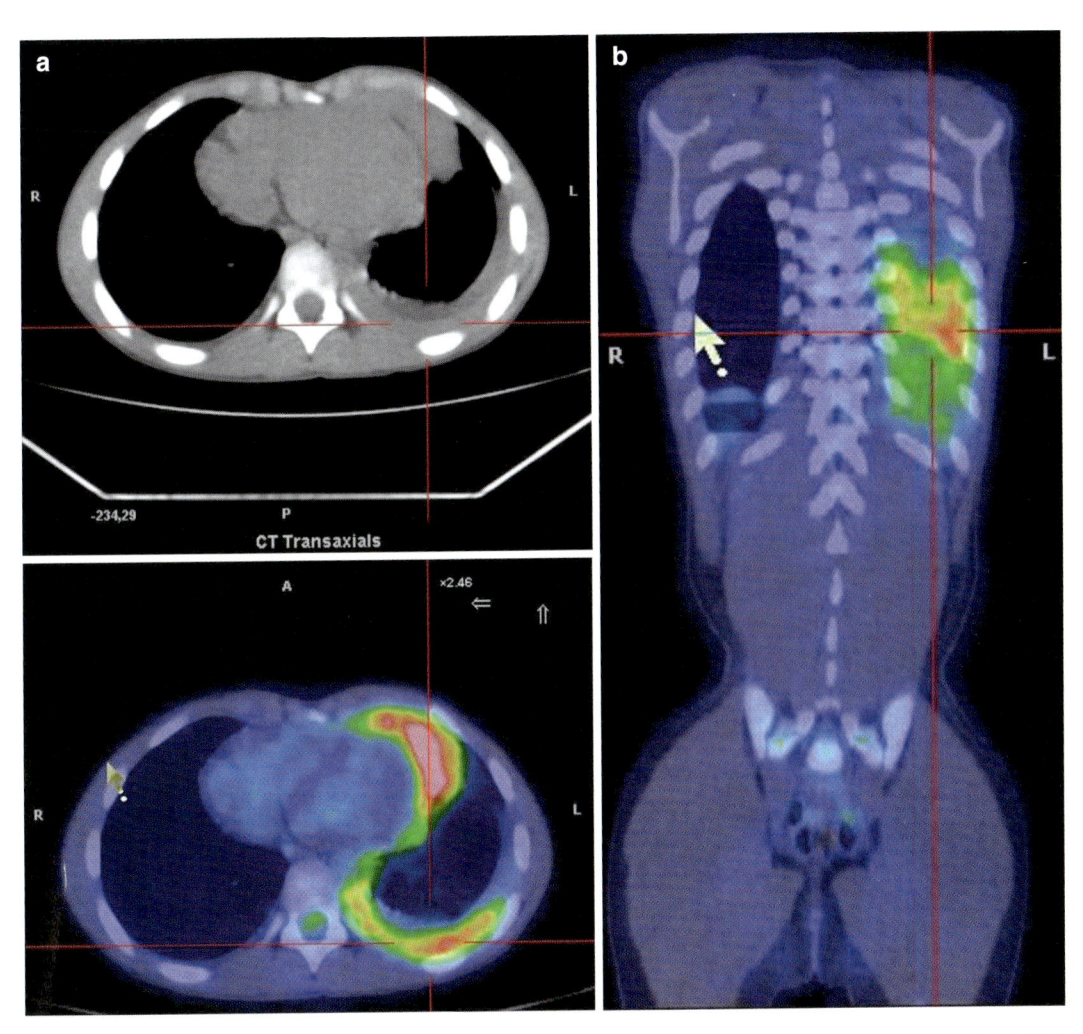

Fig. 6.5 A 9-year-old boy with stage IV Hodgkin's disease. (**a, b**) Axial CT together with axial and coronal PET/CT fusion images show posterior left pleural involvement

Case 4

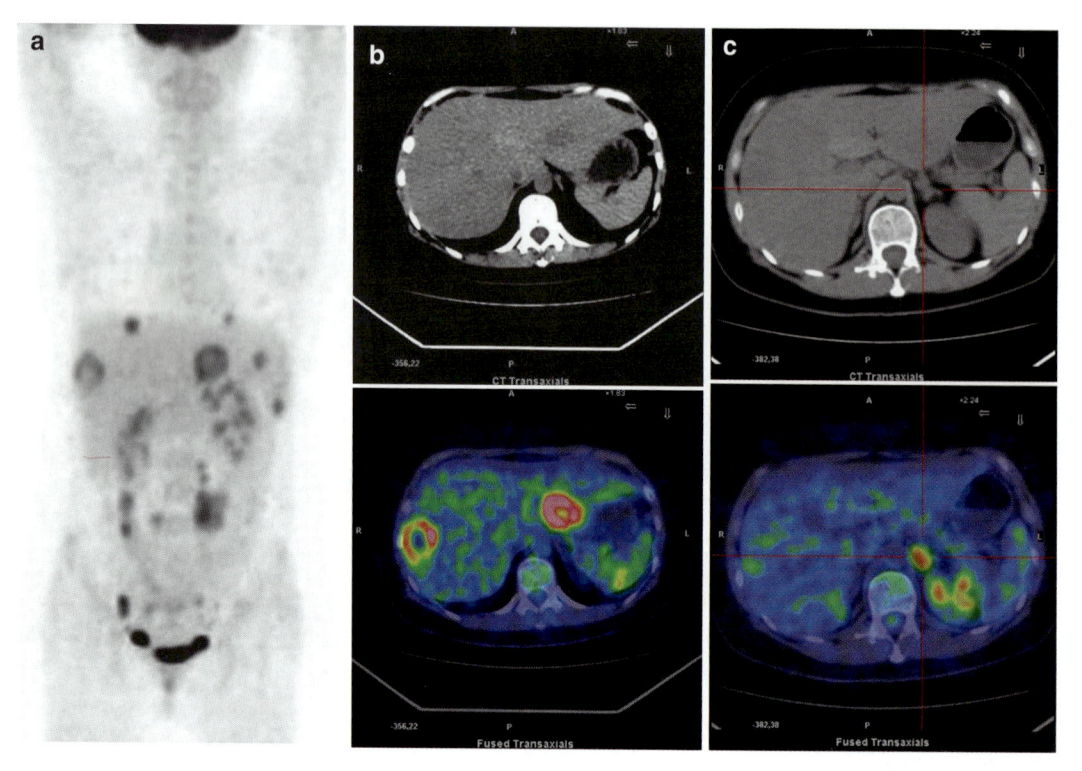

Fig. 6.6 A 17-year-old girl diagnosed with diffuse large cell lymphoma, an aggressive non-Hodgkin's lymphoma that often involves the lymph nodes, spleen, liver, bone marrow, and other organs. Maximum intensity projection (**a**) and axial CT and PET/CT fusion images (**b,c**) show liver lesions with central necrosis (**b**) and lesion of the left adrenal gland (**c**)

6 ^{18}F-FDG–PET/CT in Pediatric Lymphoma

Case 4 (continued)

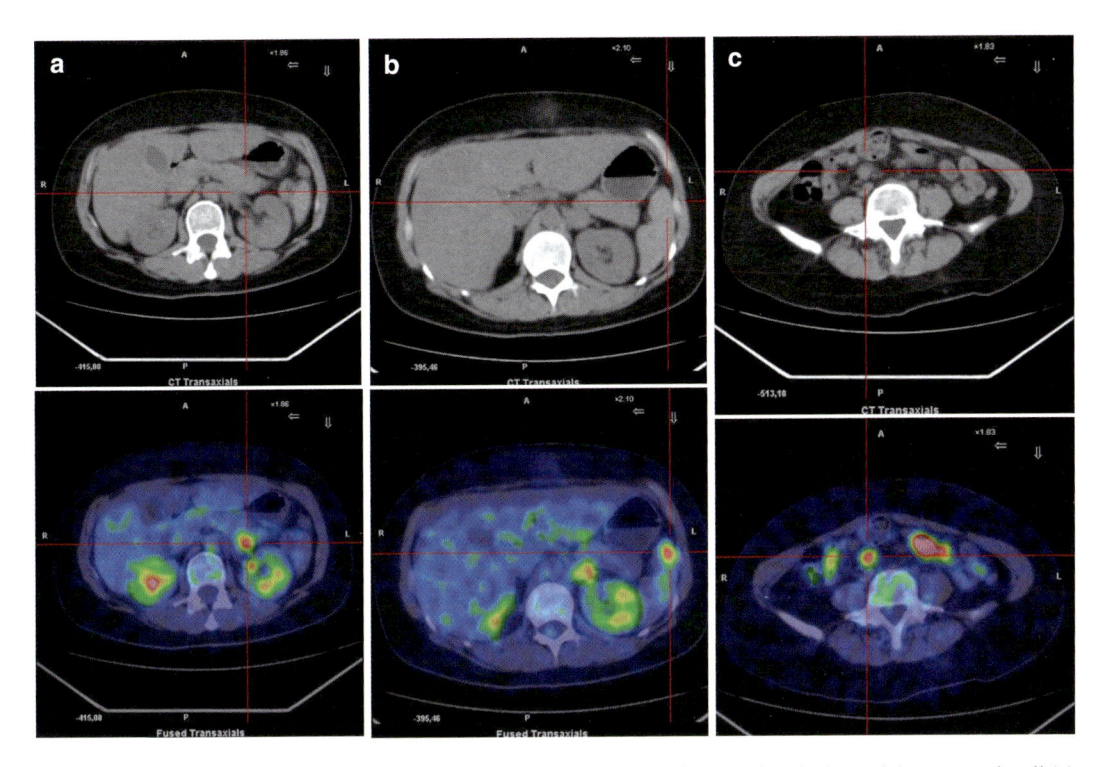

Fig. 6.7 Same patient as in Fig. 6.6. (**a–c**) Axial CT and PET/CT fusion images show lesions of the pancreatic tail (**a**) and spleen (**b**) as well as mesenteric lymph node involvement (**c**)

Case 4 (continued)

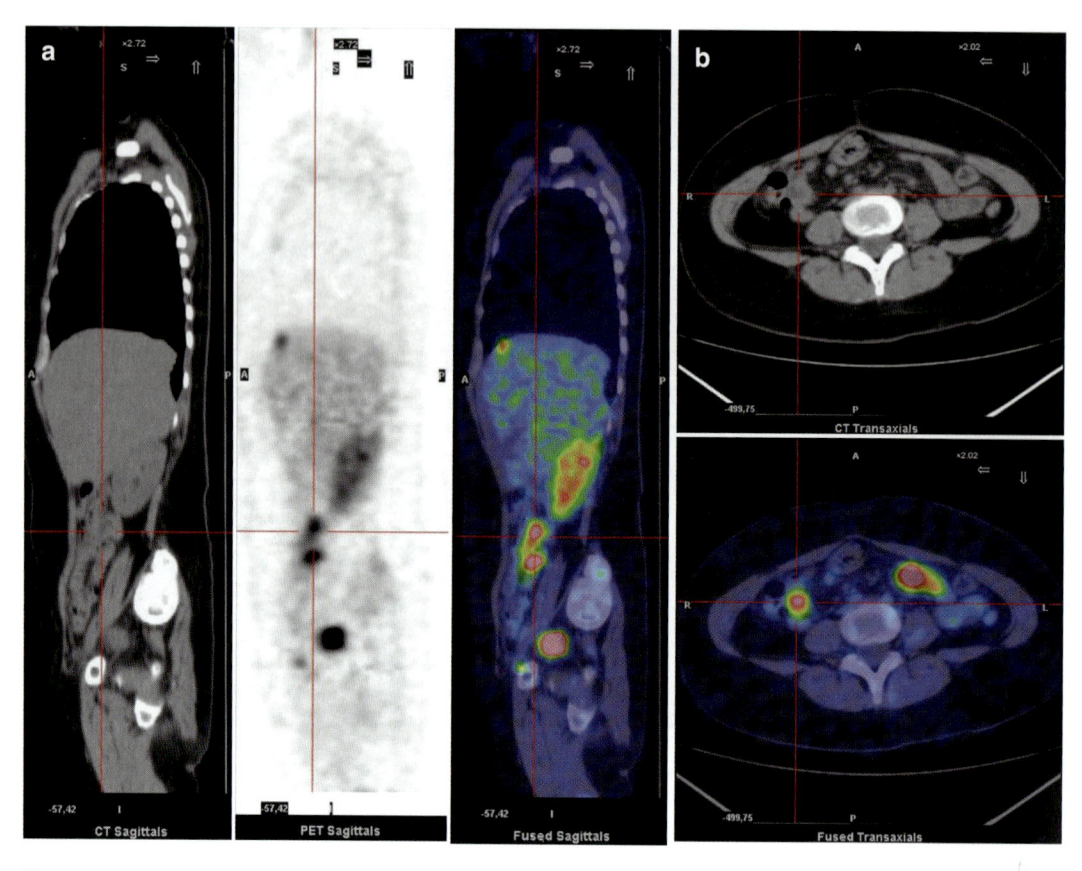

Fig. 6.8 The same patient as above. (a) Sagittal-view CT, PET, and PET/CT fusion images show bowel involvement. (b) Axial CT and PET/CT fusion images show ^{18}F-FDG uptake in the small bowel

Case 4 (continued)

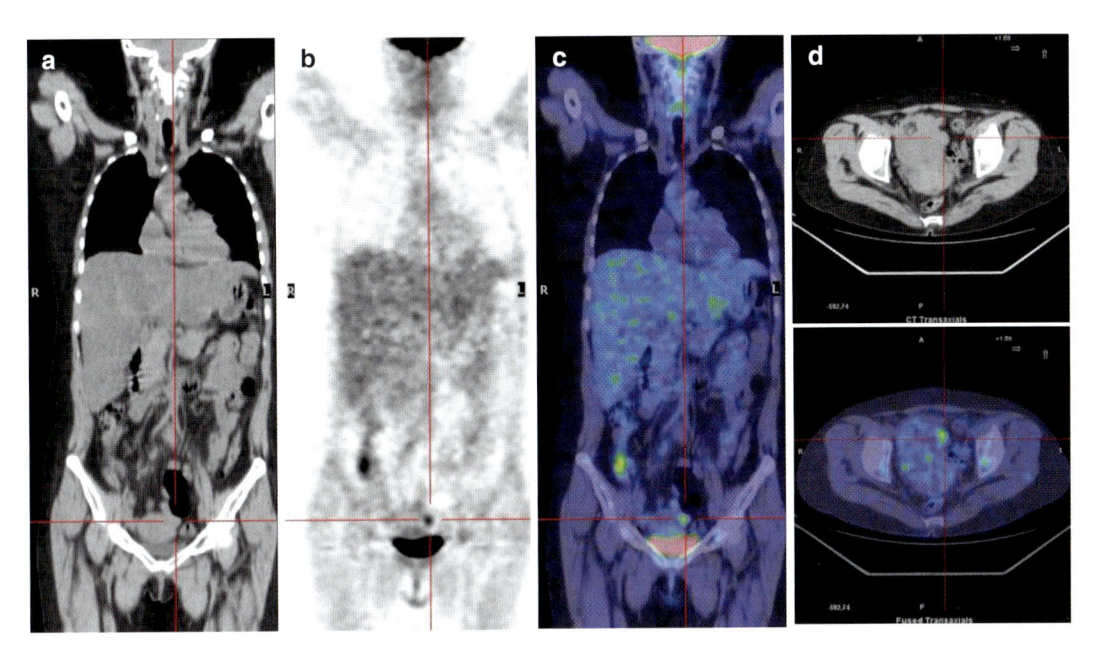

Fig. 6.9 The same patient during chemotherapy treatment. Coronal CT (**a**), PET (**b**), and PET/CT fusion images (**c**) show the disappearance of all pathological uptake. A hot spot is visible in the left pelvis (**c**), which as seen on axial CT and PET/CT fusion images (**d**) is due to a physiological ovarian follicle

Teaching Point

It is important to be aware of the patient's age and her menstrual cycle in order to correctly interpret physiological uptake in the pelvis [18, 19].

Case 5

A 2-year-old boy presented with fever, right knee pain, and lameness, previously treated with antibiotics and low-dose betamethasone. The radiological finding suggested osteoarthritis of the right hip joint with involvement of the adjacent muscles, nonresponsive to antibiotics. An arthrotomy of the right hip joint was performed: the microbiological studies were negative. Ultrasound imaging of the soft tissue of the neck showed small laterocervical bilateral lymph node adenopathy, without colliquation. A PET/CT study was requested to metabolically characterize both the hip lesions and the laterocervical lymph adenopathy (Figs. 6.10, 6.11, 6.12, 6.13, 6.14, 6.15, and 6.16).

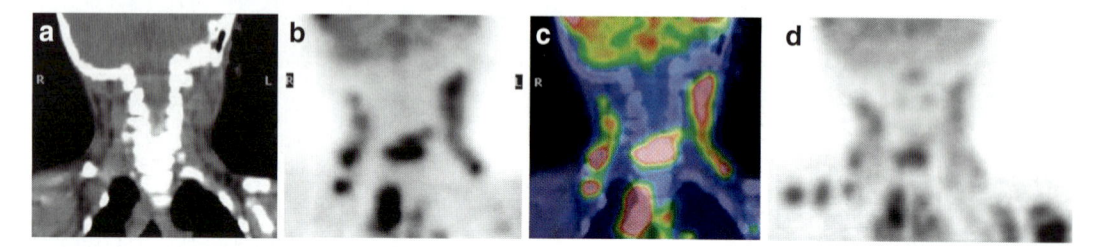

Fig. 6.10 Coronal CT (**a**), PET (**b**), PET/CT fusion images (**c**), and maximum intensity projection (**d**) of the head–neck region showing extensive ^{18}F-FDG uptake in the laterocervical lymph nodes and a lesion in the fifth cervical vertebra

6   ^{18}F-FDG–PET/CT in Pediatric Lymphoma

Case 5 (continued)

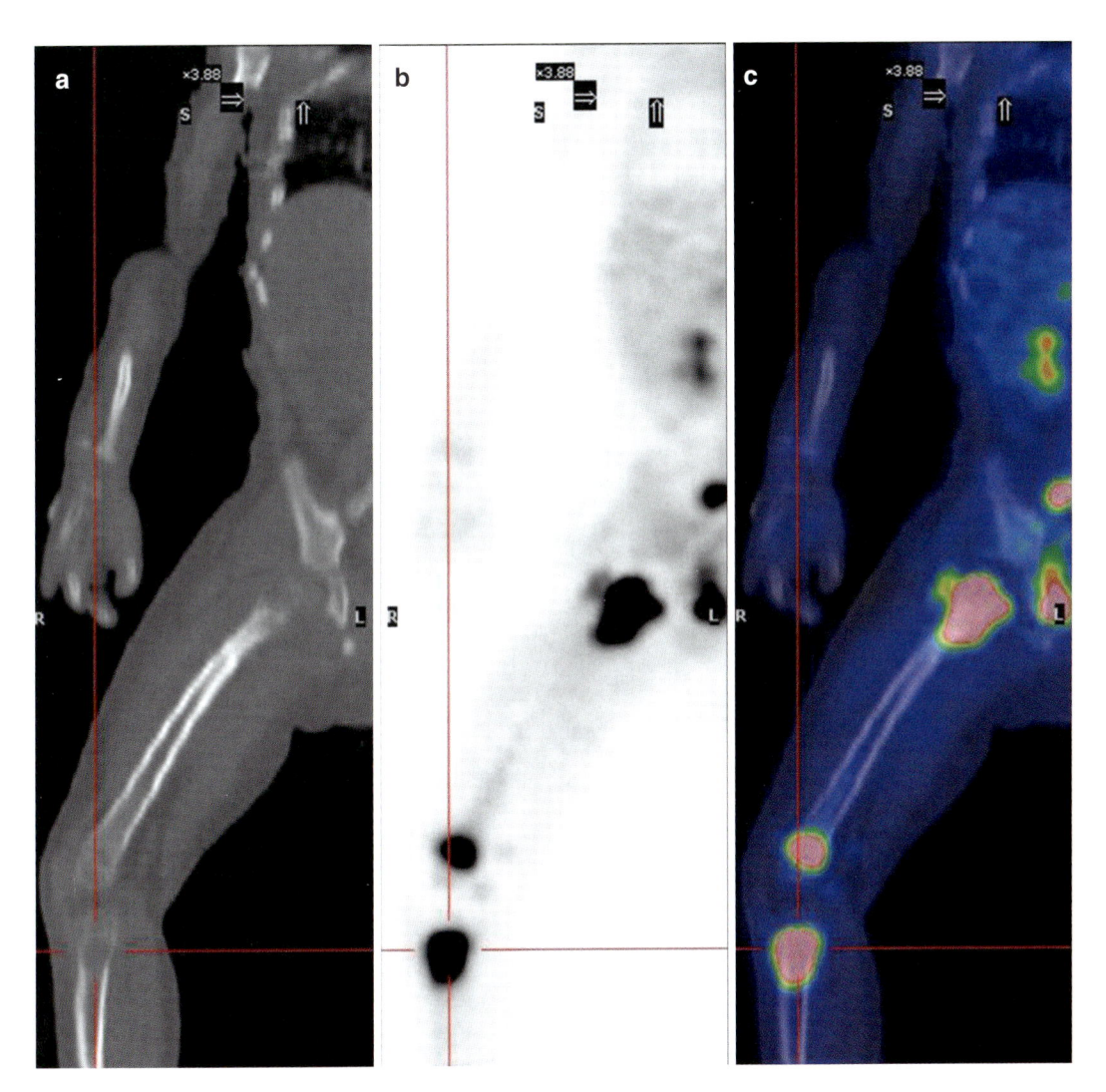

Fig. 6.11 Same patient as in Fig. 6.10. Coronal CT (**a**), PET (**b**), and PET/CT fusion (**c**) images show intense uptake in the proximal and distal right femur as well as in the proximal right tibia

Case 5 (continued)

Fig. 6.12 Same patient as above. Maximum intensity projection (**a**) and coronal PET/CT fusion (**b**) images show multiple sites of uptake in the pelvic bone, proximal humerus, right scapula, and sternum. Multiple pathological supra- and subdiaphragmatic lymph nodes are also present. A PET-guided biopsy of a laterocervical lymph node confirmed the diagnosis of t(2;5)-positive anaplastic large cell lymphoma, stage IV

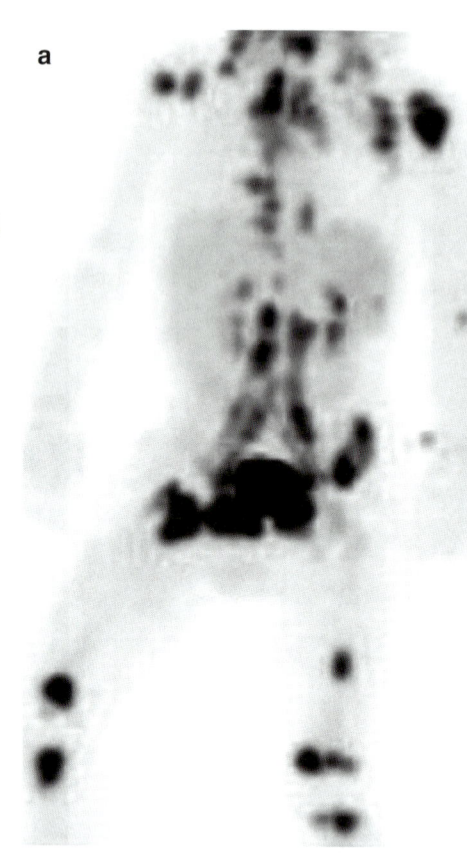

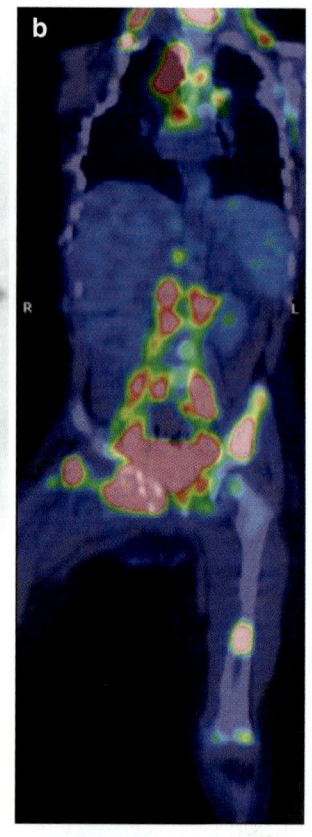

Teaching Point

Non-Hodgkin's lymphoma may have a silent onset and involve several organ systems, including bone. In this patient, the condition was initially suspected to be benign. Conventional imaging methods, generally used to evaluate the extent of non-Hodgkin's lymphoma, did not identify the malignant characteristics of the hip joint lesion. PET/CT can be a useful tool in the metabolic characterization of lesions of unknown origin. It improves their localization, and allows a guided biopsy, by identifying the more accessible and active sites, and thus increases the diagnostic success rate.

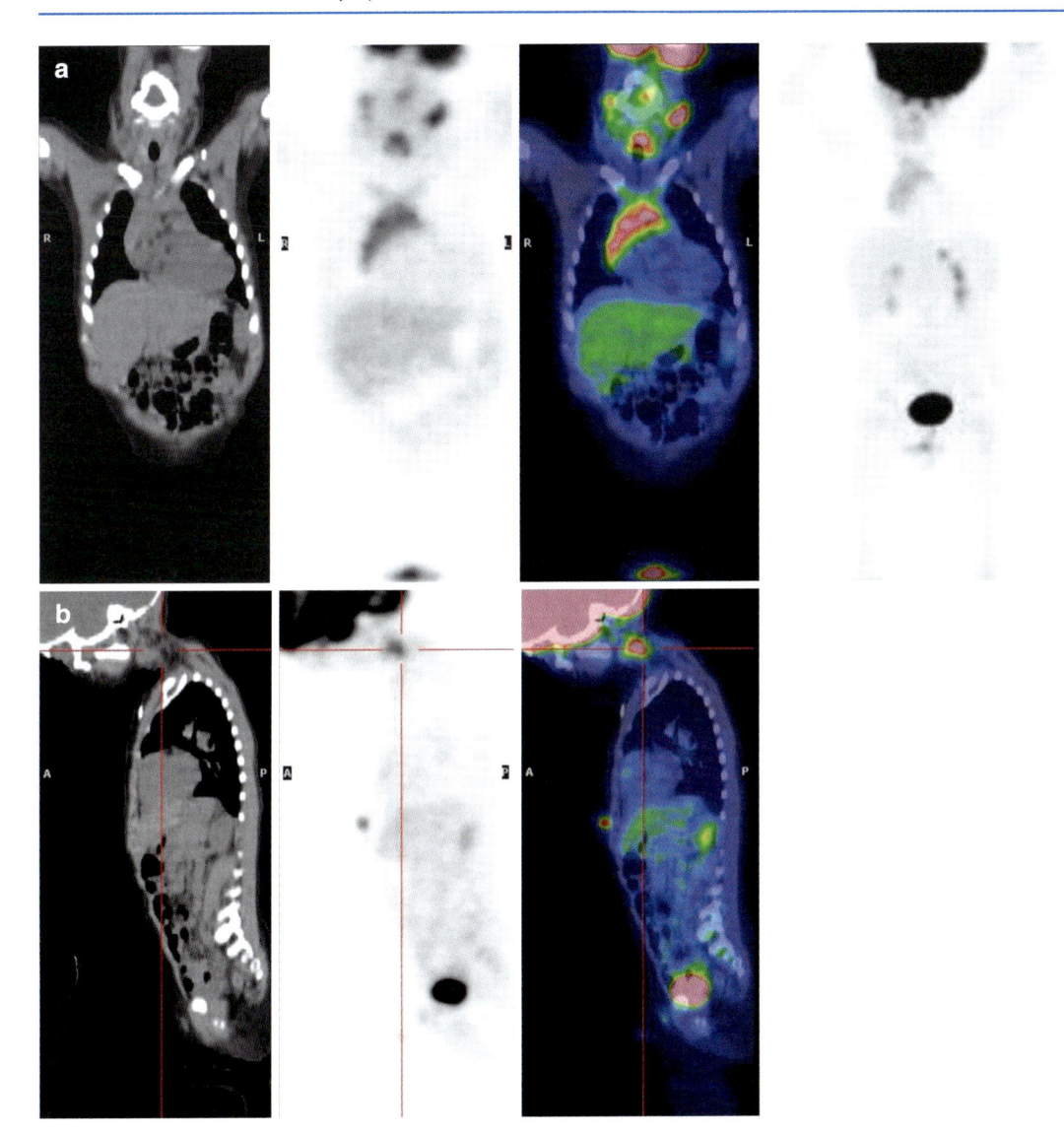

Fig. 6.13 The same patient at the end of the therapy according to the Italian chemotherapy protocol for non-Hodgkin's lymphoma (ALCL AIEOP 99). (**a**) Coronal CT, PET, and PET/CT fusion images and maximum intensity projection show complete disease remission, with the disappearance of all bone and lymph node uptake. Note the intense uptake in the anterior mediastinum, due to hyperplasia of the thymus. (**b**) Asymmetric uptake is visible in the left laterocervical region but without corresponding morphological alterations on CT. This site corresponds to brown fat activation

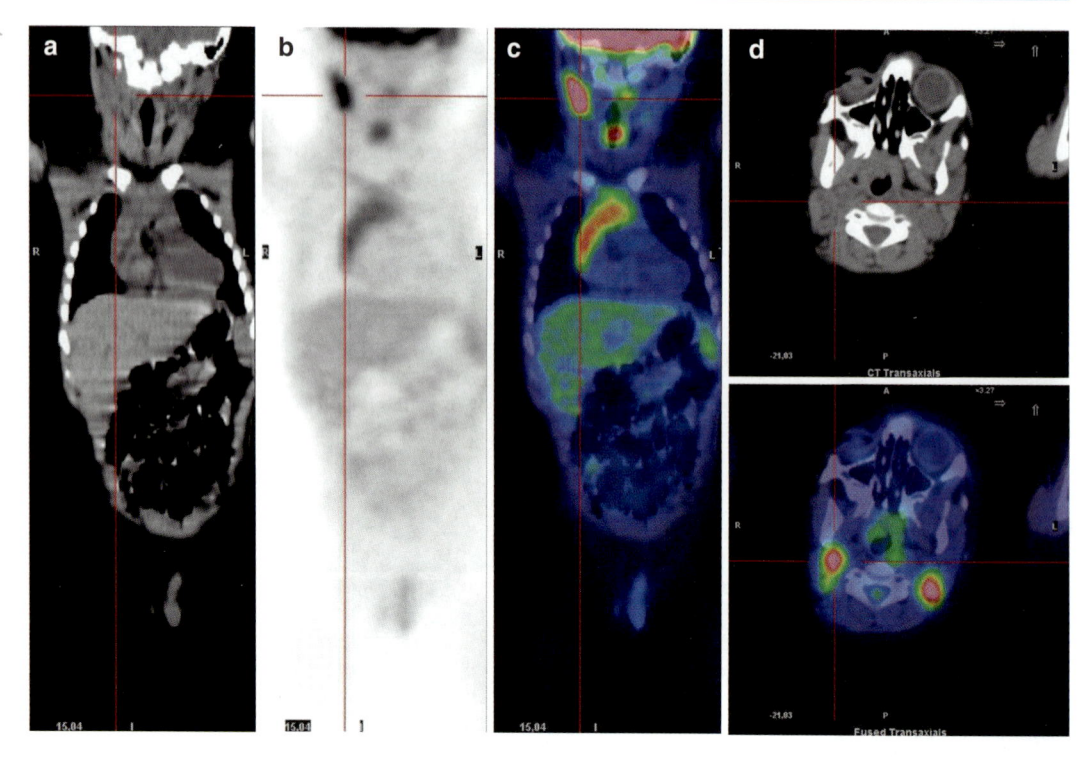

Fig. 6.14 Same patient 1 month later. Coronal CT (**a**), PET (**b**), and PET/CT fusion (**c**) images show disease relapse in the right laterocervical lymph nodes and the persistence of thymic hyperplasia. (**d**) Axial CT and PET/CT fusion images show bilateral lymphonodal recurrence of the lymphoma

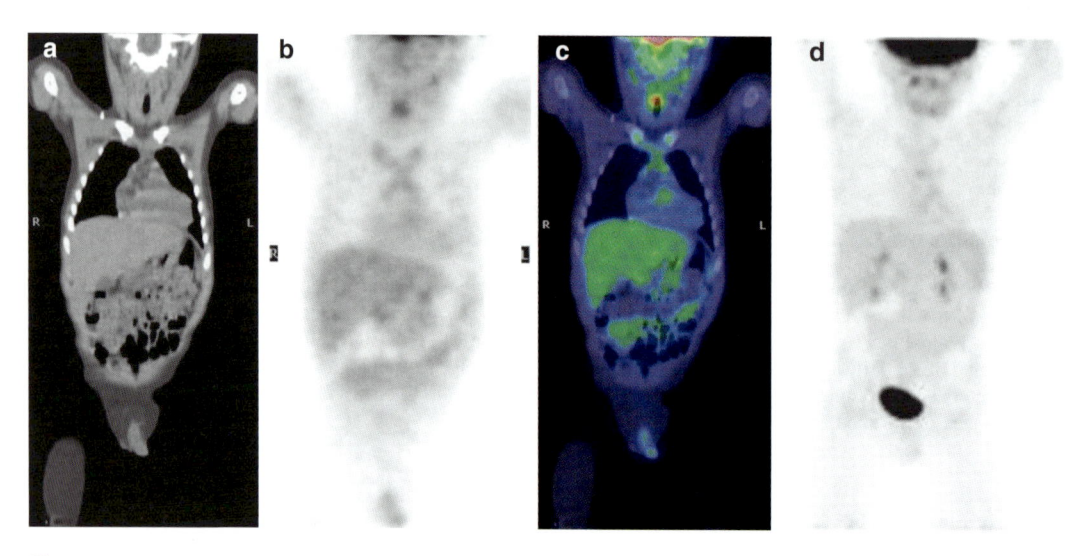

Fig. 6.15 Same patient, 9 months after allo-hematopoietic stem cell transplant and stop therapy. Coronal CT (**a**), PET (**b**), and PET/CT fusion (**c**) images and maximum intensity projection (**d**). The PET study shows normal FDG distribution. Noted the disappearance of the anterior mediastinal uptake at the site of the thymic hyperplasia. Following ^{18}F-FDG injection, the patient spent the waiting time in a warm room in order to prevent brown fat activation

6 ^{18}F-FDG–PET/CT in Pediatric Lymphoma

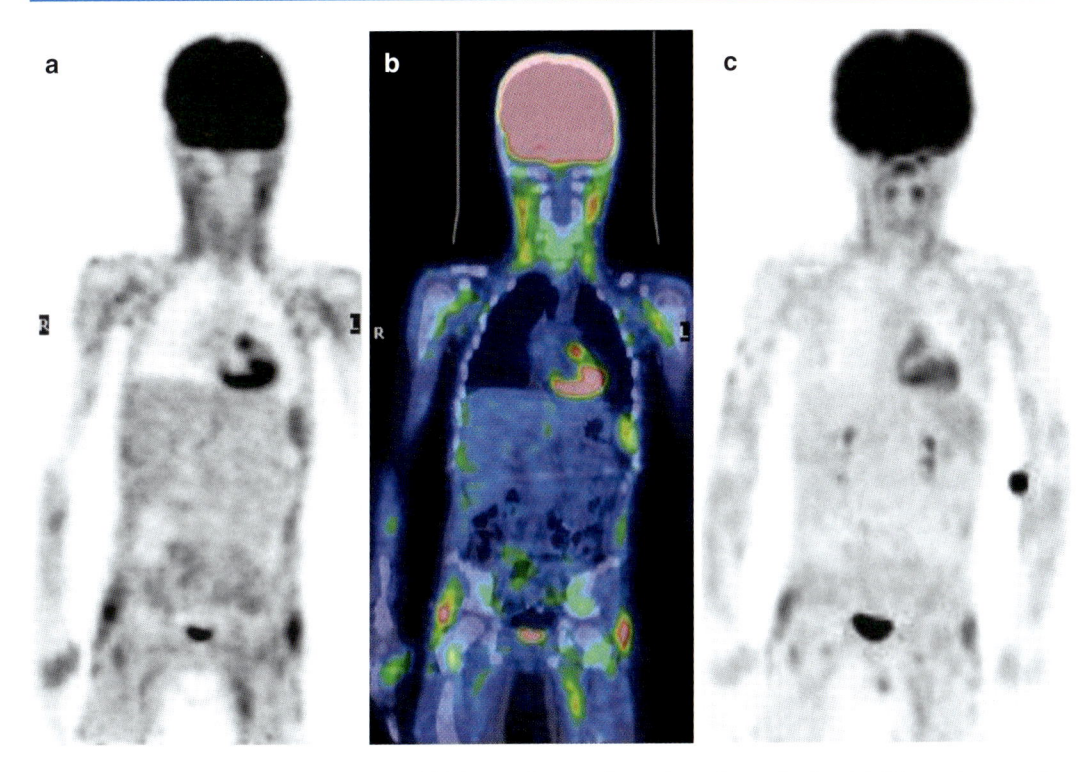

Fig. 6.16 Same patient 2 years later; the child is now 4 years old. A PET study was performed to determine the source of diffuse muscle pain, strabismus, and ocular pain, suggestive of disease recurrence in the brain. Coronal PET (**a**) and PET/CT fusion (**b**) images and maximum intensity projection (**c**) did not show uptakes consistent with NHL recurrence, but there was diffuse inhomogeneous muscular uptake. The patient underwent a muscle biopsy, which showed myositis. Serum creatine kinase was elevated

Teaching Point

Myositis refers to any condition causing inflammation in one or more muscles. Weakness, swelling, and pain are the most common symptoms. The causes of myositis include infection, injury, autoimmune conditions, and drug side effects. This condition should be kept in mind for patients undergoing PET studies, performed after other conditions that can result in increased FDG by the muscles have been excluded, such as elevated serum glucose or insulinemia, the absence of a fasting condition, or prolonged muscular activity.

Case 6

A 7-year-old boy who 5 years earlier underwent bilateral nephrectomy for Denys–Drash syndrome, followed by kidney transplantation and hypospadias repair. He was placed on immunosuppression therapy. Three years ago, he was diagnosed with an Epstein–Barr virus infection followed 2 years later by the appearance of axillary lymph node enlargement. A biopsy confirmed the suspected posttransplantation lymphoproliferative disorder (PTLD), CD20 and CD79a positive, Ki67 = 80 % (Burkitt's lymphoma B phenotype) (Figs. 6.17, 6.18, 6.19, and 6.20).

Denys–Drash syndrome is a rare disorder consisting of the triad of congenital nephropathy, Wilms' tumor, and gonadal dysgenesis, resulting from mutations in the Wilms' tumor suppressor (*WT1*) gene on chromosome band 11p13.

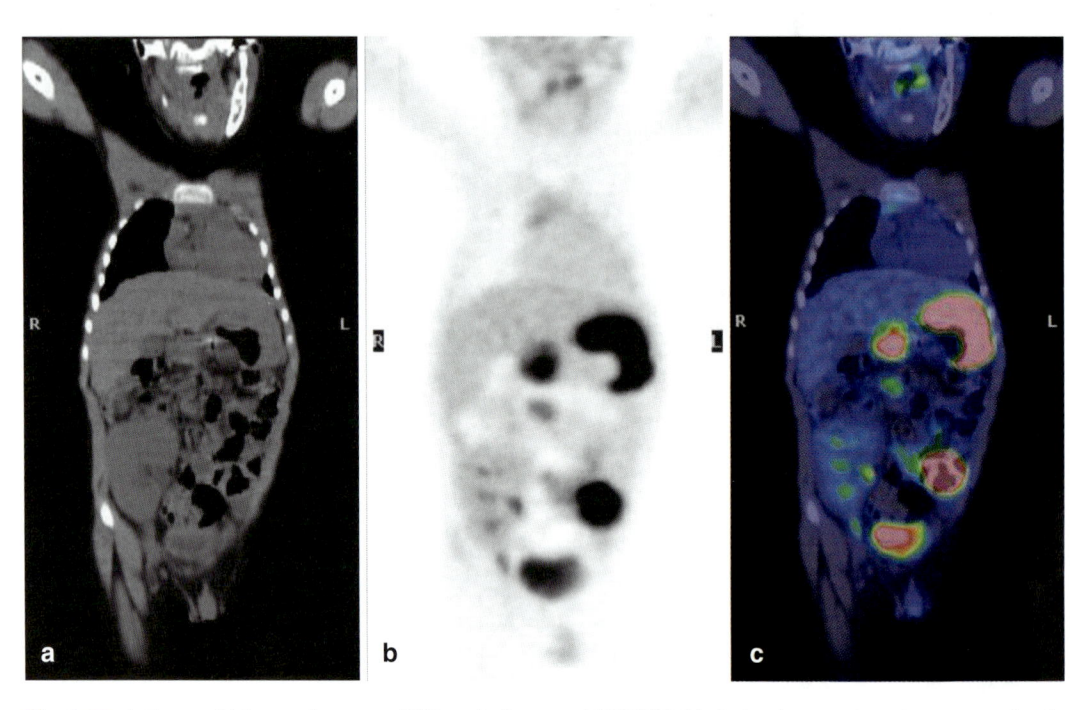

Fig. 6.17 A 7-year-old boy underwent a PET study for EBV-associated posttransplantation lymphoproliferative disorder (PTLD-EBV) staging. Coronal CT (**a**), PET (**b**), and PET/CT (**c**) fusion images show intense uptakes in the stomach and left colon in addition to a large lymphadenopathy of the celiac region

6 ^{18}F-FDG–PET/CT in Pediatric Lymphoma

Case 6 (continued)

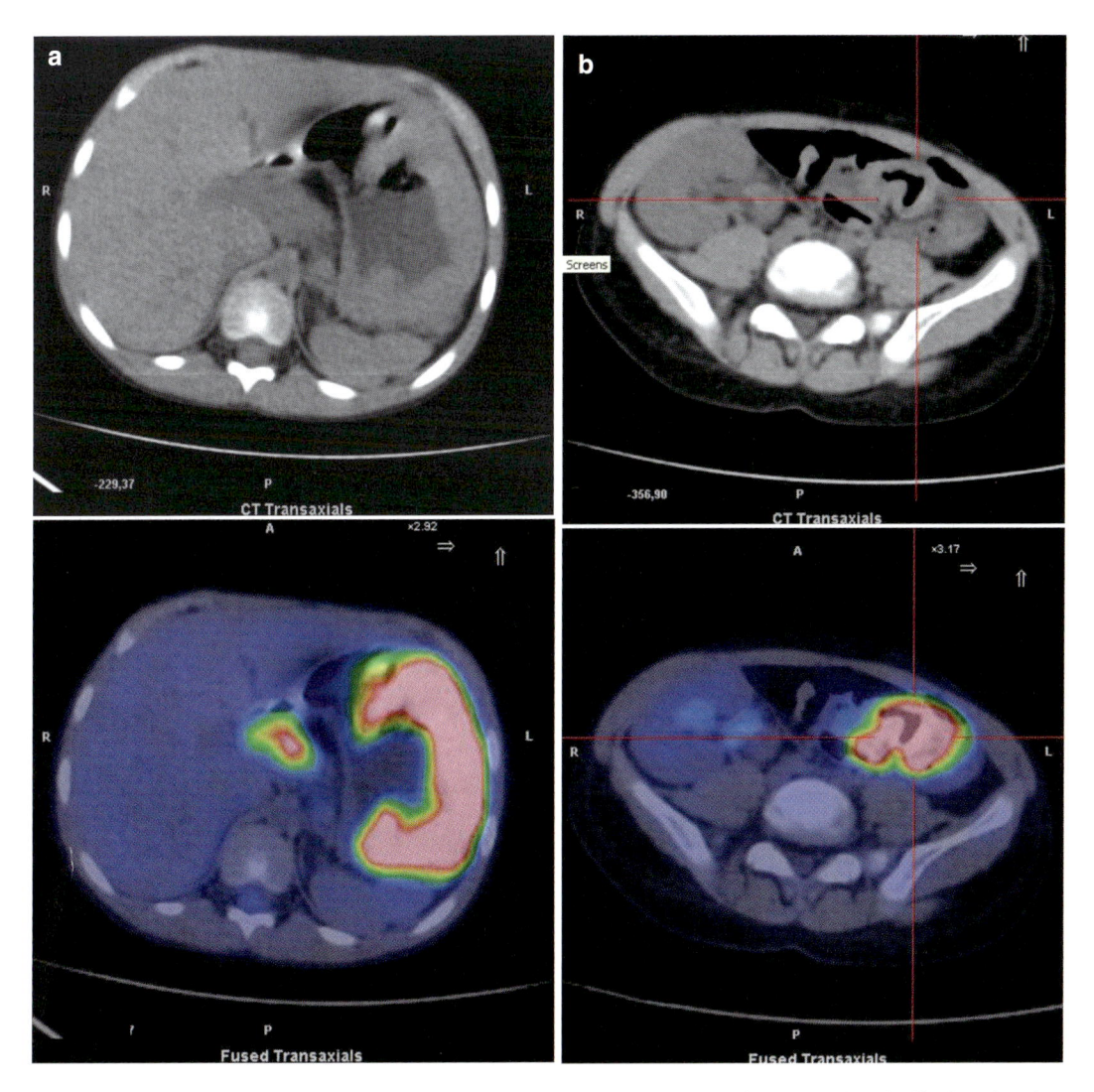

Fig. 6.18 Same patient as in Fig. 6.18. (**a**) Axial CT and PET/CT fusion images of the stomach and celiac lymph nodes. (**b**) Axial CT and PET/CT fusion images show intense uptake also in the left colon

Case 6 (continued)

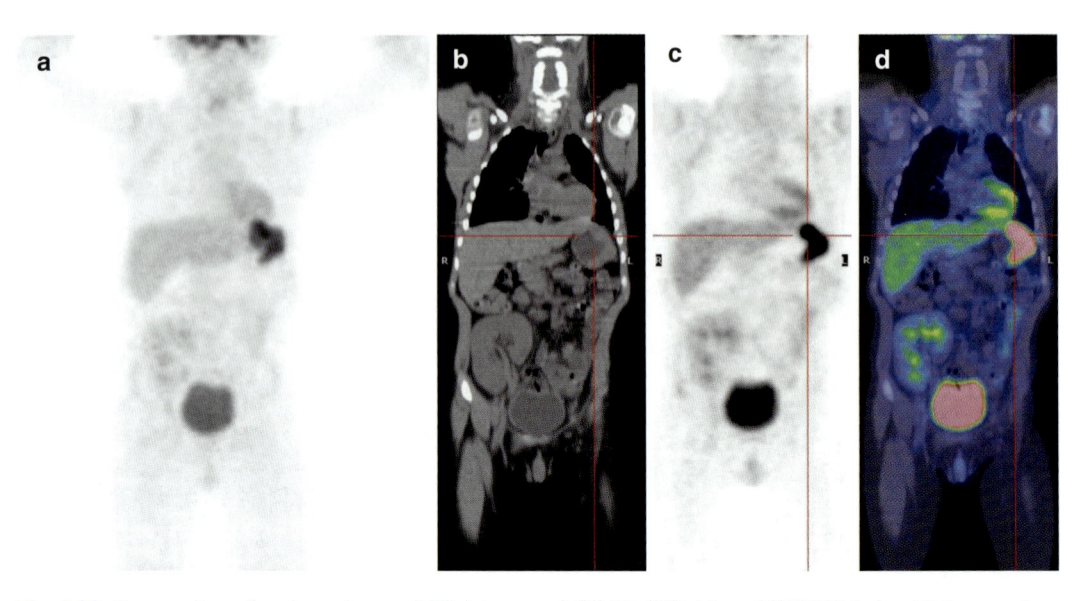

Fig. 6.19 Same patient after chemotherapy. MIP (**a**), coronal CT (**b**), PET (**c**), and PET/CT fusion (**d**) images show gastric disease persistence

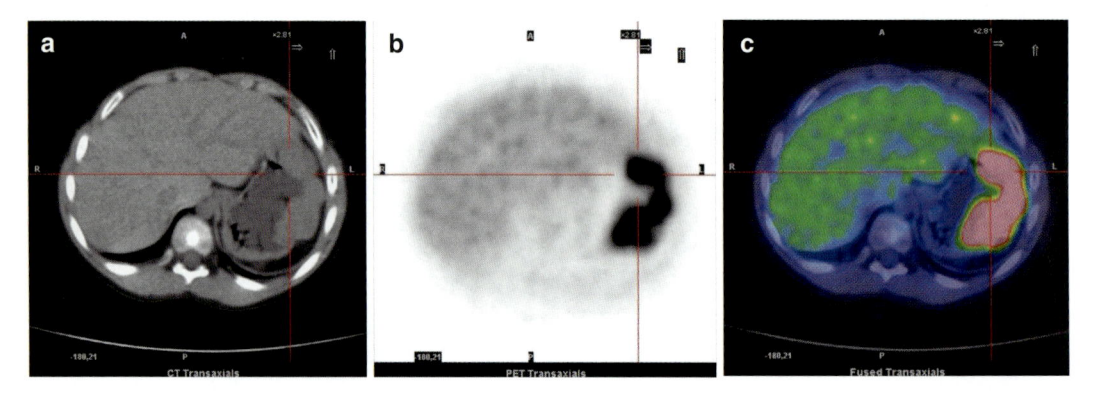

Fig. 6.20 Same patient as above. Axial CT (**a**), PET (**b**), and PET/CT fusion (**c**) images show a thickened gastric fundus, corresponding to elevated metabolic activity indicative of disease persistence

Teaching Point

PTLD occurs as a direct sequela of chronic immunosuppression [20]. It is a well recognized, although relatively uncommon complication of both solid-organ and allogeneic bone marrow transplantation. EBV, a member of the herpes virus family and one of the most common human viruses, is believed to induce PTLD. B cells are typically infected, as a consequence of either reactivation of the virus posttransplantation or primary posttransplantation EBV infection via the donor. While T-cell lymphoproliferative disorders are not associated with EBV infection, they have been documented after solid-organ and bone marrow transplantations. The vast majority are B-cell proliferations, as in this patient [21].

Case 7

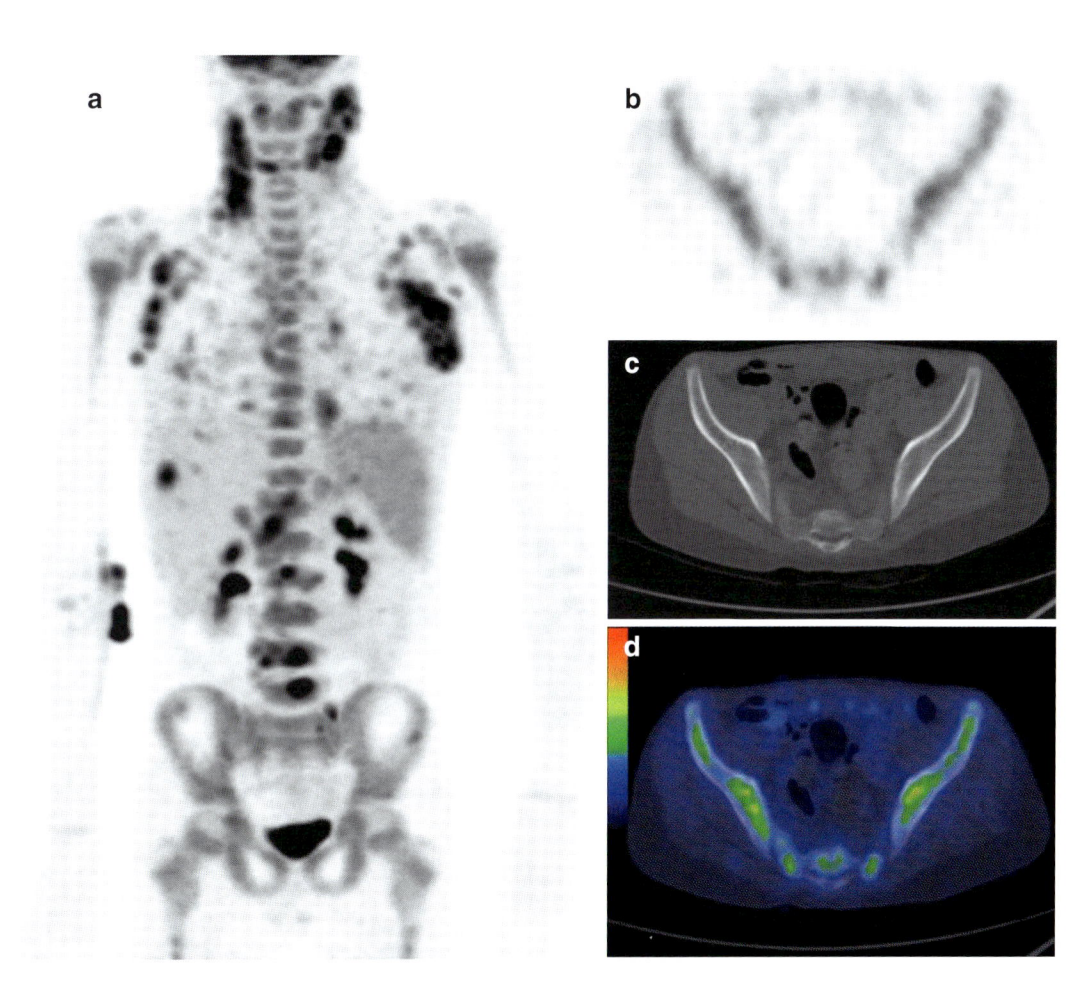

Fig. 6.21 A 10-year-old boy with Hodgkin's lymphoma nodular sclerosis type, stage IV (lungs, bone marrow, and bone involvement). (**a**) In the MIP image acquired in a basal study, multiple areas of pathological tracer uptake are evident in the supradiaphragmatic and subdiaphragmatic regions. Transaxial PET (**b**), CT (**c**), and PET/CT fusion (**d**) images show diffuse tracer uptake in the bone, with no evidence of focal uptake in the sacrum and in particular in the S3 vertebra

Case 7 (continued)

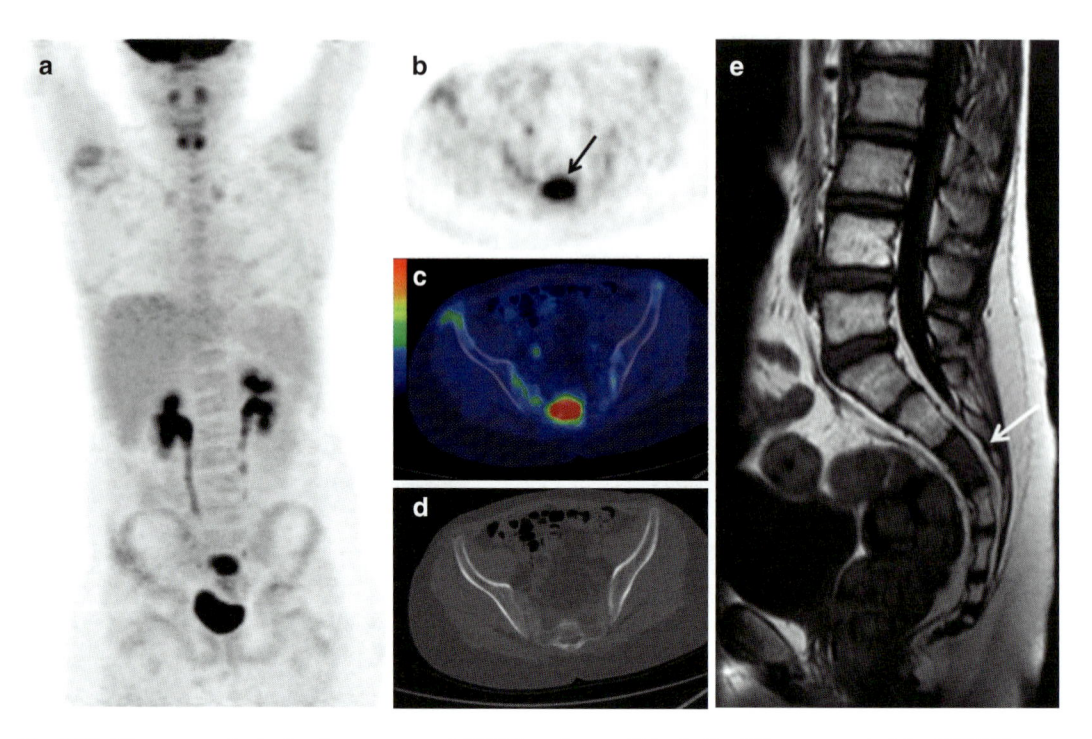

Fig. 6.22 The same patient after four courses of ABVD chemotherapy. Posttreatment evaluation. MIP (**a**), PET (**b**), PET/CT fusion (**c**), CT (**d**), and MRI sagital (**e**), images. There is complete regression of all previously described areas of pathological nodal and extranodal tracer uptake (**a**), but a new site of uptake is seen in the body of S3 vertebra (*black arrow* in **b**), not evident in the baseline study and without corresponding structural abnormalities in the CT component of the PET/CT scan. This finding, although suspicious for Hodgkin's lymphoma, was further investigated, as the patient had suffered a sacral trauma 3 weeks earlier. MRI (**e**) showed an abnormal T1 signal in the body of S3 (*white arrow*), concordant with the PET/CT findings. The S3 lesions were subsequently biopsied, which confirmed the presence of Hodgkin's lymphoma

Teaching Point
The peculiarity of this case was the complete response of the disease foci to the chemotherapy but the subsequent appearance of a new focus at a site not involved in the baseline study.

References

1. Bar-Sever Z, Keidar Z, Ben-Barak A, Bar-Shalom R, Postovsky S, Guralnik L, Ben Arush MW, Israel O (2007) The incremental value of 18F-FDG PET/CT in paediatric malignancies. Eur J Nucl Med Mol Imaging 34:630–637
2. Furth C, Denecke T, Steffen I, Ruf J, Voelker T, Misch D, Vondran F, Plotkin M, Stöver B, Henze G, Lemke AJ, Amthauer H (2006) Correlative imaging strategies implementing CT, MRI, and PET for staging of childhood Hodgkin disease. J Pediatr Hematol Oncol 28:501–512
3. Shulkin BL, Goodin GS, McCarville MB, Kaste SC, Krasin MJ, Hudson MM, Metzger M (2009) Bone and [18F]fluorodeoxyglucose positron-emission tomography/computed tomography scanning for the assessment of osseous involvement in Hodgkin lymphoma in children and young adults. Leuk Lymphoma 50:1794–1802
4. Mody RJ, Bui C, Hutchinson RJ, Frey KA, Shulkin BL (2007) Comparison of (18)F Flurodeoxyglucose PET with Ga-67 scintigraphy and conventional imaging modalities in pediatric lymphoma. Leuk Lymphoma 48:699–707
5. Hines-Thomas M, Kaste SC, Hudson MM, Howard SC, Liu WA, Wu J, Kun LE, Shulkin BL, Krasin MJ, Metzger ML (2008) Comparison of gallium and PET scans at diagnosis and follow-up of pediatric patients with Hodgkin lymphoma. Pediatr Blood Cancer 51:198–203
6. Sammer MB, Shulkin BL, Alessio A, Parisi MT (2011) Role of limited whole-body PET/CT in pediatric lymphoma. AJR Am J Roentgenol 196(5):1047–1055
7. Cheng G, Chen W, Chamroonrat W, Torigian DA, Zhuang H, Alavi A (2011) Biopsy versus FDG PET/CT in the initial evaluation of bone marrow involvement in pediatric lymphoma patients. Eur J Nucl Med Mol Imaging 38:1469–1476
8. Lopci E, Burnelli R, Guerra L, Cistaro A, Piccardo A, Zucchetta P, Derenzini E, Todesco A, Garaventa A, Schumacher F, Farruggia P, Buffardi S, Sala A, Casale F, Indolfi P, Biondi S, Pession A, Fanti S (2011) Post chemotherapy PET evaluation correlates with patient outcome in paediatric Hodgkin's disease. Eur J Nucl Med Mol Imaging 38:1620–1627
9. Furth C, Steffen IG, Amthauer H, Ruf J, Misch D, Schönberger S, Kobe C, Denecke T, Stöver B, Hautzel H, Henze G, Hundsdoerfer P (2009) Early and late therapy response assessment with [18F]fluorodeoxyglucose positron emission tomography in pediatric Hodgkin's lymphoma: analysis of a prospective multicenter trial. J Clin Oncol 27:4385–4391
10. Robertson VL, Anderson CS, Keller FG, Halkar R, Goodman M, Marcus RB, Esiashvili N (2011) Role of FDG-PET in the definition of involved-field radiation therapy and management for pediatric Hodgkin's lymphoma. Int J Radiat Oncol Biol Phys 80:324–332
11. Metwally H, Courbon F, David I, Filleron T, Blouet A, Rives M, Izar F, Zerdoud S, Plat G, Vial J, Robert A, Laprie A (2011) Coregistration of prechemotherapy PET-CT for planning pediatric Hodgkin's disease radiotherapy significantly diminishes interobserver variability of clinical target volume definition. Int J Radiat Oncol Biol Phys 80:793–799
12. Pommier P, Dussart S, Girinsky T, Chabaud S, Lagrange JL, Nguyen TD, Beckendorff V, D'Hombres A, Artignan X, Bondiau PY, Carrie C, Giammarile F (2011) Impact of 18F-fluoro-2-deoxyglucose positron emission tomography on treatment strategy and radiotherapy planning for stage I-II Hodgkin disease: a prospective multicenter study. Int J Radiat Oncol Biol Phys 79(3):823–828
13. Rhodes MM, Delbeke D, Whitlock JA, Martin W, Kuttesch JF, Frangoul HA, Shankar S (2006) Utility of FDG-PET/CT in follow-up of children treated for Hodgkin and non-Hodgkin lymphoma. J Pediatr Hematol Oncol 28:300–306
14. Edeline V, Bonardel G, Brisse H, Foehrenbach H, Pacquement H, Maszelin P, Gaillard JF, Michon J, Neuenschwander S (2007) Prospective study of 18F-FDG PET in pediatric mediastinal lymphoma: a single center experience. Leuk Lymphoma 48:823–826
15. Riad R, Omar W, Sidhom I, Zamzam M, Zaky I, Hafez M, Abdel-Dayem HM (2010) False-positive F-18 FDG uptake in PET/CT studies in pediatric patients with abdominal Burkitt's lymphoma. Nucl Med Commun 31:232–238
16. Pagano M, Berta M, Postini AM et al (2011) Nonossifying fibroma: a possible pitfall in F18-FDG PET/CT imaging of Hodgkin's disease. Radiol Case Rep 6(2):1–4
17. Goodin GS, Shulkin BL, Kaufman RA, Mc Carville MB (2006) PET/CT characterization of fibroosseous defects in children: 18F-FDG uptake can mimic metastatic disease. AJR Am J Roentgenol 187:1124–1128
18. Khademi S, Westphalen AC, Webb EM et al (2009) Frequency and etiology of solitary hot spots in the pelvis at whole-body positron emission tomography/computed tomography imaging. Clin Imaging 33(1):44–48
19. Zhu ZH, Cheng WY, Cheng X, Dang YH (2007) Characteristics of physiological uptake of uterus and ovaries on 18F-fluorodeoxyglucose positron emission tomography. Zhongguo Yi Xue Ke Xue Yuan Xue Bao 29(1):124–129
20. Andrade JG, Guaragna MS, Soardi FC et al (2008) Clinical and genetic findings of five patients with WT1-related disorders. Arq Bras Endocrinol Metabol 52(8):1236–1243
21. Vrachliotis TG, Vaswani KK, Davies EA et al (2000) CT findings in posttransplantation lymphoproliferative disorder of renal transplants. AJR Am J Roentgenol 175(1):183–188

Other Hematological Diseases (Leukemia)

Angelina Cistaro

Acute lymphoblastic leukemia (ALL) is the most frequent malignant neoplasm in childhood, accounting for approximately 30 % of pediatric cancers [1]. Common sites of either primary involvement or recurrence are the testicles (2 %) and central nervous system (CNS) (5–11 %), but other organs, particularly the ovaries, breast, eye, skin, and lymph nodes, are also possible sites of the disease. In some patients, a clinical suspicion of ALL recurrence may be difficult to confirm since many other conditions, such as infection and drugs, induce similar symptoms, including cytopenia, hepatosplenomegaly, and lymphadenopathy.

A. Cistaro, MD
Department of Nuclear Medicine,
Positron Emission Tomography Center IRMET
S.p.A., Euromedic Inc., Via Onorato Vigliani 89,
Turin 10100, Italy

Institute of Cognitive Sciences and Technologies,
National Research Council, Rome, Italy
e-mail: a.cistaro@irmet.com

Case 1

An 11-year-old girl treated for acute myeloid leukemia 1 year earlier presented with pain in the big toe of the right foot, then at the back of the foot, and in the calf. MRI of the spine demonstrated diffuse signal alteration. Both lumbar puncture and fine needle aspirations of the bone marrow were negative for leukemic cells. The outcome is shown in Fig. 7.1.

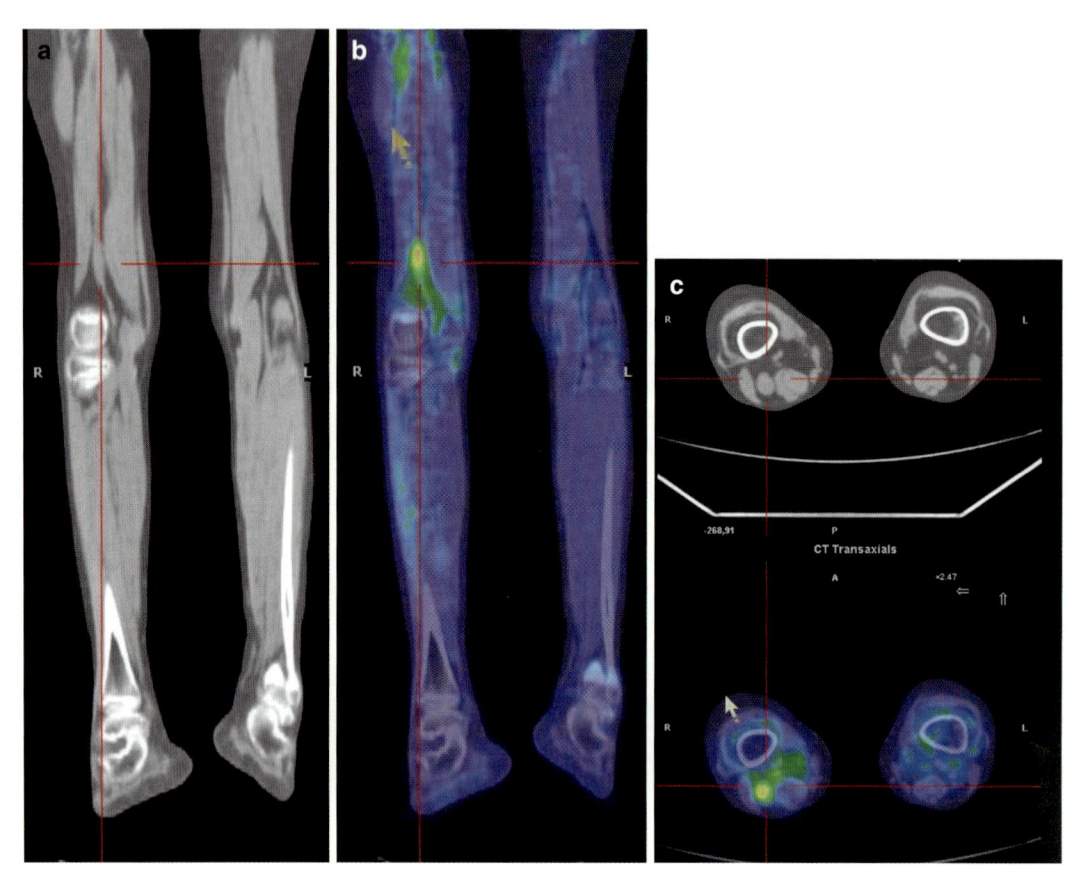

Fig. 7.1 Coronal CT (**a**), PET/CT fusion (**b**), and axial CT and PET/CT fusion (**c**) images of the legs show focal [18F-FDG] uptake in the upper right popliteal cavity, lateral to the femoral biceps muscle. A PET-guided biopsy proved the recurrence of acute myeloid leukemia

7 Other Hematological Diseases (Leukemia)

Case 2

A 5-year-old boy was diagnosed and treated for pre-B ALL. Four years later, he was reevaluated for an isolated lymphadenopathy of the head–neck region, without signs of inflammation on the overlying skin. There was no serological evidence of a recent infection nor were there any notable changes after empirical antibiotic and anti-inflammatory therapy. The outcome is shown in Figs. 7.2 and 7.3.

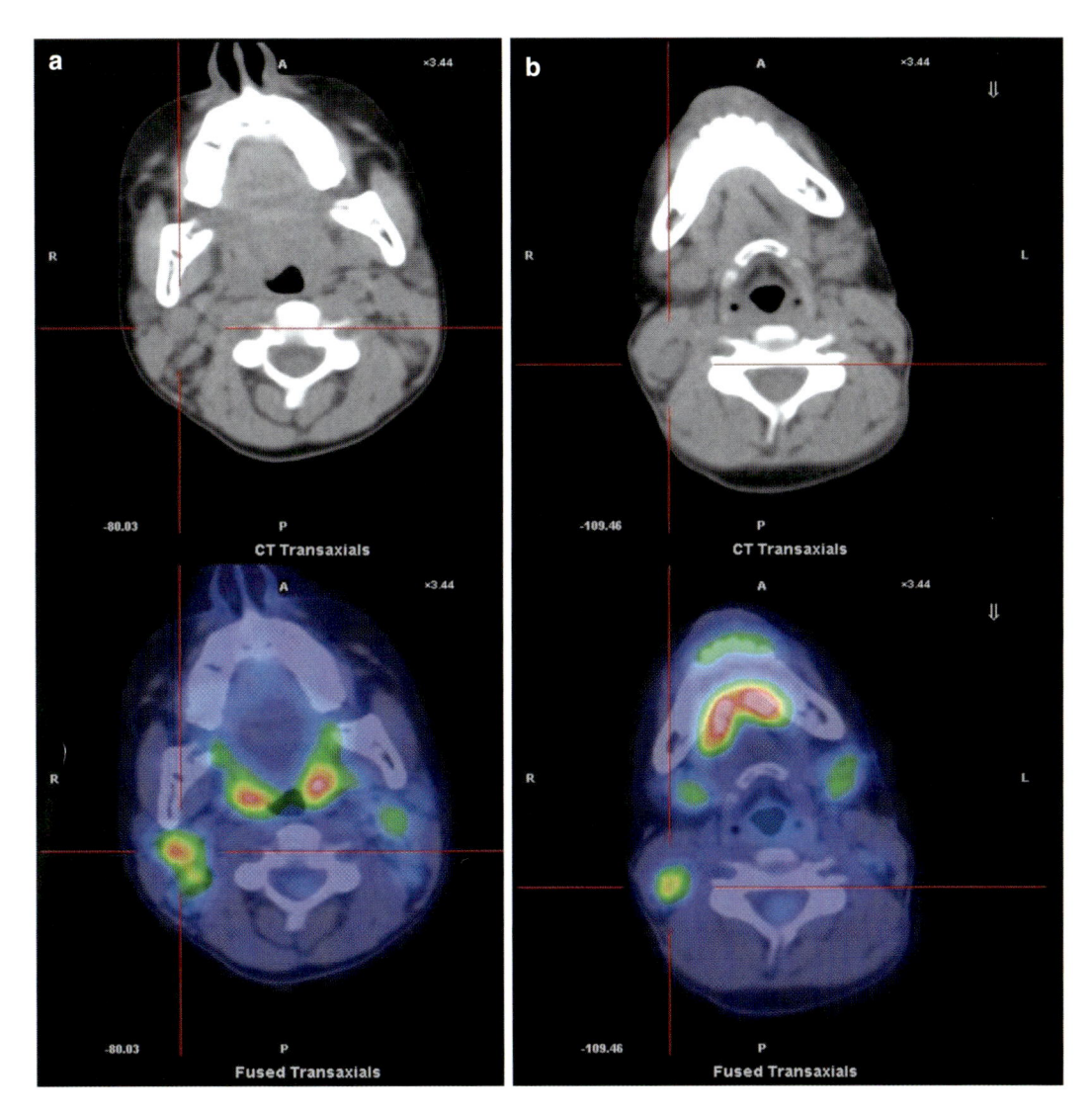

Fig. 7.2 Pretreatment PET/CT scan. (**a**, **b**) Axial CT and PET/CT fusion images show pathological ^{18}F-FDG uptake by the right laterocervical lymph nodes

Case 2 (continued)

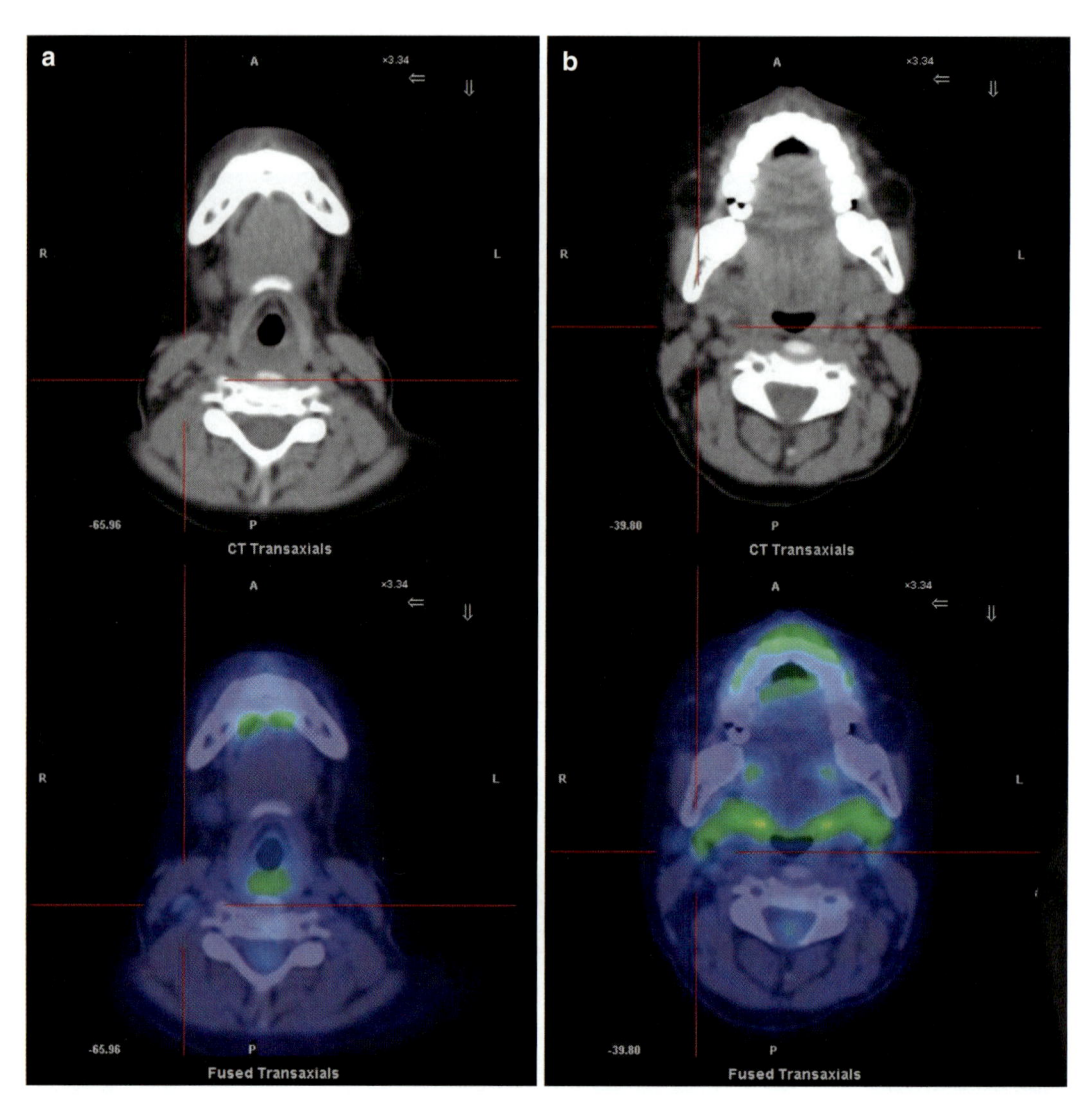

Fig. 7.3 The boy was treated with a second-line therapy. (**a**, **b**) Posttreatment ^{18}F-FDG–PET/CT scan shows no pathological uptake in previously involved sites, suggesting a complete response to therapy

Teaching Points

^{18}F-FDG–PET/CT is not a cancer-specific examination and false-positive findings have been reported, given that enhanced FDG uptake is also a feature of infectious diseases (mycobacterial, fungal, and bacterial), sarcoidosis, radiation pneumonitis, and postoperative surgical conditions. However, ^{18}F-FDG–PET/CT still has several advantages in the cancer setting, especially in guiding further diagnostic intervention at probable sites of disease recurrence [2]. It also allows the staging of other potentially involved tissues with just a single examination. In fact, a whole-body scan, obtained in a single session, increases the likelihood of finding unsuspected disease sites. Finally, during the course of therapy, ^{18}F-FDG–PET/CT can be useful in assessing the efficacy of treatment, considered to be one of the most important prognostic factors in ALL, by focusing on the identified lesions [3].

References

1. Pui C-H, Evans WE (2006) Acute lymphoblastic leukemia. N Engl J Med 354:166–178
2. Stölzel F, Röllig C, Radke J et al (2011) 18F-FDG-PET/CT for detection of extramedullary acute myeloid leukemia. Haematologica 96(10):1552–1556
3. Koh H, Nakamae H, Hagihara K, Nakane T, Manabe M, Hayashi Y et al (2011) Factors that contribute to long-term survival in patients with leukemia not in remission at allogeneic hematopoietic cell transplantation. J Exp Clin Cancer Res 30:36

Primary Bone Tumors

Natale Quartuccio and Angelina Cistaro

8.1 Introduction

Several benign bone tumors may be seen in the pediatric population [1]. The wide spectrum of benign conditions includes osteoma, enchondroma, osteoblastoma, osteochondroma, chondroblastoma, chondromyxoid fibroma, hemangioma, and tumorlike disorders such as nonossifying fibroma, eosinophilic granuloma, simple bone cyst, aneurysmal bone cyst, and fibrous dysplasia [1, 2]. Osseous malignancies, by contrast, are very rare, accounting for 6 % of all pediatric cancers [3, 4]. The most frequent primary malignant tumors are osteosarcoma and Ewing's sarcoma, followed by chondrosarcoma and fibrosarcoma [5].

Osteogenic sarcoma (OS), also called osteosarcoma, derives from primitive bone-forming mesenchymal stem cells and most often involves the metaphyseal portions of the long bones (distal femur, proximal tibia, and proximal humerus) although flat bones and the spine are affected in 10 % of OS patients [6]. The incidence peaks in the second decade of life and is rare in children younger than 10 years. OS can be caused by radiation exposure, sarcomatous transformation of Paget's disease, or in relation to hereditary retinoblastoma or rare syndromes (Werner syndrome, Li–Fraumeni, and Rothmund–Thomson). However, secondary OS is most often seen in the elderly. The clinical presentation includes pain (dull, aching, constant, worse at night) and the possible presence of a mass effect. The overall survival and event-free survival (EFS) at 5 years for patients with nonmetastatic OS are approximately 75 and 65 %, respectively [7]. The prognosis is related to the presence of metastases at diagnosis, patient age, tumor location, response of the primary tumor to neoadjuvant chemotherapy, and tumor grade [6, 8]. There is evidence suggesting that histological subtypes and variants also impact survival [9, 10]. For example, chondroblastic OS responds poorly to chemotherapy and the outcome of these patients is worse than those with other histotypes [6]. By contrast, patients with periosteal OS have a favorable outcome [11].

N. Quartuccio, MD
Nuclear Medicine Unit, Department of Biomedical Sciences and Morphological and Functional Images, University of Messina, Via Consolare Valeria 1, Messina 98125, Italy
e-mail: natale.quartuccio84@hotmail.it

A. Cistaro, MD (✉)
Department of Nuclear Medicine, Positron Emission Tomography Center IRMET S.p.A., Euromedic Inc., Via Onorato Vigliani 89, Turin 10100, Italy

Institute of Cognitive Sciences and Technologies, National Research Council, Rome, Italy
e-mail: a.cistaro@irmet.com

8.2 Ewing's Sarcoma

Ewing's sarcoma (EWS), a member of the Ewing family of tumors (ESFT), is the second most frequent pediatric bone tumor, with a peak of incidence in the second decade of life. The incidence of ESFT is 1–3 per million people per year [12]. Molecular diagnostic techniques play a key diagnostic role, as 85 % of patients are positive for the [t(11;22)(q24;q12)] translocation, between the EWSR1 gene of chromosome 22 and an ETS family gene, usually FLI1, of chromosome 11 [13]. The [t(21;22)(q22;q12)] translocation is found in only 10 % of EWS tumors and other translocations are extremely rare [14]. Translocations generate the EWS-FLI-1 fusion protein, which is thought to act as an aberrant transcriptional activator [15].

The preferential locations of EWS are the pelvis (26 %), femur (20 %), tibia/fibula (18 %), chest wall (16 %), upper extremity (9 %), and spine (6 %) [2]. The symptoms are not pathognomonic as they include pain and swelling, fever, and weight loss. The main prognostic factors at diagnosis are tumor stage, distant disease, primary location in the axial skeleton, and primary tumor size exceeding 8 cm [16]. At diagnosis, approximately 20 % of EWS patients present with metastases, most often in the bones (51 %) and lungs (44 %) but also in other sites (5 %) [17]. The 5-year survival of patients with localized disease is 68 %, whereas for those with metastatic disease, it is 39 % [18].

An imaging diagnostic work-up of pediatric bone sarcomas generally starts with the inexpensive plain film, but lytic lesions are detected on X-ray only when the loss of mineralization reaches 30–50 %. To evaluate the primary tumor site, MRI is a fundamental tool as it defines the local extent, bone marrow involvement, and the presence of skip lesions. Currently, 99mTc whole-body scintigraphy is used in most nuclear medicine departments to detect osseous metastases, while high-resolution CT is still the gold standard in evaluating the extent of chest disease [19]. However, peritumoral edema can complicate MRI-based assessments of the bone marrow and both CT and MRI are limited by potential artifacts and significant beam hardening in the presence of metallic prostheses, e.g., in patients who have undergone limb salvage procedures.

In the last decade, the utility of FDG–PET/CT as an imaging tool in malignant osseous tumors has been established based on its ability to visualize the bones and soft tissues in a single examination (Figs. 8.1, 8.2, and 8.3). In addition, FDG–PET/CT, by overcoming some of the typical limitations of morphological imaging, is an emerging powerful tool in the assessment of metastatic disease at diagnosis as well as at follow-up [1, 20]. A particular advantage of FDG–PET/CT over conventional imaging is its ability to differentiate between disease recurrence and the post-therapeutic distortions of the normal anatomy and tissues following radiotherapy and surgery. In these cases, a normal FDG–PET/CT may prevent biopsies. In detecting distant tumor recurrence, FDG–PET/CT, with its whole-body imaging capabilities, is the preferred imaging approach, whereas MRI and CT may better depict local recurrence in the primary tumor bed due to their small fields of view [21]. Therefore, the recommended imaging strategy in the pediatric population would be the more extensive use of whole-body MRI or the introduction of hybrid PET/MRI into clinical practice.

Low-grade sarcomas can be falsely negative on FDG–PET/CT [22] but they are less frequent in pediatric patients [23, 24]. Nonetheless, the measure of sarcoma metabolism by means of standard uptake value (SUV) has been also proposed as a predictor of pathological grade of the tumor and a guide for biopsy toward the most biologically significant regions of large masses [25].

8 Primary Bone Tumors

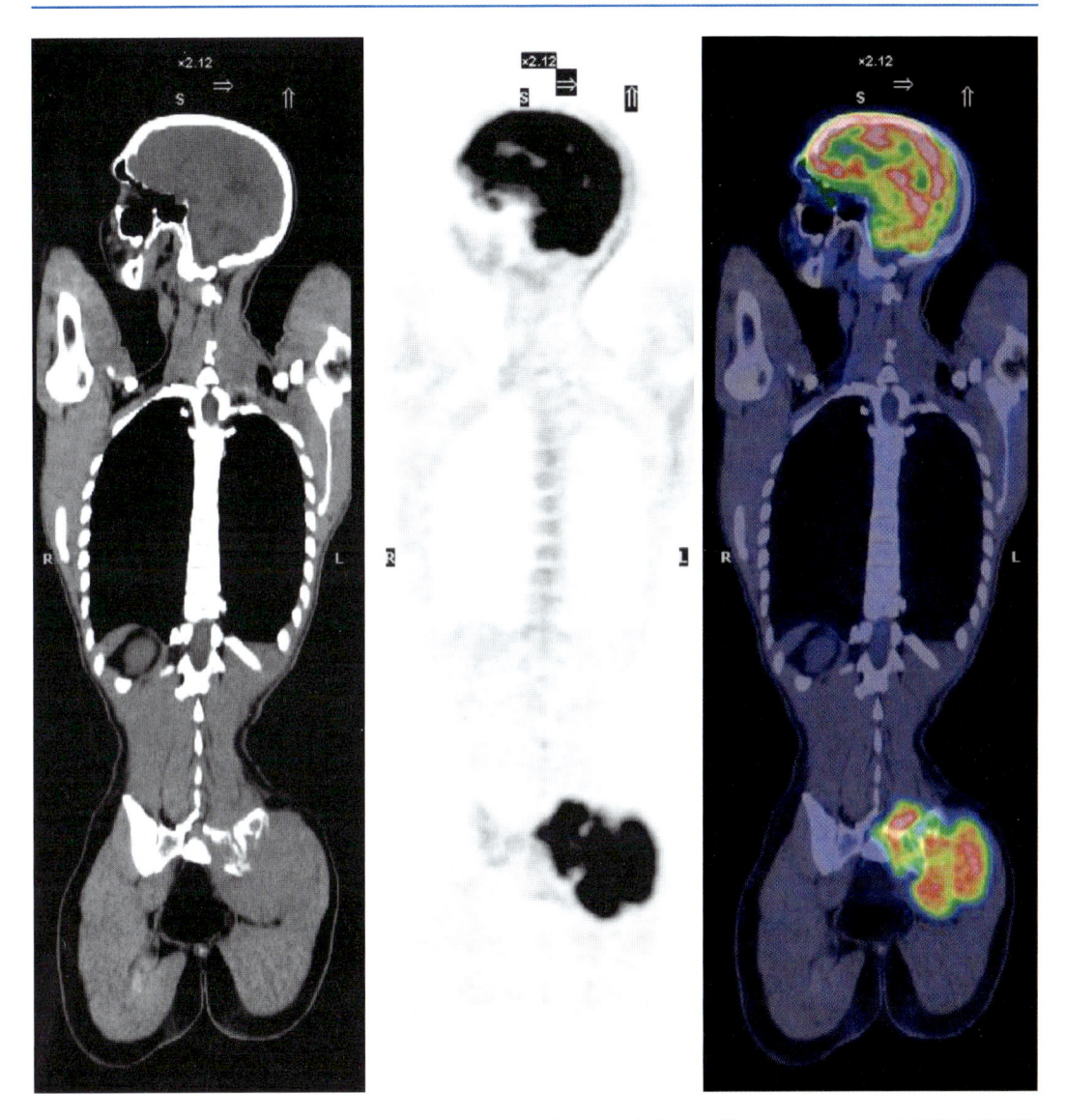

Fig. 8.1 A 17-year-old boy with Ewing's sarcoma of the left pelvis, with extension into the iliac bone, acetabulum, gluteus, and piriformis muscles. As the patient suffered intense pain in the affected areas, the study FDG–PET/CT was done with the patient prone rather than supine

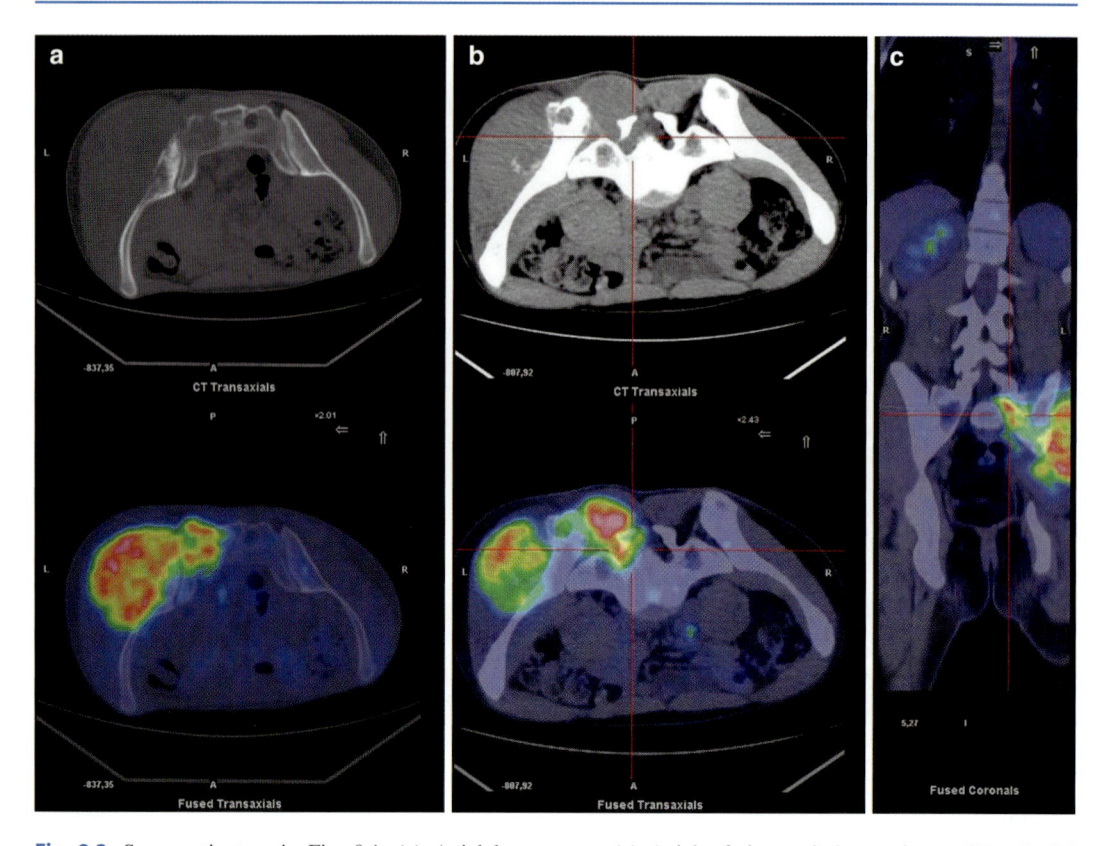

Fig. 8.2 Same patient as in Fig. 8.1. (**a**) Axial bone window CT and PET/CT fusion images of the prone pelvis show pathological uptake in the left sacrum and iliac bone. On CT, interruption of the posterior cortical bone of the sacrum, a sign of the lesion's aggressiveness, can be seen (**a**). Axial soft tissue window setting on CT and axial (**b**) and coronal PET/CT fusion (**c**) images of the prone pelvis show pathological uptake in the foramen of the sacral nerve and in the erector muscle of the spine

8 Primary Bone Tumors

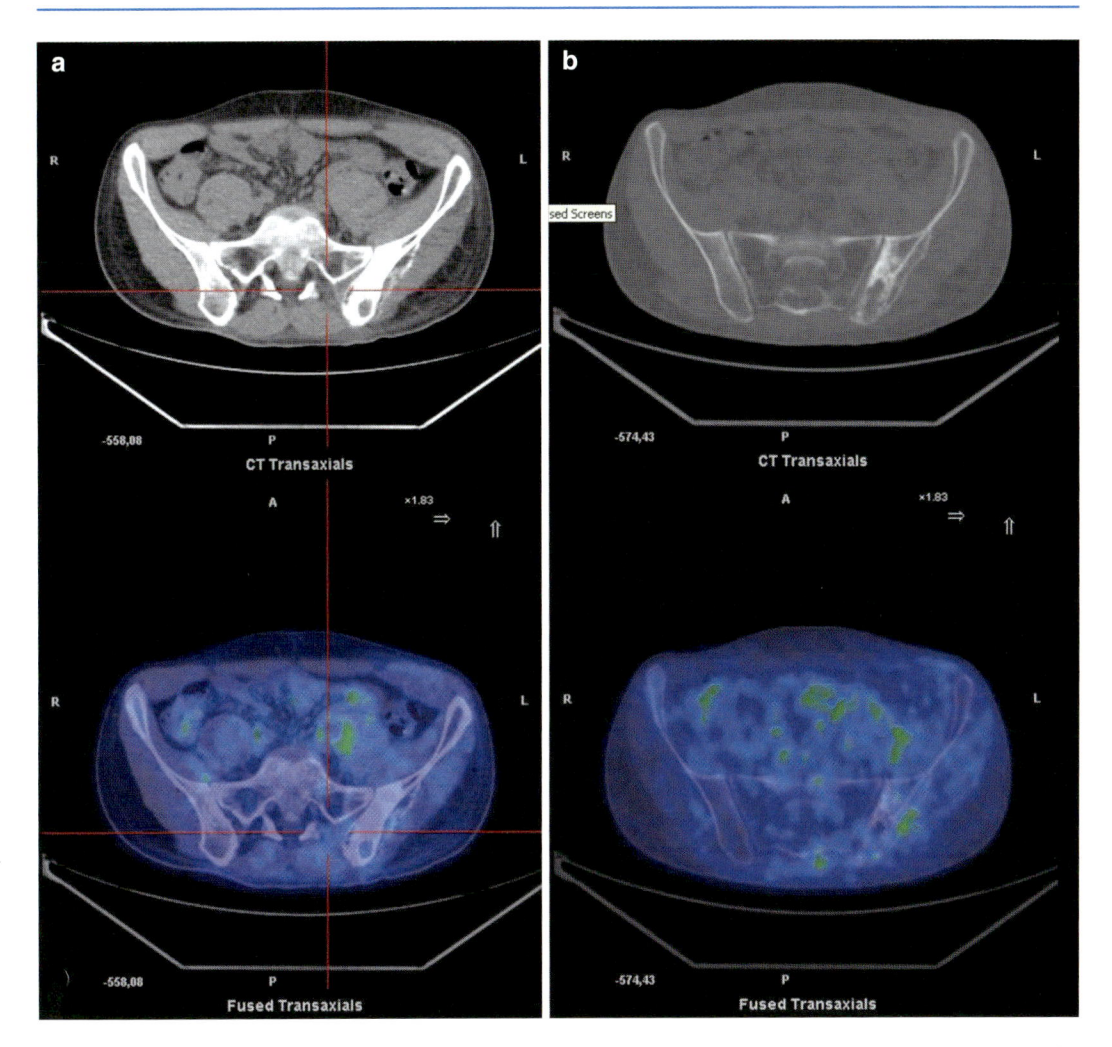

Fig. 8.3 Axial mediastinal (**a**) and bone (**b**) windows CT and PET/CT fusion images posttreatment show the complete disappearance of the pathological soft tissue and bone uptake. Reduction of the sarcoma mass reduced the patient's pain, which allowed image acquisition in the conventional (supine) position

8.3 Lung Metastases in Primary Bone Sarcoma

In up to 20 % of patients with OS or EWS, clinically evident metastatic disease is already present at the time of diagnosis. Among these patients, the lungs will be involved in 92 % [26]. In patients who do not initially present with metastases, the probability of lung metastasis is 28 % after 5 years [27]. Early detection of lung metastases enables disease control by metastasectomy [28–30], which results in a more favorable prognosis (5-year disease-free and overall survival of 10–35 %). By contrast, in patients treated with combination chemotherapy, a complete response is obtained in <10 % of the cases and the prognosis is poor [31].

High-resolution CT, due to its high sensitivity, remains the gold standard in detecting lung metastases, although difficulties are encountered in defining the true nature of lung nodules in these patients. FDG–PET/CT has good specificity in the assessment of suspicious nodules and better diagnostic performance than other imaging methods when the diameter of the lung lesion is >6 mm [20] because of the limited resolution of PET or CT alone and the artifacts that arise in these studies from partial volume effects and respiratory movement. Instead, the higher specificity of ^{18}F-FDG–PET/CT reinforces the complementary roles of these other modalities in the assessment of lung lesions (Figs. 8.4, 8.5, and 8.6) such that indiscriminate use of surgical biopsies and nodulectomies is often avoided [20].

Lung nodules, frequently small in size and multiple, must be evaluated with a semiquantitative or qualitative approach. The classical SUV_{max} cutoff value (2.5) used to discriminate between benign and malignant lung nodules is not suitable in pediatric oncology patients because their lung lesions differ from those of adults with respect to glucose metabolism. Furthermore, in the clinical history, several conditions must be considered, such as recent cough, fever, and infections, all of which can generate benign pulmonary nodules with high glucose metabolism that are mistakenly interpreted as tumors. Cistaro et al. attempted to establish an SUV_{max} cutoff value that allowed the correct diagnosis of pulmonary nodules in pediatric patients with bone sarcomas. Whereas for lesions <5 mm significant SUV_{max} (and the SUV ratio) values could not be defined, an SUV_{max} threshold >1.09 was found to be consistent with malignancy for nodules >6 mm in diameter. The authors concluded that knowledge of the patient's clinical history combined with the use of a semiquantitative approach may diminish the number of false-positive malignant nodules. Overall, ^{18}F-FDG–PET had an accuracy of 88.9 %, a sensitivity of 90.3 %, a specificity of 87.5 %, and a PPV and NPV of 90.3 and 87.5 %, respectively [30].

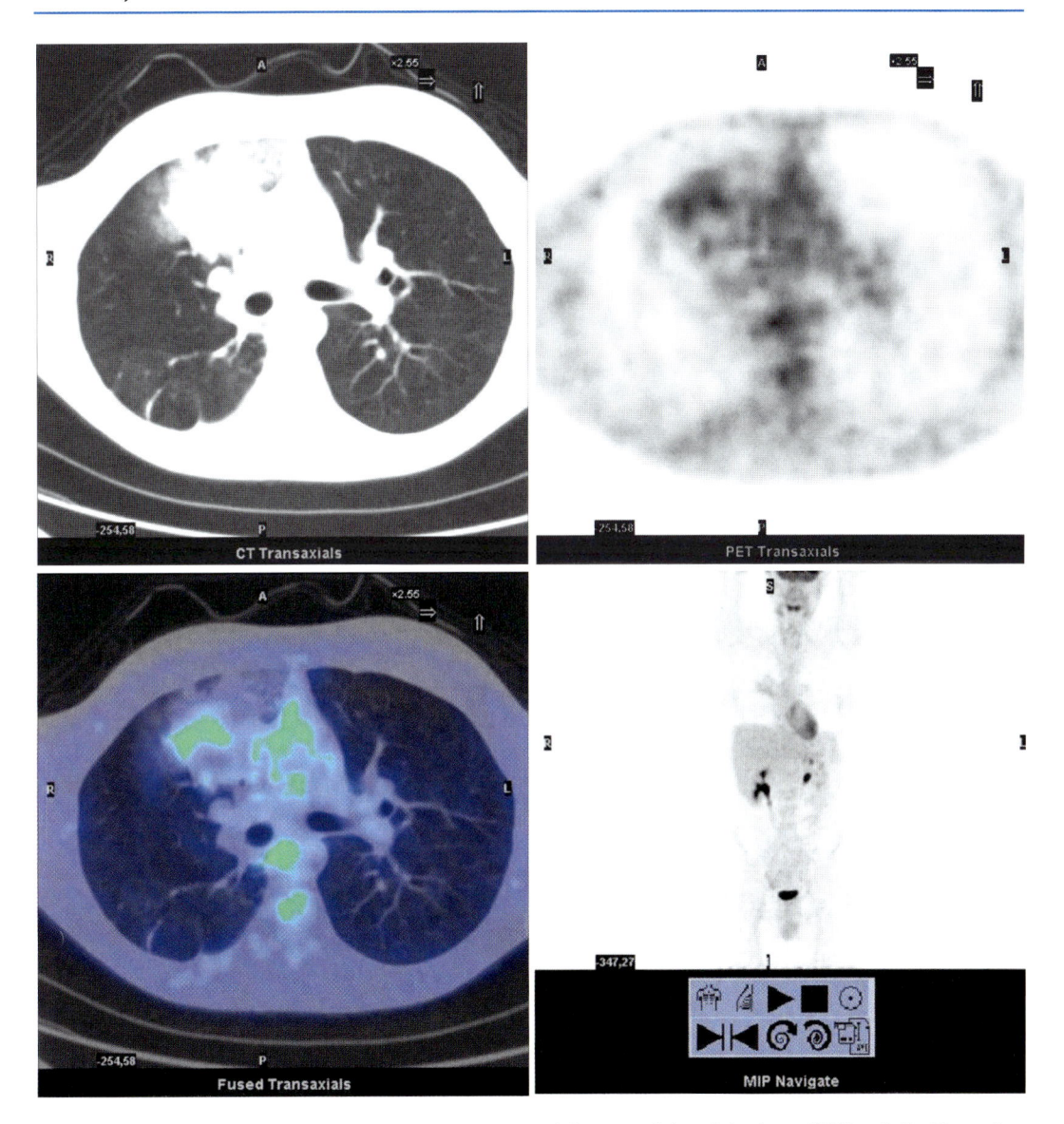

Fig. 8.4 A 14-year-old boy with Fraumeni syndrome who was treated for bilateral retinoblastoma and osteoblastic osteosarcoma of the right femur. The PET restaging study showed inhomogeneous uptake in the right upper lobe of the lung (SUV_{max} 2.4). The patient underwent resection of the lesion, subsequently diagnosed as a metastasis without necrosis

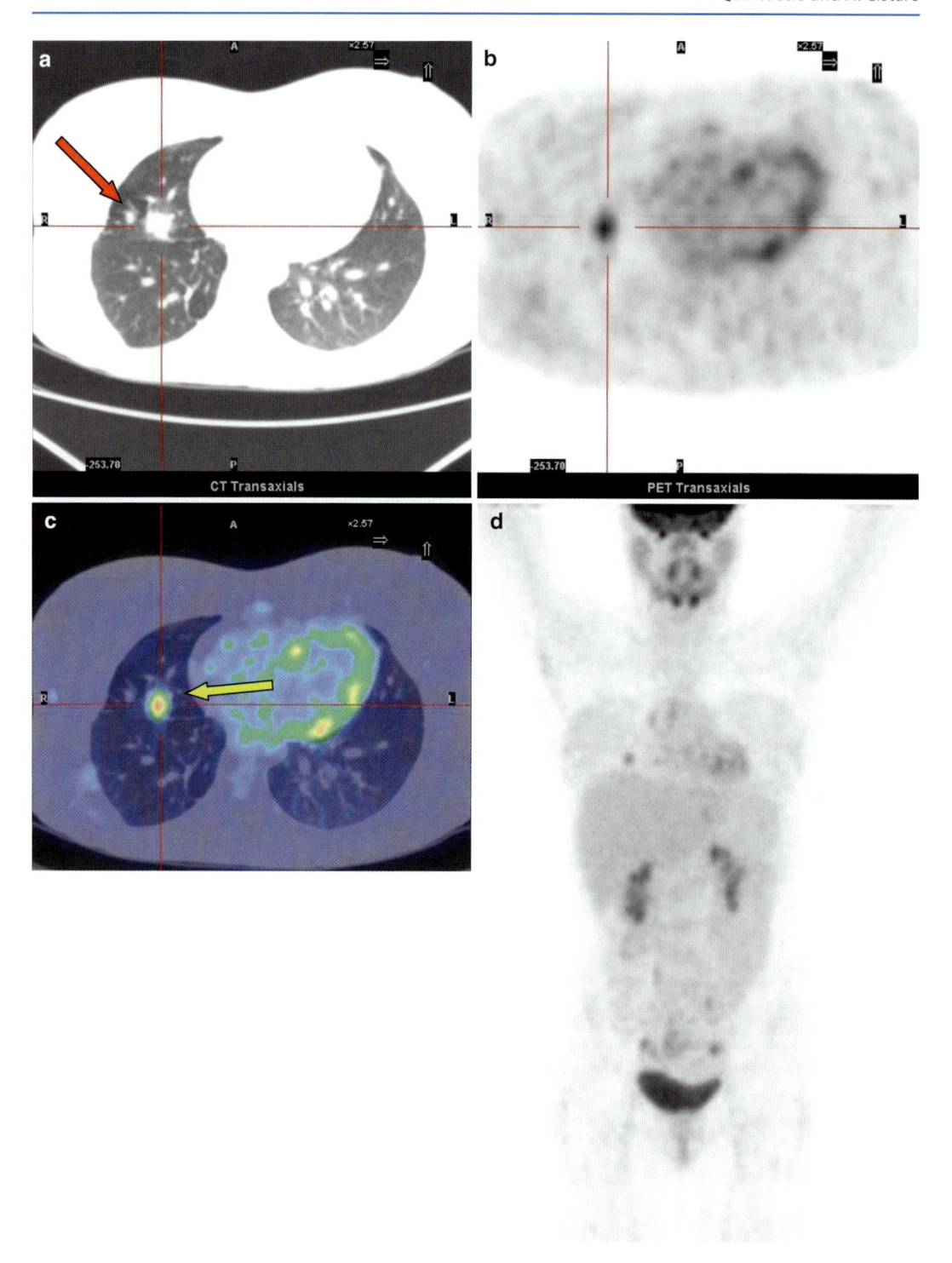

Fig. 8.5 A 21-year-old female treated 7 years earlier for osteosarcoma of the humerus, including seven pulmonary metastasectomies. (**a**–**d**) Axial lung windows on CT and PET/CT fusion images show focal FDG uptake corresponding to a nodule on the right upper lobe of the lung ($SUV_{max}=5:7$) (*yellow arrow* in **c**). The nodule was interpreted as of inflammatory origin and the patient was treated with antibiotics. A chest CT 15 days later confirmed the inflammatory nature of the lesion. On CT, another small nodule (*red arrow* in **a**) initially detected 2 years earlier is seen

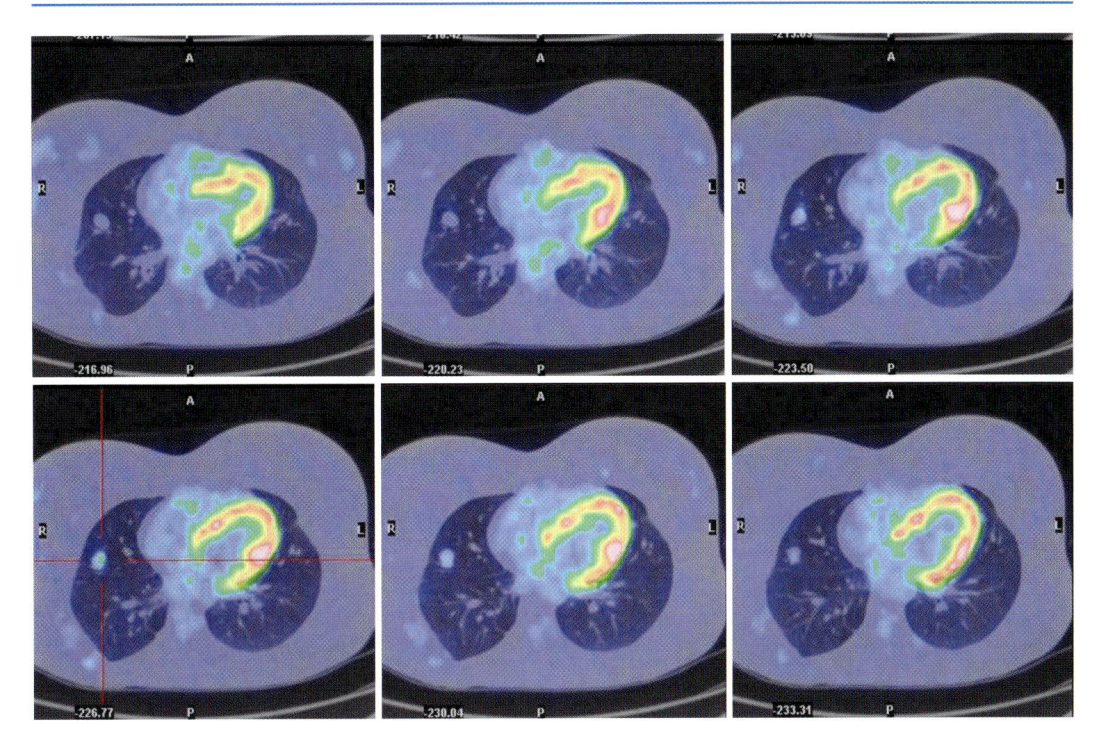

Fig. 8.6 The same patient 6 months later. Axial PET/CT fusion images show a mild increase in the dimensions and degree of ^{18}F-FDG uptake by the small nodule (SUV_{max}=2.3). The patient underwent lung surgery. The final diagnosis was metastasis with poor necrosis

8.4 Bone Metastases

No consistent data on the risk and sites of extrapulmonary metastasis from bone sarcomas are available. However, the bones seem to be the more frequent site of extrapulmonary metastases, as bone metastases develop in 33 % of patients (Fig. 8.7) [31]. Since the bones are not connected to the lymphatic system, tumor dissemination is almost exclusively through the blood.

FDG–PET/CT directly identifies bone lesions on the basis of their glucose metabolism and is thus better able to detect the osseous metastases of EWS than 99mTc bone scintigraphy [32]. Nonetheless, despite its lower resolution, bone scintigraphy has a high detection rate for skeletal OS metastases. This most likely reflects the intense osteoid production and osteoblastic activity of OS. EWS tends to infiltrate the bone marrow rather than mineralized bone such that osteodestruction is dominated by osteoclastic activity [33, 34].

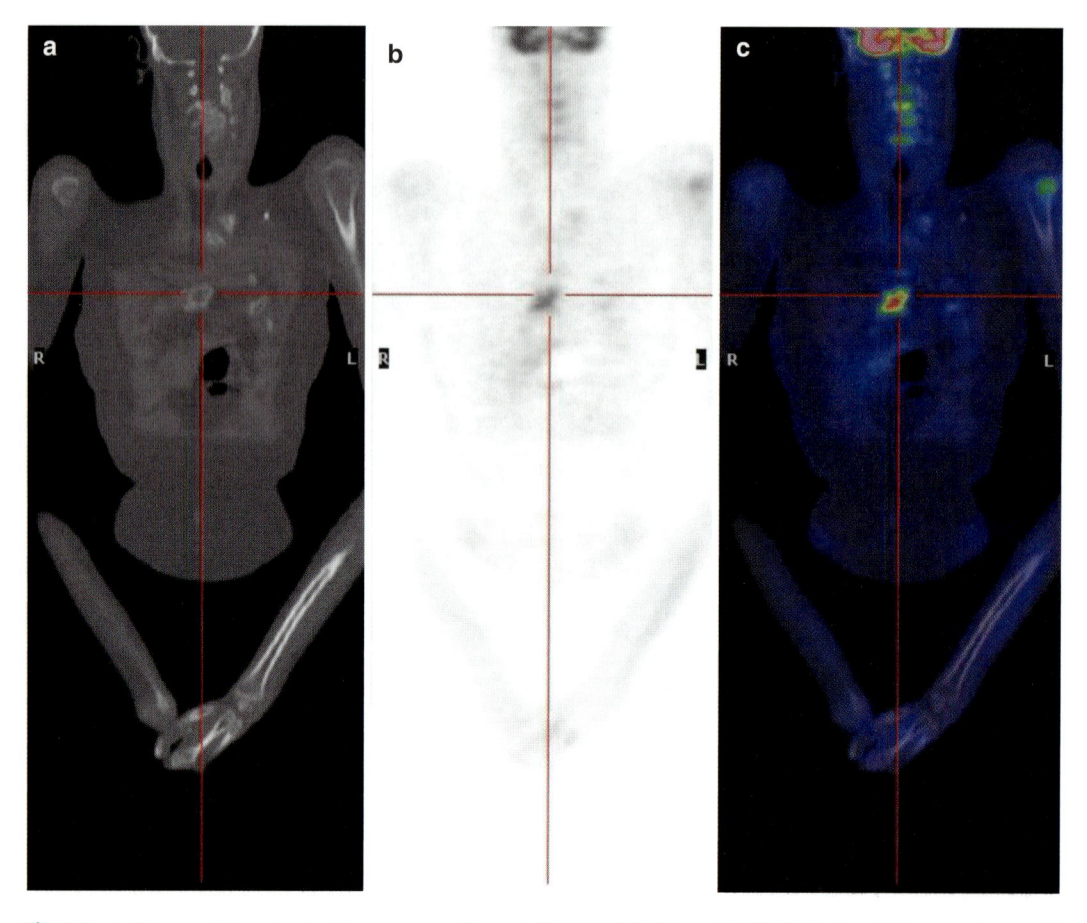

Fig. 8.7 A 17-year-old boy treated for sarcoma. Coronal CT (**a**), PET (**b**), and PET/CT fusion (**c**) images show mild FDG uptake in the left humeral head and another, more intense accumulation in the sternum

8.5 Other Sites of Metastases

Extrapulmonary and extraosseous lesions are extremely rare. According to the limited data on lymph node involvement, metastatic lymph nodes are seen in 10 % of the OS cases at autopsy [35]. FDG–PET/CT effectively detects lymph node metastases (Fig. 8.8) as well as metastases in other, more unusual sites (<3 % of patients with metastatic disease), e.g., brain, liver, muscles, abdomen, and scalp [20, 26]. A large retrospective study by the Cooperative German–Austrian–Swiss Osteosarcoma Study Group yielded detailed data on the distribution of OS metastases; in 12.4 % of the 1702 OS patients, metastases were present at the time of diagnosis. The lungs were involved in 86.7 % patients, distant bones in 21.2 %, and other sites in 0.09 % (lymph nodes in 15 patients, other soft tissues in 3, skin, brain, and liver in 1 patient each) [36]. The European Intergroup Cooperative Ewing's Sarcoma Study Group collected data from 975 EWS patients. In 179 (18.4 %), metastases were detected at initial presentation. In 79 of those patients, the lungs were the only site involved by metastasis, while in 92 patients, bone with or without lung involvement was present. Eight patients had metastases at other sites, and in one patient, the metastatic site was not specified [17]. In patients with metastatic disease, FDG–PET/CT can identify extrapulmonary lesions with a higher sensitivity, specificity, and accuracy than provided by conventional imaging (83.3 vs. 77.8%, 98.1 vs. 96.7 %, 96.9 vs. 95.2 %, respectively) [20].

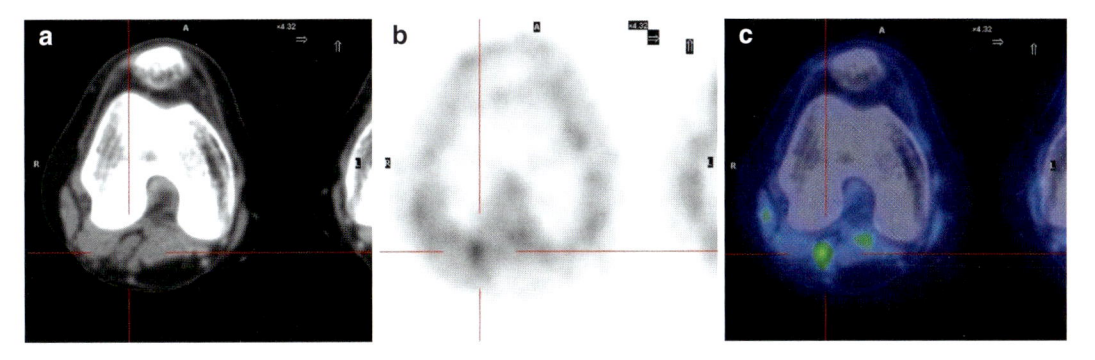

Fig. 8.8 A 15-year-old girl treated for Ewing's sarcoma of the right fibula. Axial CT (**a**), PET (**b**), and PET/CT (**c**) fusion images show a small focal area of uptake in the left popliteal fossa, indicating recurrence of the disease in the lymph nodes

8.6 Local Recurrence

Since pediatric patients with bone sarcoma usually undergo surgery in combination with robust chemotherapy and radiotherapy protocols, they are likely to develop tissue scarring, fibrosis, and inflammation that on imaging can simulate recurrent disease. Assessment of local recurrence by means of morphological imaging can be difficult because of tissue changes following previous treatment. In addition, metallic prostheses can cause significant artifacts on MRI. In these settings, FDG–PET/CT may be diagnostically useful as it is able to differentiate viable tumor from fibrosis and inflammatory tissue from malignancy (Figs. 8.9 and 8.10) [21]. The sensitivity, specificity, accuracy, NPV, and PPV of FDG–PET/CT in discriminating local recurrence from bone tumors were reported to be 100, 92, 95, 100, and 88 %, respectively [37].

Patients who suffer a relapse of primary bone cancer have a poor prognosis [38]. In a retrospective analysis of 114 OS patients, McTiernan and colleagues reported a 5-year estimate of post-relapse survival (PRS) of 19.2 ± 7.7 %. A much worse outcome (5-year PRS = 13.3 ± 8.8 %) was documented for patients with simultaneous local and distant recurrence than for patients with local recurrence alone (27.3 ± 11.6 %), but the difference was not statistically significant [37].

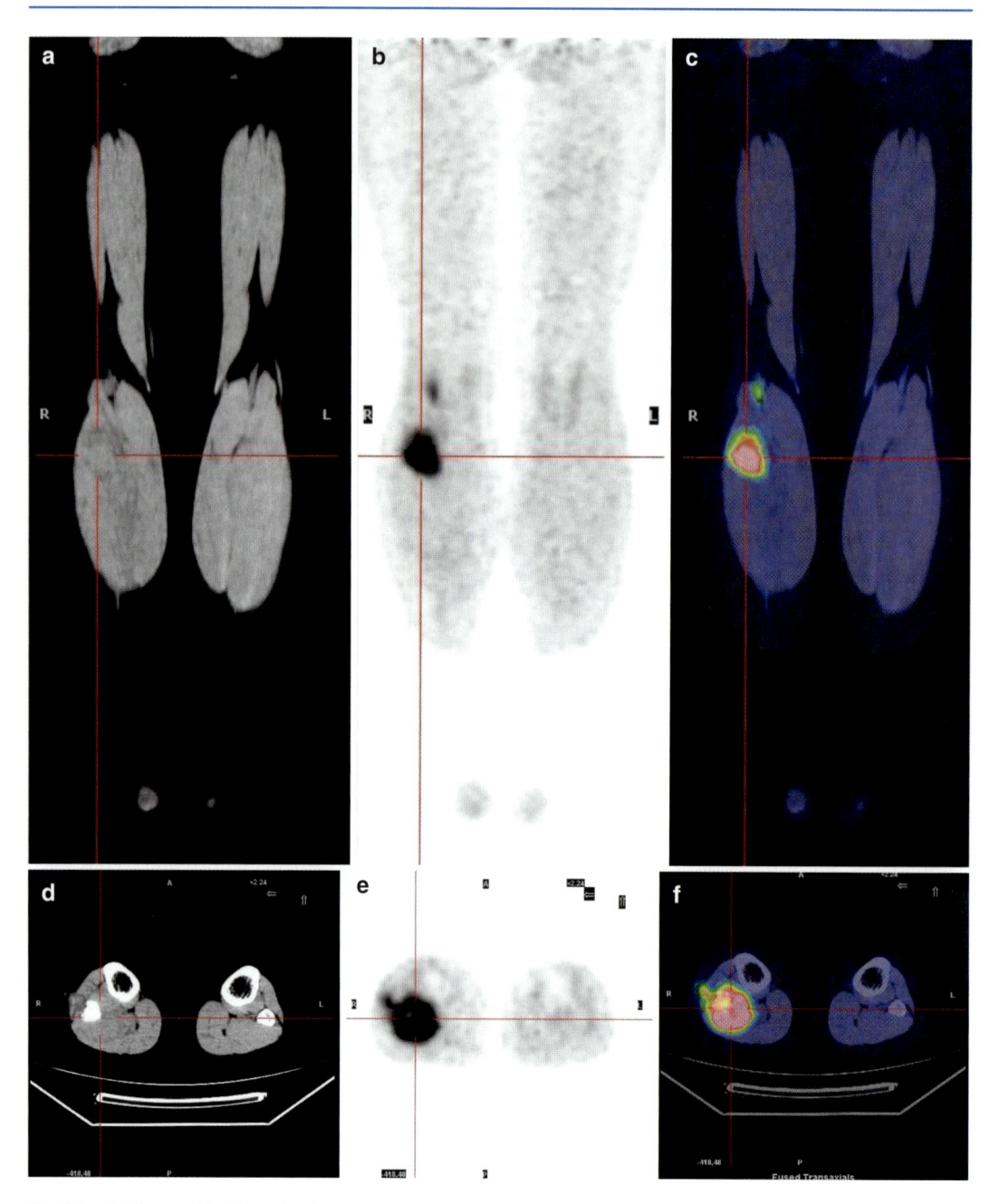

Fig. 8.9 A 15-year-old girl previously treated for Ewing's sarcoma of the right fibula. The coronal (**a–c**) and axial (**d–f**) CT (**a, d**), PET (**b, e**), and PET/CT fusion (**d, f**) images show a right soft tissue recurrence between the popliteal muscles, involving the proximal fibula

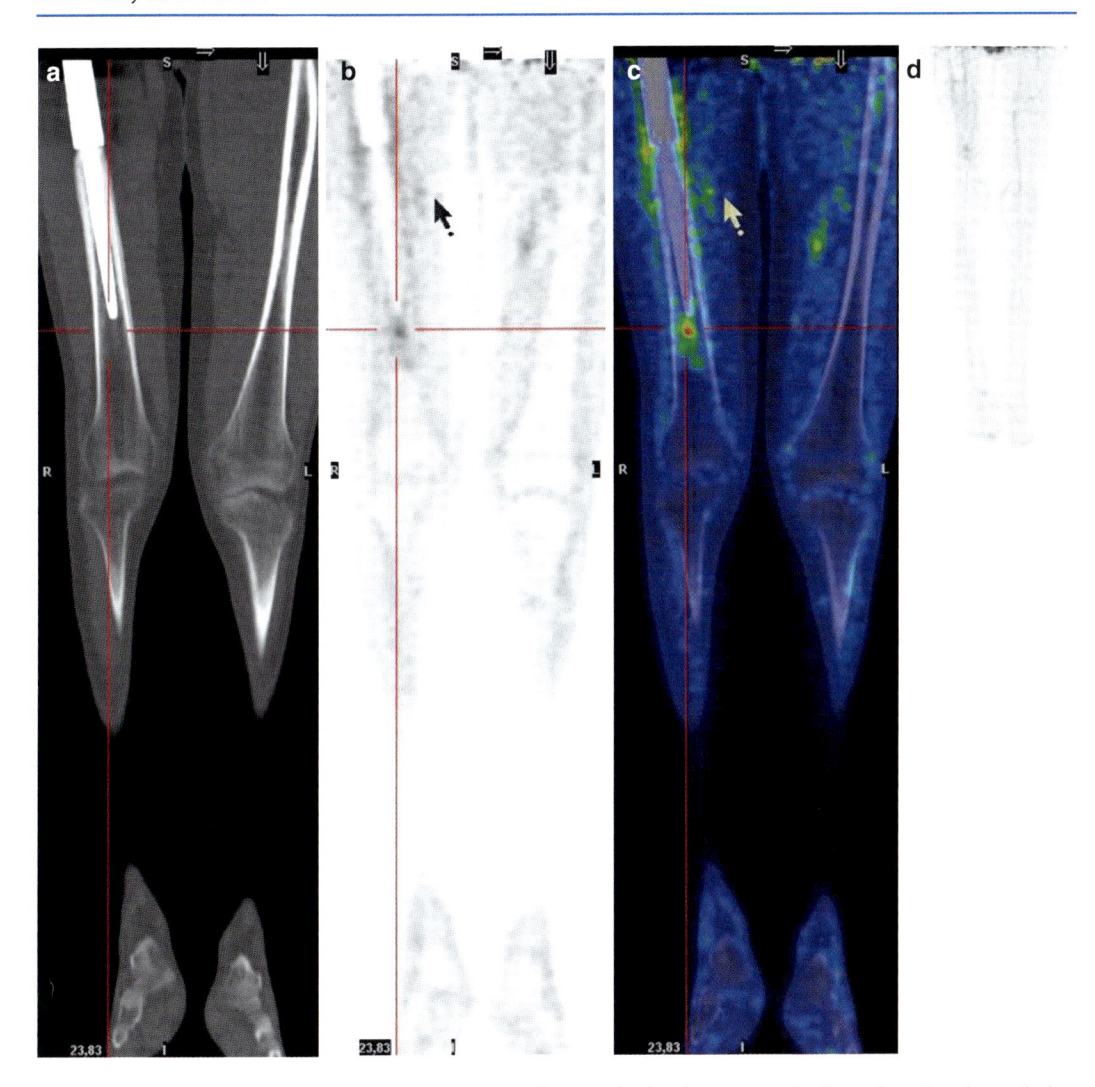

Fig. 8.10 A 15-year-old boy treated for osteosarcoma of the left femur. Coronal CT (**a**), PET (**b**), and PET/CT fusion (**c**) images show focal uptake at the apex of the prosthesis due to static–dynamic alterations during walking and standing. (**d**) MIP shows the different lengths of the legs, with the left being shorter than the right

8.7 Therapy Monitoring

In OS, a further application of FDG–PET/CT is to monitor the response of the primary tumor or the metastases to chemotherapy, including to new therapeutic protocols (Figs. 8.11, 8.12, and 8.13). While the therapeutic response of bone tumor lesions is usually assessed on the basis of morphological changes on CT and MRI, in bone tumors, a change in the size of the lesion is not always a reliable parameter. By contrast, in the follow-up of neoplastic lesions, FDG uptake is significantly related to tumor or metastatic response and, in this context, is superior to morphological assessment. In addition, identification of the most active site of the mass can also guide the clinician in choosing the best biopsy site as well as in devising a tailored radiotherapy plan [32, 39–41]. Some authors have suggested the use of a post-therapy SUV_{max} cutoff (2.5) response or an SUV_2 : SUV_1 ratio of 0.5 to discriminate between good and poor responses [42]. Differences in the therapeutic response criteria used in the evaluation of OS and EWS have also been noted. Using histological regression as the reference, Denecke et al. studied 27 patients with EWS and OS who were evaluated by FDG–PET/CT and MRI before and after neoadjuvant chemotherapy prior to tumor resection. In the subgroup of OS patients, FDG–PET/CT was superior to MRI in the noninvasive response assessment, whereas in EWS patients, neither FDG–PET nor MRI criteria enabled a reliable response assessment [41]. However, these conclusions were based on small series and further investigations are warranted.

As in soft tissue sarcomas, radiotherapy is also the suggested treatment for patients with bone sarcomas. However, because detailed investigations are lacking, PET/CT is currently not routinely used for radiotherapy planning, but as in other tumors, it may be useful to determine the correct target volume and to select a patient-tailored radiation field according to disease extent (Figs. 8.14, 8.15, and 8.16) [43].

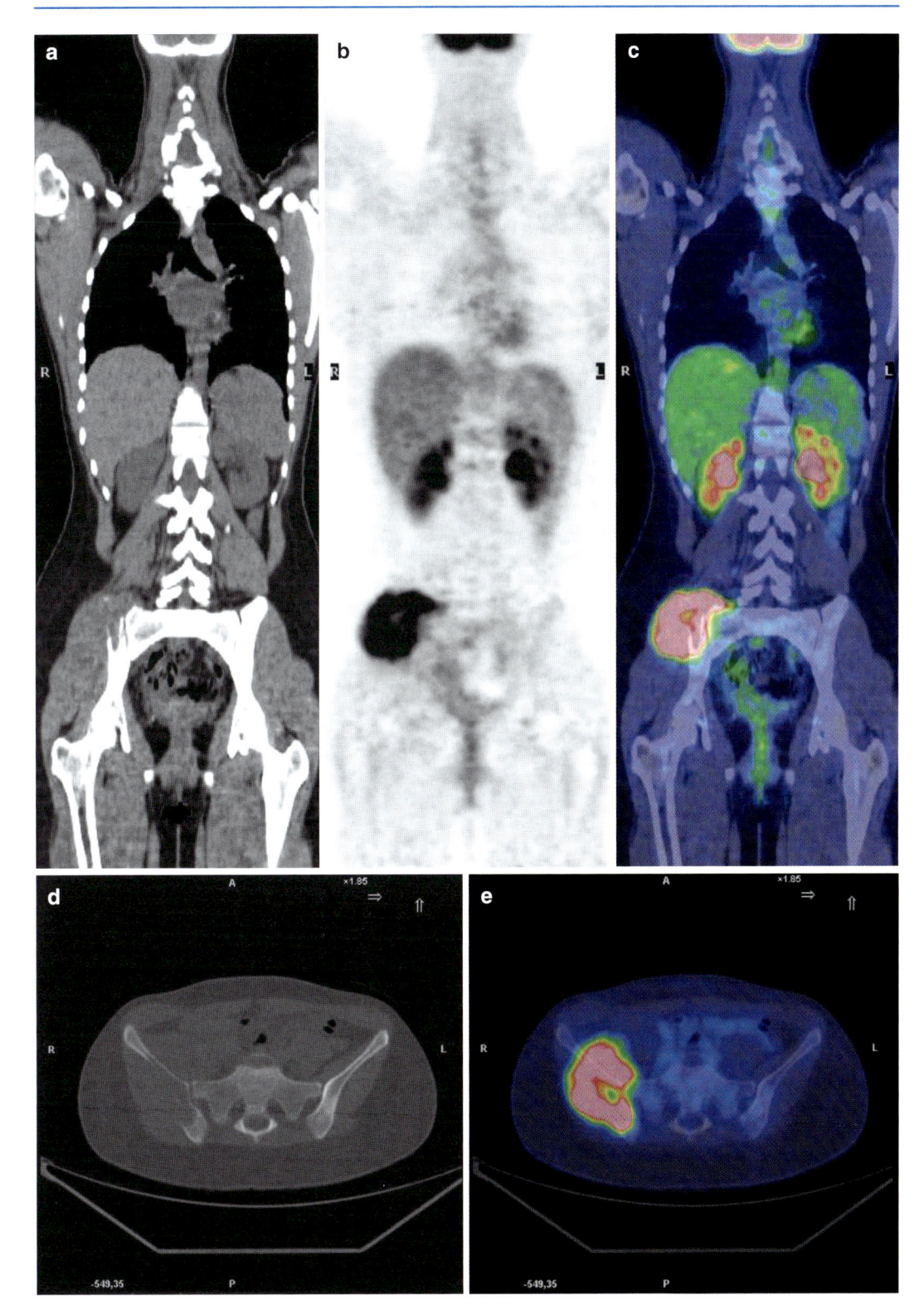

Fig. 8.11 A 17-year-old girl received chemotherapy followed by surgery for osteoblastic osteosarcoma of the distal right femur and lung metastasis. Coronal mediastinal window CT (**a**), PET (**b**), and PET/CT fusion (**c**) images show a recurrence of the osteosarcoma on the right iliac bone and peri-skeletal soft tissue. Axial bone window settings on CT (**d**) and PET/CT fusion (**e**) images show cortical erosion of the right iliac bone

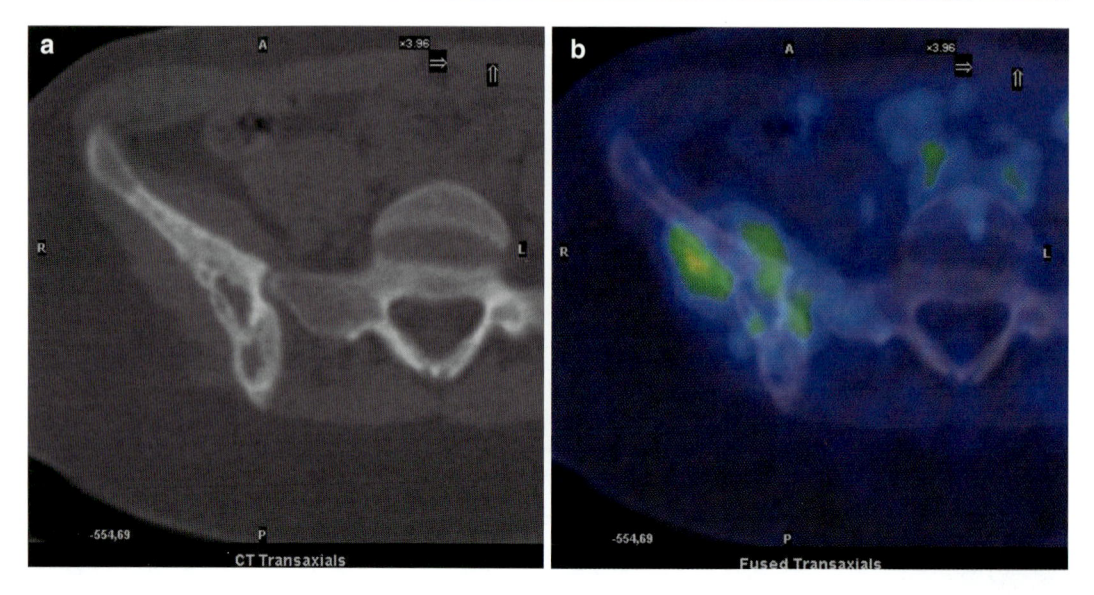

Fig. 8.12 The same patient after chemotherapy. Axial bone window settings on CT (**a**) and PET/CT fusion (**b**) images show persisting inhomogeneous ^{18}F-FDG uptake reflecting the continued presence of some vital tumor cells

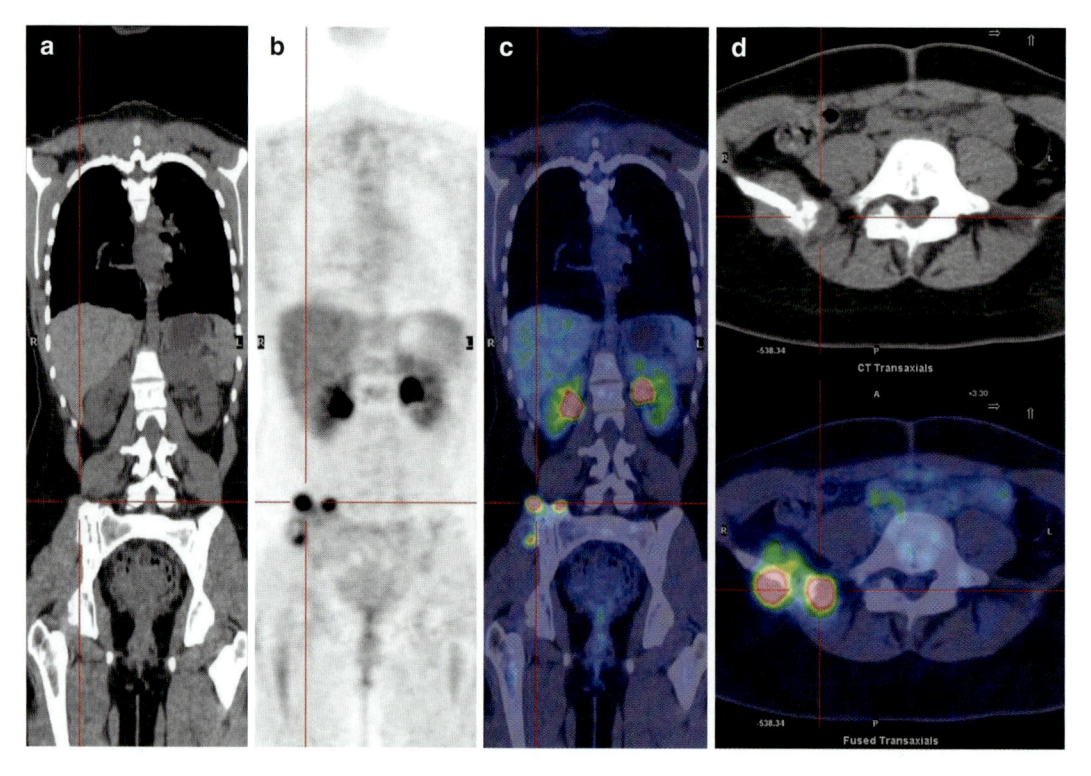

Fig. 8.13 The same patient as in Figs. 8.11 and 8.12. The decision was made to treat the patient with samarium lexidronam pentasodium. Coronal (**a–c**) and axial (**d**) CT (**a**), PET (**b**), and (**c, d**) PET/CT fusion images after radiometabolic therapy show a resumption of tumor growth. The patient died 1 year later due to local and distant disease progression

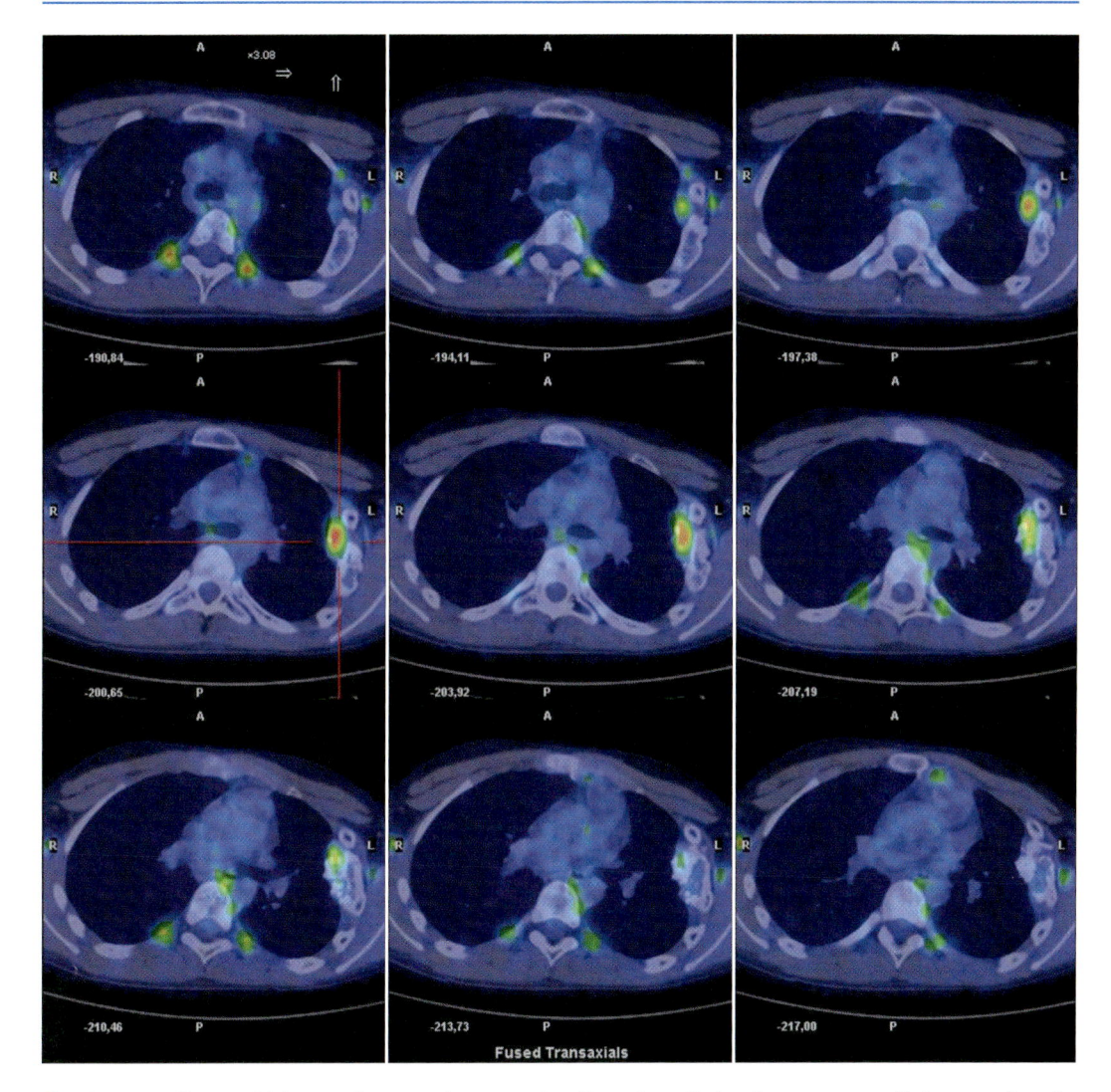

Fig. 8.14 A 13-year-old boy underwent chemo- and radiotherapy for an extensive Ewing's sarcoma of the left chest wall with pleural extension. Axial PET/CT fusion images show ^{18}F-FDG uptake at the level of ribs IV and V. Since the radiation dose was not sufficient to radiate the entire morphology of the lesion, a PET study was carried out for radiotherapy planning, focusing on the metabolic activity of the tumor

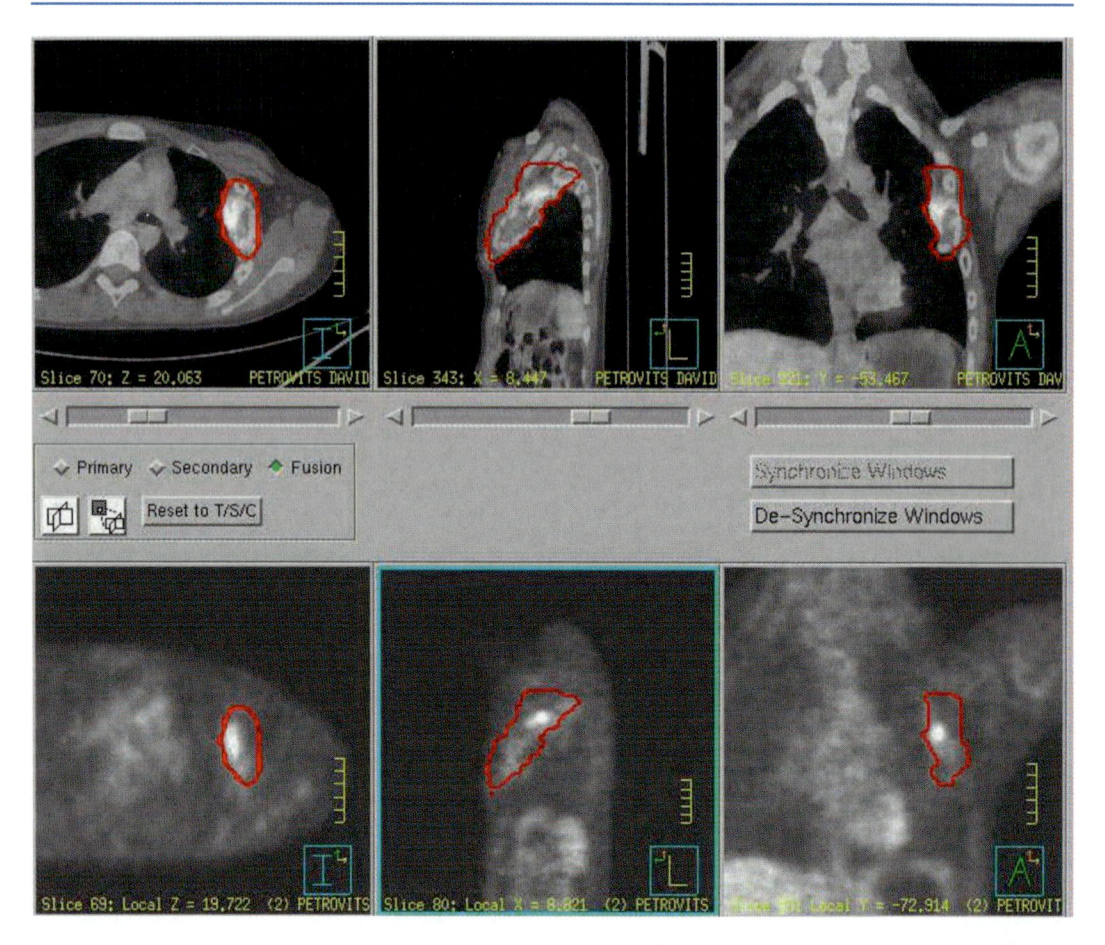

Fig. 8.15 Fusion PET/CT planning radiotherapy targeting focal ^{18}F-FDG uptake (Images provided by A. Mussano and E. Madon, Radiotherapy Unit, Regina Margherita Children's Hospital, Turin, Italy)

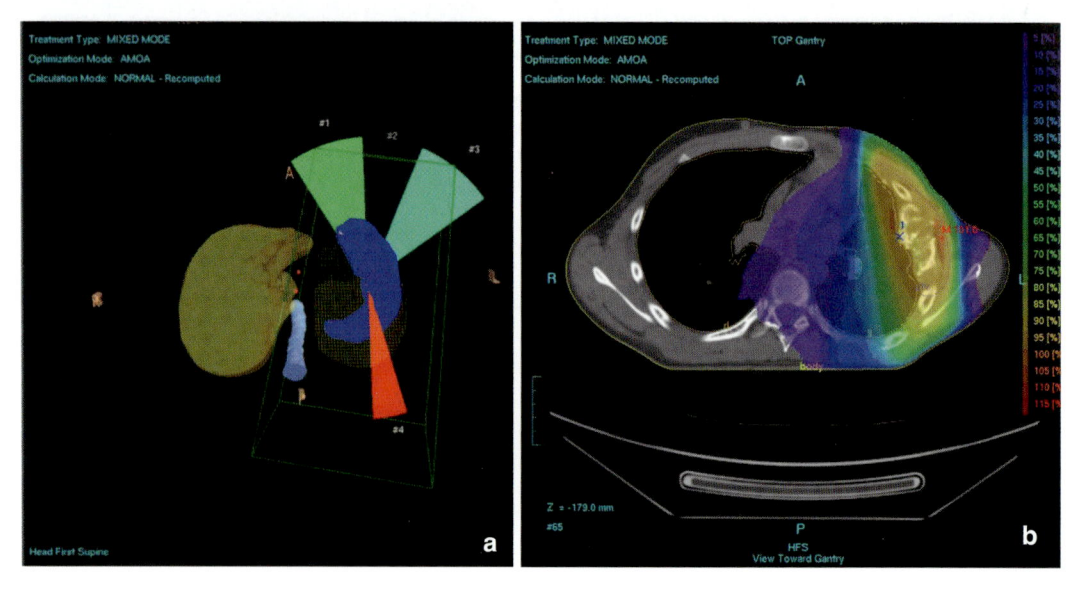

Fig. 8.16 (**a**) Geometry of irradiation. (**b**) Image at the isocenter shows the transversal dose distribution (Images provided by A. Mussano and E. Madon, Radiotherapy Unit, Regina Margherita Children's Hospital, Turin, Italy)

References

1. Vlychou M, Athanasou NA (2008) Radiological and pathological diagnosis of paediatric bone tumours and tumour-like lesions. Pathology 40:196–216
2. Wyers MR (2010) Evaluation of pediatric bone lesions. Pediatr Radiol 40:468–473
3. Quak E, van de Luijtgaarden AC, de Geus-Oei LF et al (2011) Clinical applications of positron emission tomography in sarcoma management. Expert Rev Anticancer Ther 11:195–204
4. Ludwig JA (2008) Ewing sarcoma: historical perspectives, current state of the-art, and opportunities for targeted therapy in the future. Curr Opin Oncol 20:412–418
5. Kaste SC (2011) Imaging pediatric bone sarcomas. Radiol Clin North Am 49:749–765
6. Bakhshi S, Radhakrishnan V (2010) Prognostic markers in osteosarcoma. Expert Rev Anticancer Ther 10:271–287
7. Arndt CA, Rose PS, Folpe AL et al (2012) Common musculoskeletal tumors of childhood and adolescence. Mayo Clin Proc 87:475–487
8. Quartuccio N, Treglia G, Salsano M et al (2013) The role of Fluorine-18-Fluorodeoxyglucose positron emission tomography in staging and restaging of patients with osteosarcoma. Radiol Oncol 47:97–102
9. Bacci G, Bertoni F, Longhi A et al (2003) Neoadjuvant chemotherapy for high-grade central osteosarcoma of the extremity. Histologic response to preoperative chemotherapy correlates with histologic subtype of the tumor. Cancer 97:3068–3075
10. Bacci G, Mercuri M, Longhi A et al (2005) Grade of chemotherapy-induced necrosis as a predictor of local and systemic control in 881 patients with non-metastatic osteosarcoma of the extremities treated with neoadjuvant chemotherapy in a single institution. Eur J Cancer 41:2079–2085
11. Grimer RJ, Bielack S, Flege S et al (2005) Periosteal osteosarcoma – a European review of outcome. Eur J Cancer 41:2806–2811
12. Potratz J, Dirksen U, Jürgens H et al (2012) Ewing sarcoma: clinical state-of-the-art. Pediatr Hematol Oncol 29:1–11
13. Balamuth NJ, Womer RB (2010) Ewing's sarcoma. Lancet Oncol 11:184–192
14. Randall RL, Lessnick SL, Jones KB et al (2010) Is there a predisposition gene for Ewing's sarcoma? J Oncol 2010:397632. http://www.hindawi.com/journals/jo/2010/397632/cta/
15. Treglia G, Salsano M, Stefanelli A et al (2012) Diagnostic accuracy of ^{18}F-FDG-PET and PET/CT in patients with Ewing sarcoma family tumours: a systematic review and a meta-analysis. Skeletal Radiol 41:249–256
16. Jawad MU, Cheung MC, Min ES et al (2009) Ewing sarcoma demonstrates racial disparities in incidence-related and sex-related differences in outcome: an analysis of 1631 cases from the SEER database, 1973–2005. Cancer 115:3526–3536
17. Cotterill SJ, Ahrens S, Paulussen M et al (2000) Prognostic factors in Ewing's tumor of bone: analysis of 975 patients from the European Intergroup Cooperative Ewing's Sarcoma Study Group. J Clin Oncol 18:3108–3114
18. Esiashvili N, Goodman M, Marcus RB Jr (2008) Changes in incidence and survival of Ewing sarcoma patients over the past 3 decades: Surveillance, Epidemiology, and End Results data. J Pediatr Hematol Oncol 30:425–430
19. Ferrari S, Balladelli A, Palmerini E et al (2011) Imaging in bone sarcomas. The chemotherapist's point of view. Eur J Radiol 2011 Dec 28. doi:10.1016/j.ejrad.2011.11.028
20. London K, Stege C, Cross S, Onikul E et al (2012) 18F-FDG PET/CT compared to conventional imaging modalities in pediatric primary bone tumors. Pediatr Radiol 42:418–430
21. Bredella MA, Caputo GR, Steinbach LS (2002) Value of FDG positron emission tomography in conjunction with MR imaging for evaluating therapy response in patients with musculoskeletal sarcomas. AJR Am J Roentgenol 179:1145–1150
22. Schwarzbach MH, Dimitrakopoulou-Strauss A, Willeke F et al (2000) Clinical value of [18-F] fluorodeoxyglucose positron emission tomography imaging in soft tissue sarcomas. Ann Surg 231:380–386
23. Ducimetière F, Lurkin A, Ranchère-Vince D et al (2011) Incidence of sarcoma histotypes and molecular subtypes in a prospective epidemiological study with central pathology review and molecular testing. PLoS One 6:e20294
24. Mirabello L, Troisi RJ, Savage SA (2009) Osteosarcoma incidence and survival rates from 1973 to 2004: data from the Surveillance, Epidemiology, and End Results Program. Cancer 115:1531–1543
25. Folpe AL, Lyles RH, Sprouse JT et al (2000) (F-18) fluorodeoxyglucose positron emission tomography as a predictor of pathologic grade and other prognostic variables in bone and soft tissue sarcoma. Clin Cancer Res 6:1279–1287
26. Jeffree GM, Price CHG, Sissons HA (1975) The metastatic patterns of osteosarcoma. Br J Cancer 32:87
27. Aljubran AH, Griffin A, Pintilie M et al (2009) Osteosarcoma in adolescents and adults: survival analysis with and without lung metastases. Ann Oncol 20:1136–1141
28. Letourneau PA, Shackett B, Xiao L et al (2011) Resection of pulmonary metastases in pediatric patients with Ewing sarcoma improves survival. J Pediatr Surg 46:332–335
29. Huang YM, Hou CH, Hou SM et al (2009) The metastasectomy and timing of pulmonary metastases on the outcome of osteosarcoma patients. Clin Med Oncol 3:99–105
30. Cistaro A, Lopci E, Gastaldo L et al (2012) The role of (18) F-FDG PET/CT in the metabolic characterization

of lung nodules in pediatric patients with bone sarcoma. Pediatr Blood Cancer 59:1206–10
31. Roth JA, Putnam JB, Wesley MN (1985) Deferring determinants of prognosis following resection of pulmonary metastasis from osteogenetic and soft tissue sarcoma patients. Cancer 55:1361–1366
32. Bestic JM, Peterson JJ, Bancroft LW (2009) Pediatric FDG PET/CT: physiologic uptake, normal variants, and benign conditions. Radiographics 29:1487–1500
33. Franzius C, Daldrup-Link HE, Wagner-Bohn A et al (2002) FDG-PET for detection of recurrences from malignant primary bone tumors: comparison with conventional imaging. Ann Oncol 13:157–160
34. Völker T, Denecke T, Steffen I et al (2007) Positron emission tomography for staging of pediatric sarcoma patients: results of a prospective multicenter trial. J Clin Oncol 25:5435–5441
35. Malawer MM, Helman LJ, O'Sullivan B (2011) Sarcomas of bone. In: DeVita VT Jr, Lawrence TS, Rosenberg SA (eds) Cancer: Principles and Practice of Oncology. 9th ed. Philadelphia, Pa: Lippincott Williams & Wilkins, pp 1578–1609
36. Bielack SS, Kempf-Bielack B, Delling G et al (2002) Prognostic factors in high-grade osteosarcoma of the extremities or trunk: an analysis of 1,702 patients treated on neoadjuvant cooperative osteosarcoma study group protocols. J Clin Oncol 20:776–790
37. McTiernan AM, Cassoni AM, Driver D et al (2006) Improving outcomes after relapse in Ewing's sarcoma: analysis of 114 patients from a single institution. Sarcoma 2006:83548
38. Shankar AG, Ashley S, Craft AW et al (2003) Outcome after relapse in an unselected cohort of children and adolescents with Ewing sarcoma. Med Pediatr Oncol 40:141–147
39. Hicks RJ, Toner GC, Choong PF (2005) Clinical applications of molecular imaging in sarcoma evaluation. Cancer Imaging 5:66–72
40. Anderson P (2006) Samarium for osteoblastic bone metastases and osteosarcoma. Expert Opin Pharmacother 7:1475–1486
41. Denecke T, Hundsdörfer P, Misch D et al (2010) Assessment of histological response of paediatric bone sarcomas using FDG PET in comparison to morphological volume measurement and standardized MRI parameters. Eur J Nucl Med Mol Imaging 37:1842–1853
42. Hamada K, Tomita Y, Inoue A et al (2009) Evaluation of chemotherapy response in osteosarcoma with FDG-PET. Ann Nucl Med 23:89–95
43. Sheplan LJ, Juliano JJ (2010) Use of radiation therapy for patients with soft-tissue and bone sarcomas. Cleve Clin J Med 77:S27–S29

Utility of ¹⁸F–FDG–PET/CT in Soft Tissue Sarcomas

9

Somali Gavane, Angelina Cistaro, and Heiko Schoder

9.1 Background

Pediatric soft tissue sarcomas (STS) are a heterogeneous group of mesenchymal tumors that differ in both their behavior and their treatment. The many different histological subtypes also widely vary with respect to the degree of malignancy and aggressiveness. Table 9.1 lists the tumors included in the soft tissue category according to the 2002 World Health Organization classification.

The main indications of FDG–PET/CT in STS are the staging of locally advanced high-grade tumors and the detection of suspected local recurrence.

Rhabdomyosarcoma (RMS) is the most common STS in children and adolescents, accounting for ~5 % of all pediatric cancers and about half of all STS [1]. The tumor can arise anywhere in the body and carries a high risk of locoregional lymph node extension. Survival at 5 years is improved by combining polychemotherapy with local treatment of the primary tumor and its metastases.

S. Gavane, MD • H. Schoder, MD
Nuclear Medicine Department,
Memorial Sloan-Kettering Cancer Center,
1275 York Avenue, New York, NY 10065, USA
e-mail: gavanes@mskcc.org; schoderh@mskcc.org

A. Cistaro, MD (✉)
Department of Nuclear Medicine, Positron Emission Tomography Center IRMET S.p.A., Euromedic Inc., Via Onorato Vigliani 89, Turin 10100, Italy

Institute of Cognitive Sciences and Technologies, National Research Council, Rome, Italy
e-mail: a.cistaro@irmet.com

Table 9.1 Soft tissue tumors according to the 2002 WHO classification

Adipocytic tumors
Dedifferentiated liposarcoma
Myxoid/round cell liposarcoma
Pleomorphic liposarcoma
Fibroblastic/myofibroblastic tumors
Fibrosarcoma
Low-grade myxofibrosarcoma
Low-grade fibromyxoid sarcoma
Sclerosing epithelioid fibrosarcoma
So-called fibrohistiocytic tumors
Undifferentiated pleomorphic sarcoma/malignant fibrous histiocytoma (MFH)
Smooth muscle tumors
Leiomyosarcoma
Skeletal muscle tumors
Rhabdomyosarcoma (embryonal, alveolar, and pleomorphic forms)
Vascular tumors
Epithelioid hemangioendothelioma
Angiosarcoma—deep
Tumors of peripheral nerves
Malignant peripheral nerve sheath tumor
Chondro-osseous tumors
Extraskeletal chondrosarcoma (mesenchymal and other variants)
Extraskeletal osteosarcoma
Tumors of uncertain differentiation
Synovial sarcoma
Epithelioid sarcoma
Alveolar soft part sarcoma
Clear cell sarcoma of soft tissue
Extraskeletal myxoid chondrosarcoma

(continued)

Table 9.1 (continued)

Primitive neuroectodermal tumor (PNET)/extraskeletal Ewing's tumor
Desmoplastic small round cell tumor
Extrarenal rhabdoid tumor
Undifferentiated sarcoma; sarcoma, not otherwise specified (NOS)

^{18}F-FDG–PET/CT provides important additional information in the initial staging of RMS, mainly by evaluating the lymph nodes and metastases, with a significant impact on therapeutic management (Figs. 9.1, 9.2, 9.3, 9.4, 9.5, 9.6, 9.7, 9.8, 9.9, and 9.10). There is also a high prognostic impact of ^{18}F-FDG–PET/CT in the early assessment of the therapeutic response [2, 3].

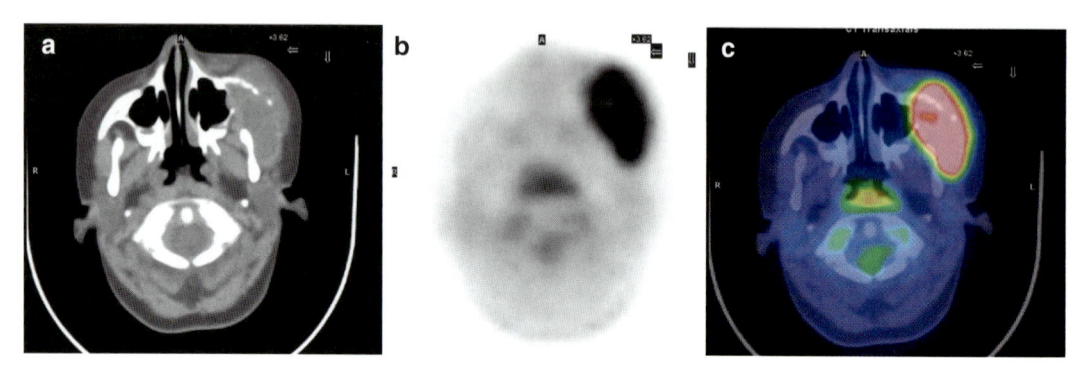

Fig. 9.1 A 6-year-old girl with embryonal rhabdomyosarcoma of the left zygomatic region. Axial CT (**a**), PET (**b**), and PET/CT fusion (**c**) images show large and intense ^{18}F-FDG uptake in the zygomatic arch, masseter and temporal muscles

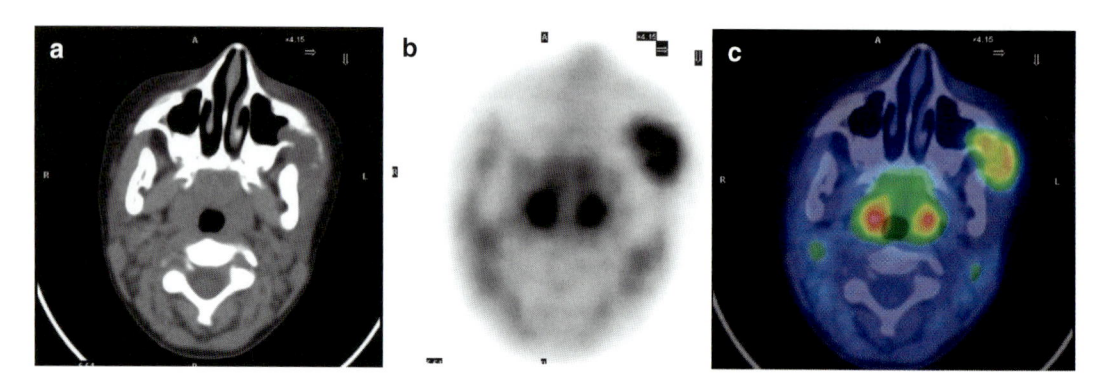

Fig. 9.2 The same patient as in Fig. 9.1, after chemotherapy for embryonal rhabdomyosarcoma of the left zygomatic region. Axial CT (**a**), PET (**b**), and PET/CT fusion (**c**) images show persisting disease, indicative of only a partial response to treatment

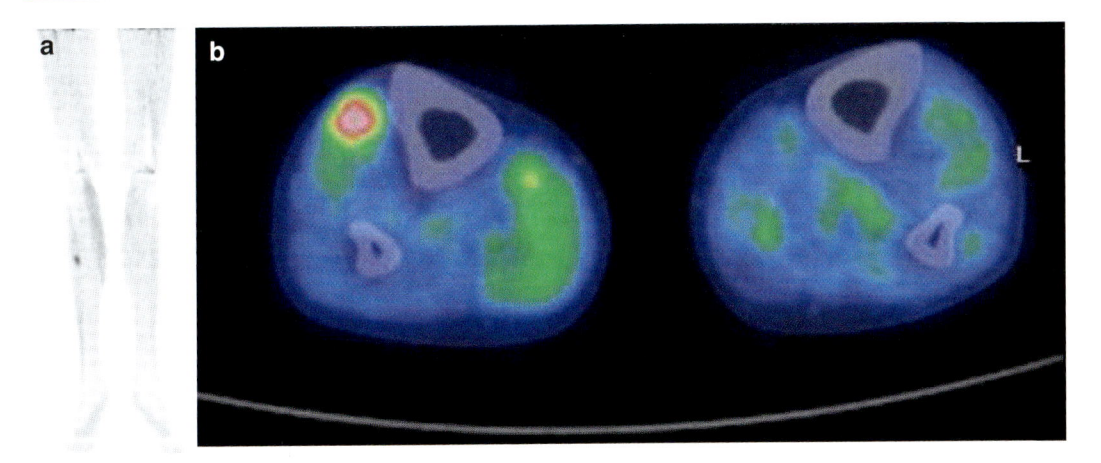

Fig. 9.3 A 17-year-old boy with rhabdomyosarcoma of the right anterior tibial muscle. Maximum intensity projection (**a**) and axial PET/CT fusion images (**b**) of the legs

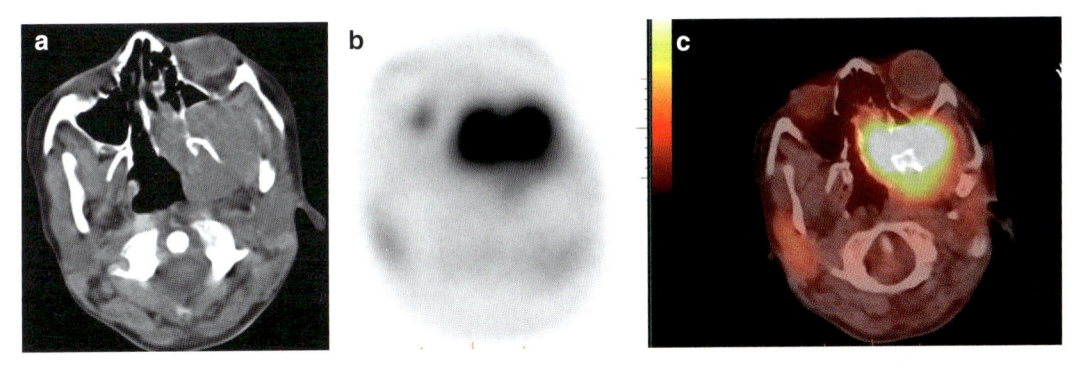

Fig. 9.4 A 7-year-old girl presented with turning of the left eye and double vision. Her ophthalmologist prescribed antibiotics. After a week, her chief complaint was headache. She had also suffered a nosebleed followed by the sudden loss of vision in her left eye. CT scan of the head and paranasal sinuses (**a**) revealed a large irregular infiltrative process involving the base of the central skull and the floor of the left middle cranial fossa, with intracranial extension into the left orbit and left subtemporal fossa. ^{18}F-FDG–PET/CT (**b, c**) demonstrated a large hypermetabolic mass (SUV = 8.4) in the left nasopharynx and extending to the left orbit and left ethmoid sinus. Biopsy of the mass suggested an embryonal rhabdomyosarcoma

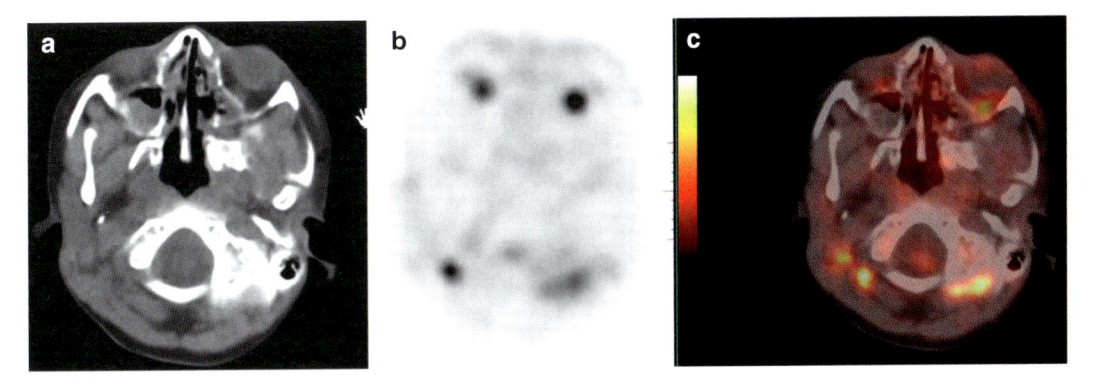

Fig. 9.5 Same patient as in Fig. 9.4; posttreatment evaluation. The patient received 12 cycles of irinotecan, vincristine, adriamycin, cytoxan, ifosfamide, and carboplatin along with 5,040 cGy of radiation to the primary tumor site. (**a–c**) At the end of treatment, ^{18}F-FDG–PET/CT showed complete resolution of the primary mass

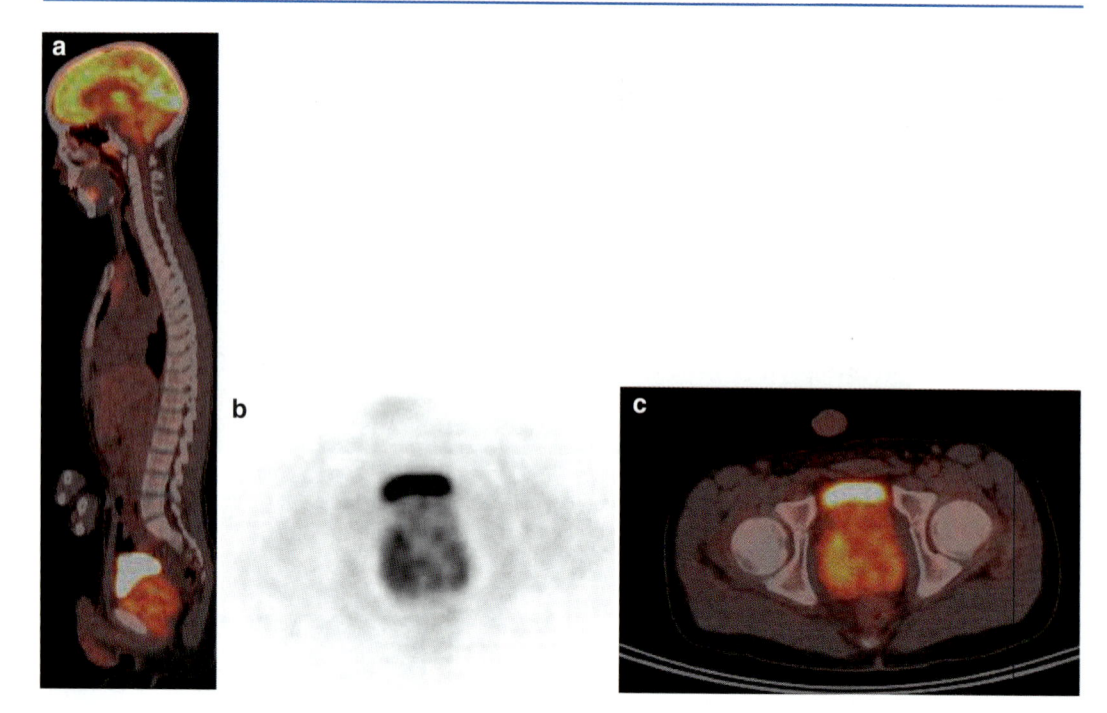

Fig. 9.6 A 12-year-old boy presented with dysuria, hesitancy, dribbling, and urgency while urinating. His pediatrician performed a urine analysis and an ultrasound, with the latter showing enlargement of the prostate gland. A CT scan of the pelvis showed a large prostatic mass extending inferiorly into the base of the penis (**a**, **c**). ^{18}F-FDG–PET/CT demonstrated a large heterogeneous hypermetabolic mass (SUV 6) of the prostate gland that compressed the posterior wall of the urinary bladder (**b**). Biopsy of the mass suggested a high-grade rhabdomyosarcoma of the prostate

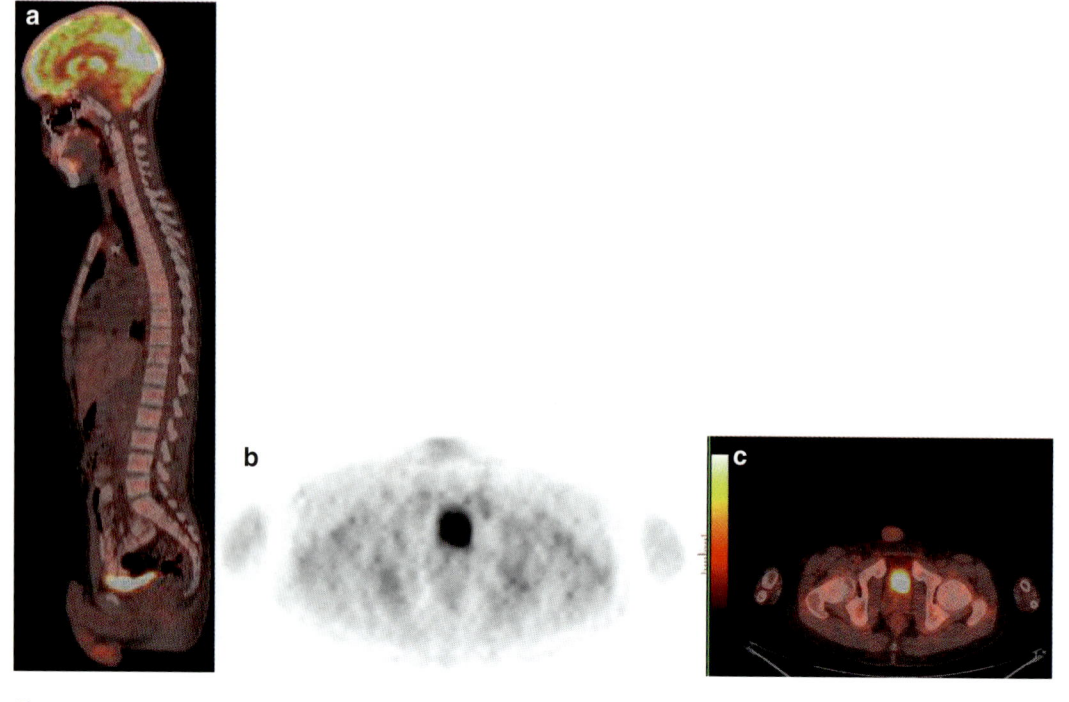

Fig. 9.7 Same patient as in Fig. 9.6; posttreatment evaluation. The patient received 12 cycles of irinotecan, vincristine, and carboplatin along with 5,040 cGy radiation to the primary tumor site. (**a–c**) At the end of treatment, ^{18}F-FDG–PET/CT showed complete resolution of the primary mass

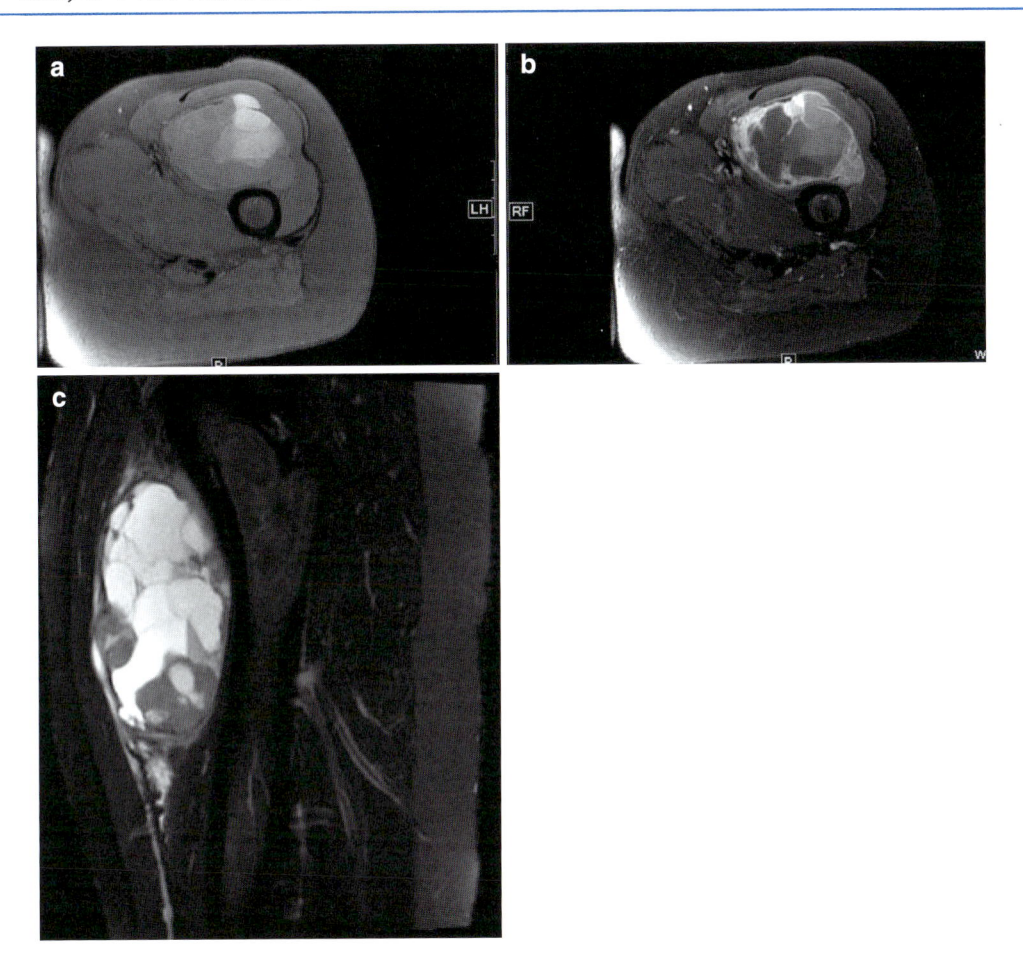

Fig. 9.8 A 22-year-old girl presented with pain and swelling in the left thigh. (**a–c**) A dedicated MRI of the lower extremity showed an 8.0 × 5.7 × 9.0 cm mixed solid cystic tumor, a large proportion of which consisted of blood fluid levels, located within the vastus intermedius muscle of the proximal thigh. Possible focal cortical thinning and probable slight permeation of the femoral cortex subjacent to the tumor were noted. Biopsy showed a spindle-cell sarcoma, consistent with synovial sarcoma

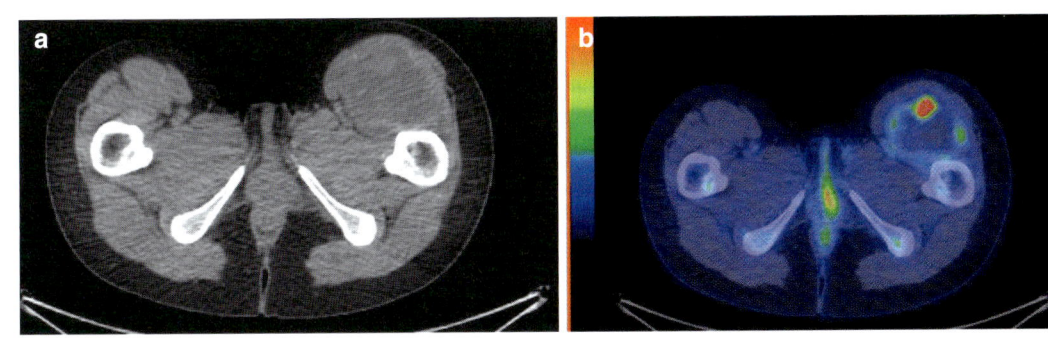

Fig. 9.9 Same patient as in Fig. 9.8. (**a, b**) Axial CT and FDG–PET/CT, performed for staging, showed a large mixed-attenuation mass in the left vastus intermedius muscle with a peripheral rim of mild FDG uptake, central photopenia, and a nodular, intensely hypermetabolic solid component (SUV = 23.8). There was no evidence of metastatic disease elsewhere in the body

Fig. 9.10 Same patient as in Figs. 9.8 and 9.9. Surgical excision of the synovial sarcoma was performed, together with periosteal stripping with prophylactic internal fixation of the left femur. The patient received six cycles of ifosfamide and doxorubicin and 6,300 cGy of radiation to her left thigh. (**a**, **b**) The end of treatment FDG–PET/CT showed resolution of the disease

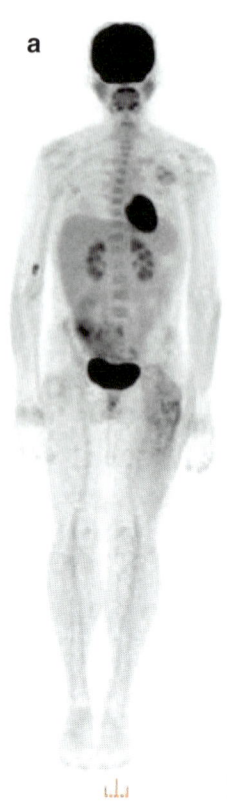

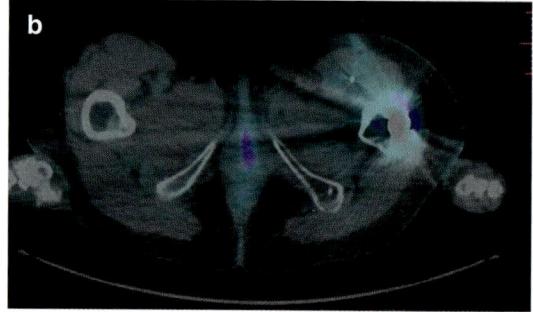

9.2 Discussion

Synovial sarcoma is a common STS in children [4, 5], with males and females equally affected. Although these tumors mainly occur in the extremities, predominantly the lower extremities, in rare cases, they originate in the head and neck, thorax, or abdomen [5]. For primary staging, MRI is the initial imaging modality of choice and in particular for planning the surgical approach. Chest CT is necessary to assess possible lung metastasis [6]. FDG–PET is useful in risk assessment, in diagnosis, and in assessing response to chemoradiation therapy [7].

References

1. Paulino AC, Okcu MF (2008) Rhabdomyosarcoma. Curr Probl Cancer 32:7–34
2. Baum SH, Frühwald M, Rahbar K, Wessling J, Schober O, Weckesser M (2011) Contribution of PET/CT to prediction of outcome in children and young adults with rhabdomyosarcoma. J Nucl Med 52:1535–1540
3. Samuel AM (2010) PET/CT in pediatric oncology. Indian J Cancer 47(4):360–370
4. Brennan MF, Singer S, Maki RG et al (2005) Sarcomas of the soft tissues and bone. In: DeVita VT, Hellmann S, Rosenberg SA (eds) Cancer: principles and practice of oncology, vol 35. Lippincott Williams & Wilkins, Philadelphia, p 1584
5. Kransdorf MJ (1995) Malignant soft-tissue tumors in a large referral population: distribution of diagnoses by age, sex, and location. AJR Am J Roentgenol 164:129–134
6. Kransdorf MJ, Murphey MD (2011) Radiologic evaluation of soft-tissue masses: a current perspective. AJR Am J Roentgenol 175:575–587
7. Lisle JW, Eary JF, O'Sullivan J, Conrad EU (2008) Risk assessment based on FDG-PET imaging in patients with synovial sarcoma. Clin Orthop Relat Res 467:1605–1611

Primary Hepatic Tumors

10

Natale Quartuccio and Angelina Cistaro

10.1 Hepatoblastoma

Liver tumors account for 1–4 % of all solid tumors in the pediatric population. Among the subgroup of primary liver tumors, 60 % are malignant, with hepatoblastoma (HB) as the most common (1.3 cases per million children per year) but also including hepatocellular carcinoma (HCC), rhabdomyosarcoma, angiosarcoma, rhabdoid tumor, undifferentiated sarcoma of the liver (USL), and other rare tumors [1]. The term "hepatoblastoma" refers to a group of liver tumors of embryonal origin [2]. They can be divided into pure epithelial and mixed (formed by epithelial and mesenchymal components) types depending on their histology [3, 4]. Most HBs are sporadic, although familial cases arise in association with Beckwith–Wiedemann syndrome, familial adenomatous polyposis and other syndromes [5]. The clinical onset is characterized by an abdominal mass, while in advanced disease, anorexia and weight loss also may be present. An increased serum alpha-fetoprotein (α-FP) concentration is typical, occurring in 90 % of HB patients [6]. Up to 20 % of patients present at diagnosis with advanced disease, including secondary lesions in the lungs. Brain and bone metastases are less frequent and are most often seen during disease relapse [2]. At follow-up, increased serum α-FP is indicative of disease recurrence and predicts a poor prognosis [3].

To date, the treatment of choice is neoadjuvant chemotherapy, to reduce the mass, followed by tumor resection. Patients with unresectable lesions have a poor prognosis [7, 8]. The International Society of Paediatric Oncology Liver Tumour Group (SIOPEL) recommends neoadjuvant chemotherapy followed by delayed surgery. Assessment is based on SIOPEL's PRETEXT staging system (PRE Treatment EXTent of disease), which considers liver anatomy and radiological findings at diagnosis to predict the feasibility of tumor resection and the outcome [9]. Liver transplantation has been proposed as an option in patients with unresectable tumors [10]. With the introduction of these innovative, potentially curative strategies, the 5-year survival rate of HB patients has increased from 35 to 75 % in the last 30 years [9, 10].

Conventional imaging techniques to evaluate HB include ultrasound (US), computed tomography (CT), and magnetic resonance imaging (MRI). US has the advantage that it does not

---

N. Quartuccio, MD
Nuclear Medicine Unit, Department of Biomedical Sciences and Morphological and Functional Images, University of Messina, Via Consolare Valeria 1, Messina 98125, Italy
e-mail: natale.quartuccio84@hotmail.it

A. Cistaro, MD (✉)
Department of Nuclear Medicine, Positron Emission Tomography Center IRMET S.p.A., Euromedic Inc., Via Onorato Vigliani 89, Turin 10100, Italy

Institute of Cognitive Sciences and Technologies, National Research Council, Rome, Italy
e-mail: a.cistaro@irmet.com

expose children to radiation. In addition, color Doppler is very sensitive in assessing tumor vascularization. Percutaneous biopsy has been successfully performed under US guidance. However, anatomic details are much better presented by CT [3], which is currently the gold standard for the diagnosis, preoperative evaluation, and follow-up of pediatric liver tumors [11]. Its disadvantage is that after liver resection, postoperative changes resulting in fibrosis and post-treatment necrosis in the liver are frequent and may affect CT accuracy [12]. Instead, in this setting, MRI is more sensitive than CT in discriminating between disease recurrence and postoperative abnormalities, but it often requires the child's sedation such that it is reserved for cases of suspected HB recurrence [13]. In the literature, there have been a few reports on the utility of ^{18}F-FDG–PET/CT in HB [14–19]. Uptake of the ^{18}F-FDG tracer is thought to reflect the ability of HB cells to store large amounts of glycogen granules in their cytoplasm [20]. Thus far, the main role of ^{18}F-FDG–PET/CT is twofold: disease restaging in patients who have undergone chemotherapy and surgery and their follow-up (Figs. 10.1 and 10.2). The ability of this imaging modality to detect early recurrence and metastatic disease has been reported [21].

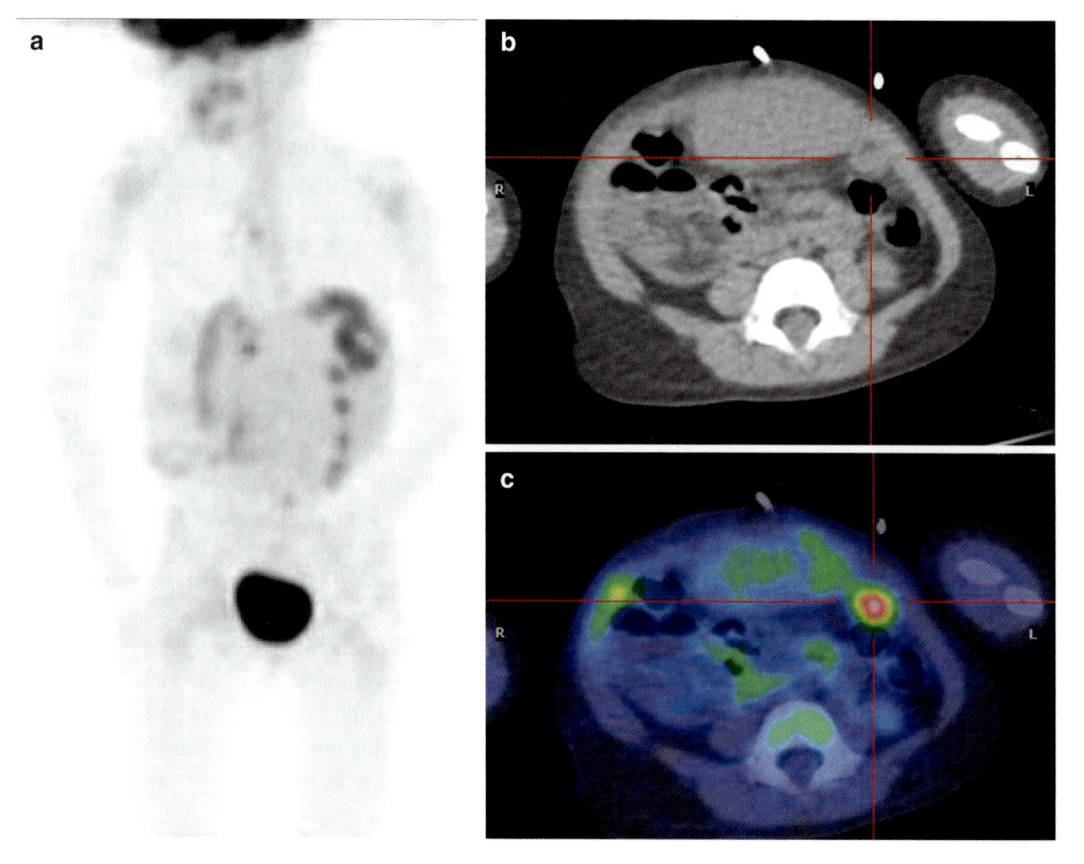

Fig. 10.1 A 3-year-old girl who underwent liver transplantation for mixed hepatoblastoma. PET evaluation following increased serum alpha-fetoprotein. Maximal intensity projection (**a**), axial CT (**b**, **d**), and PET/CT (**c**, **e**) fusion images show the FDG-avid peritoneal lesions

10 Primary Hepatic Tumors 95

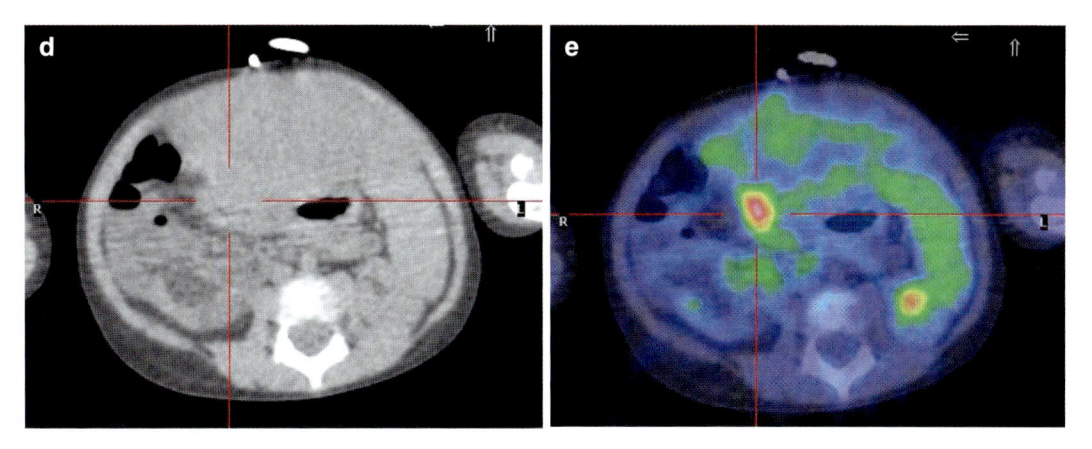

Fig. 10.1 (continued)

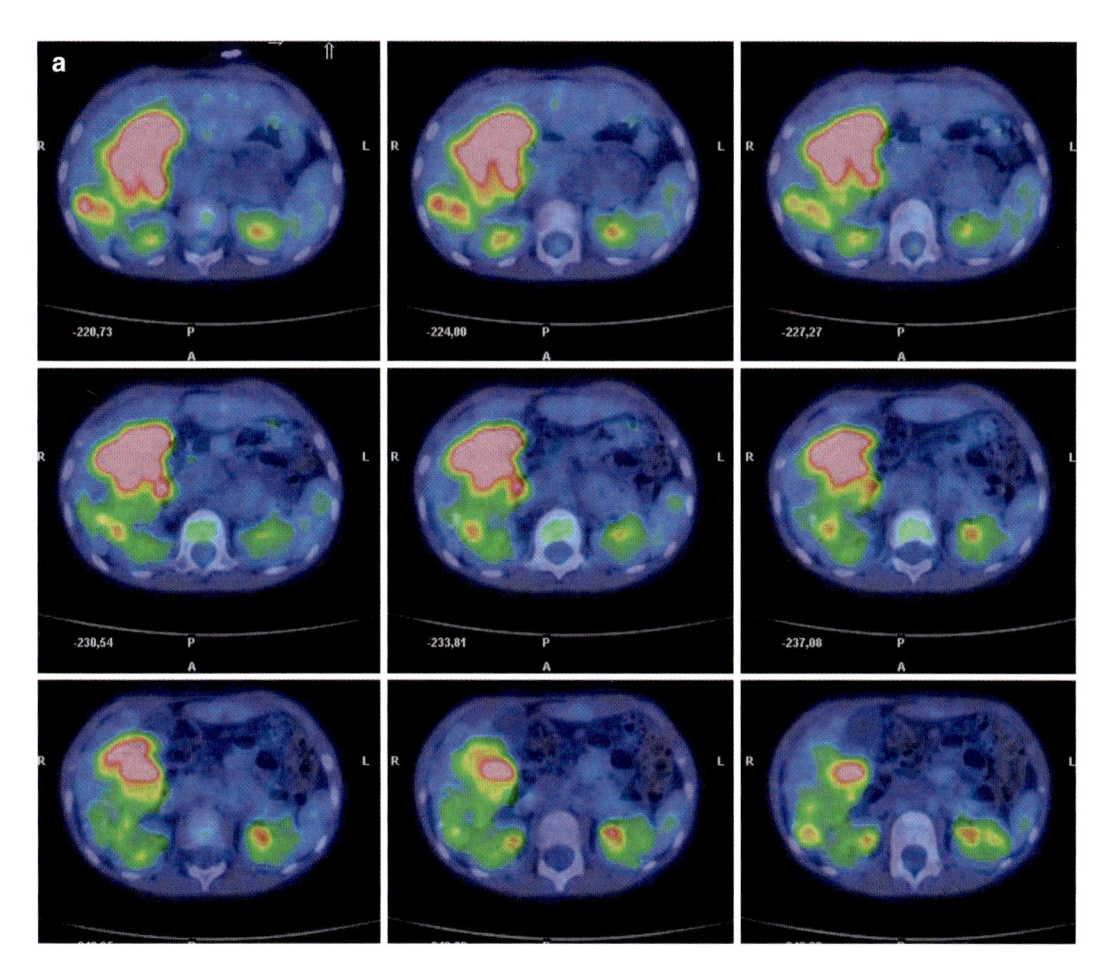

Fig. 10.2 A 4-year-old boy with hepatoblastoma. PET evaluation to determine liver transplantation eligibility. Axial PET/CT fusion images show FDG-avid lesions in the liver (**a**) and lungs (**b**). The patient was referred for chemotherapy

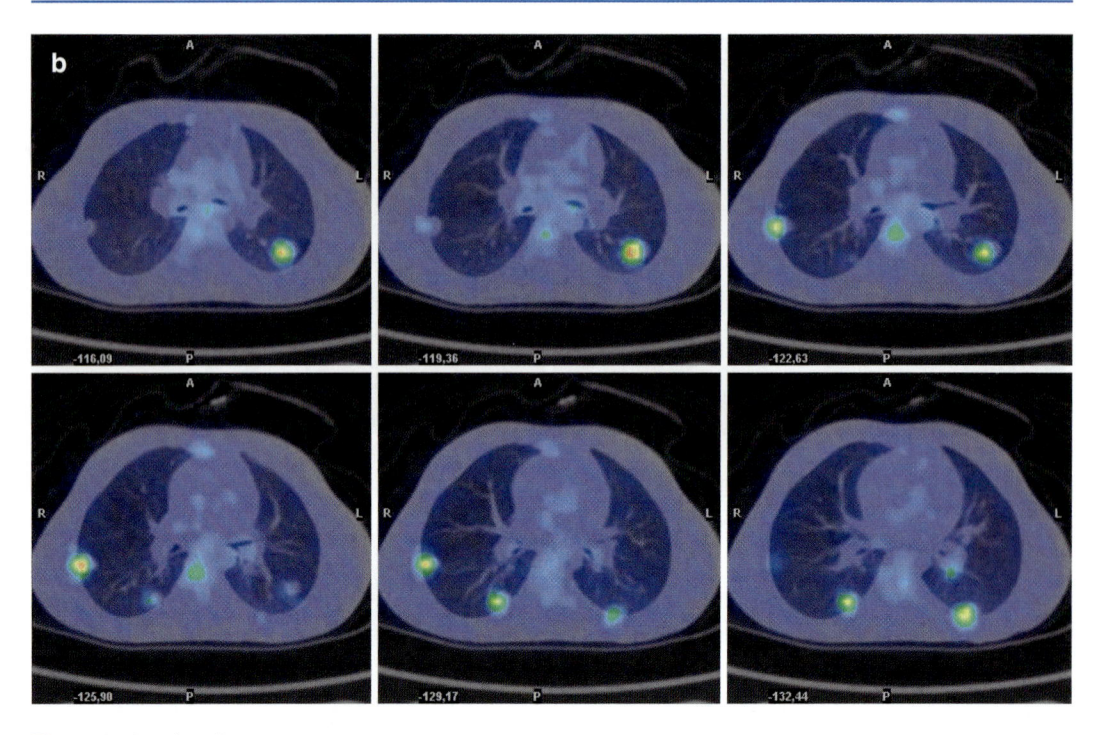

Fig. 10.2 (continued)

10.2 Hepatocarcinoma

As the second most common malignant liver tumor in childhood, HCC comprises 35 % of all hepatic malignancies in children [22]. HCC is histologically divided into classical and fibrolamellar types. Fibrolamellar HCC is the most frequent histological variation and is commonly observed in children and adolescents [23]. Conditions associated with a high risk for HCC development are α-1-antitrypsin deficiency, Wilson's disease, hemochromatosis, hereditary tyrosinemia, Fanconi's anemia, familial adenomatous polyposis and Gardener's syndrome [1]. As in HB, α-FP is increased in HCC in the majority of patients [24]. Since the tumor is chemoresistant, surgical resection and liver transplantation (in case of unresectable HCC confined to the liver) are the only therapeutic options [25]. At diagnosis, 50 % of patients present with metastases [26], mostly in the lungs (31 %). Extrahepatic tumor extension and vascular invasion are also frequently seen (39 %) [27]. The US echogenicity of HCC is similar to that of the liver, and the CT characteristics are highly variable, either homogeneous or heterogeneous, solitary or multifocal, and well- or ill defined. While in adults the presence of underlying cirrhosis may help in the differential diagnosis, it is rare in the pediatric population [28]. CT is generally used to evaluate the response to treatment, but it cannot be used to estimate tumor viability (Fig. 10.3).

Several articles on the impact of PET/CT in adult HCC have been published, but there are no reports on the use of this imaging technique in pediatric patients. Lee et al. evaluated 138 adult patients with low-grade or high-grade HCC, either newly diagnosed or reevaluated after treatment (tumor resection, transcatheter arterial chemoembolization, radiofrequency ablation, systemic

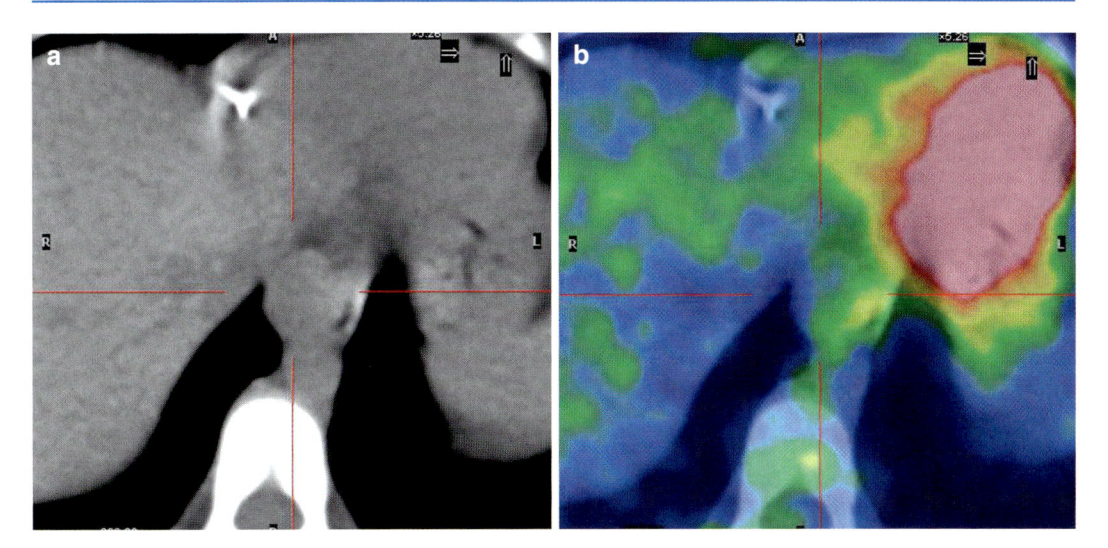

Fig. 10.3 An 8-year-old boy treated for hepatoblastoma. PET evaluation following increased alpha-fetoprotein levels. Axial CT (**a**) and CT/PET fusion (**b**) images show no FDG uptake in a small cardiac lesion seen on CT. The patient underwent surgery; the histological finding was hepatocarcinoma

chemotherapy), who underwent ^{18}F-FDG–PET/CT or conventional imaging modalities [29]. The detection rate for lung metastases by ^{18}F-FDG–PET/CT was lower than that obtained with CT, and for lesions below 1 cm, it diminished dramatically, probably because of the limited resolution. In the detection of lymph node lesions, by contrast, there were no differences between CT and ^{18}F-FDG–PET/CT. Moreover, ^{18}F-FDG–PET/CT was significantly superior to bone scan in patients with bone metastases, depicting all bone lesions [29].

Talbot et al. [30] compared ^{18}F-FDG with ^{18}F-fluorocholine in the detection and staging of HCC in patients with chronic liver disease and suspected liver nodules. FDG was shown to be significantly more sensitive, especially in the detection of well-differentiated tumors. Although ^{18}F-FDG was unable to demonstrate focal nodular hyperplasia, it was more sensitive than ^{18}F-fluorocholine for other malignancies. Consequently, the authors suggested performing PET/CT with both radiopharmaceuticals as the best option [30]. Another study proposed the use of FDG–PET/CT in the assessment of tumor response and tumor viability after interventional therapy (transcatheter arterial chemoembolization) but further investigations on the benefits of this application are warranted [31].

10.3 Undifferentiated Sarcoma of the Liver

Undifferentiated sarcoma of the liver is the third most frequently occurring hepatic malignancy of childhood. Unlike HB and HCC, in this rapidly growing tumor [2], α-FP levels are usually normal and thus are of no diagnostic relevance. On US but also on CT and MRI, USLs are generally large and solid in appearance. While FDG–PET has been suggested as a valuable method in the evaluation of USL patients during postoperative chemotherapy, it has yet to be confirmed in the literature (Figs. 10.4 and 10.5) [32]. The treatment of choice is chemotherapy followed by resection. Preferential sites of metastases are the lungs and bones [33].

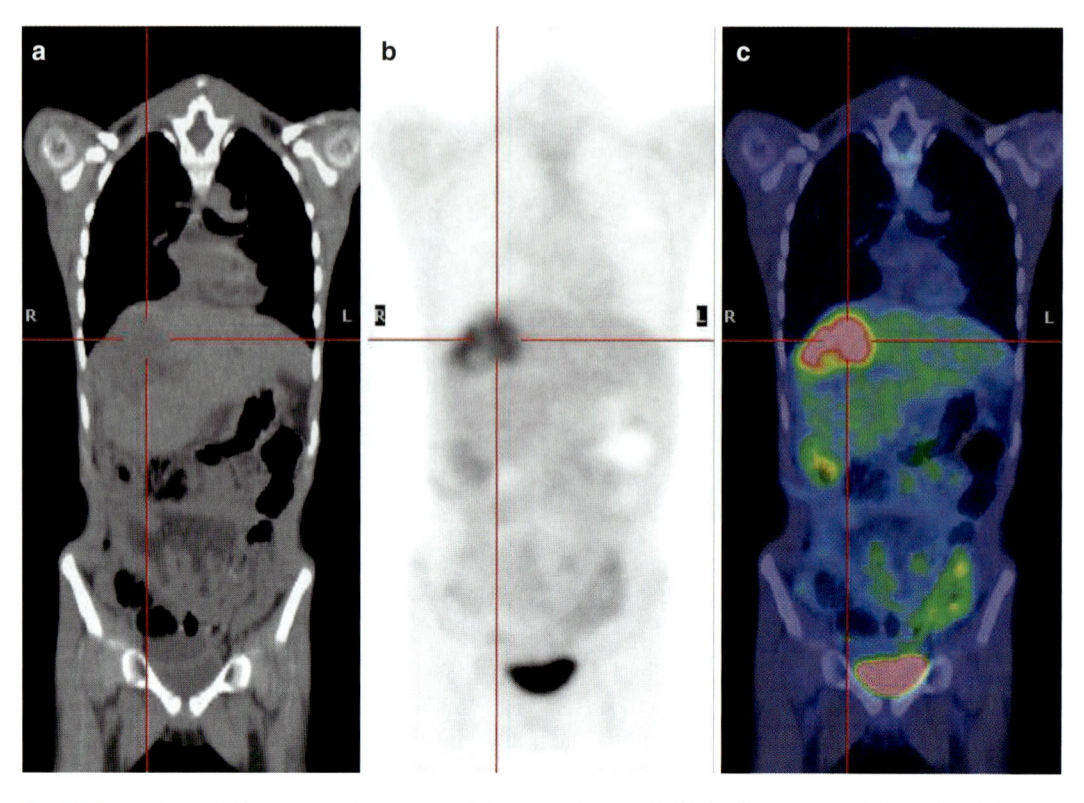

Fig. 10.4 An 8-year-old boy treated for sarcoma of the liver. Coronal CT (**a**), PET (**b**), and PET/CT fusion (**c**) images show a large FDG-avid lesion of the right hepatic lobe, corresponding to disease recurrence

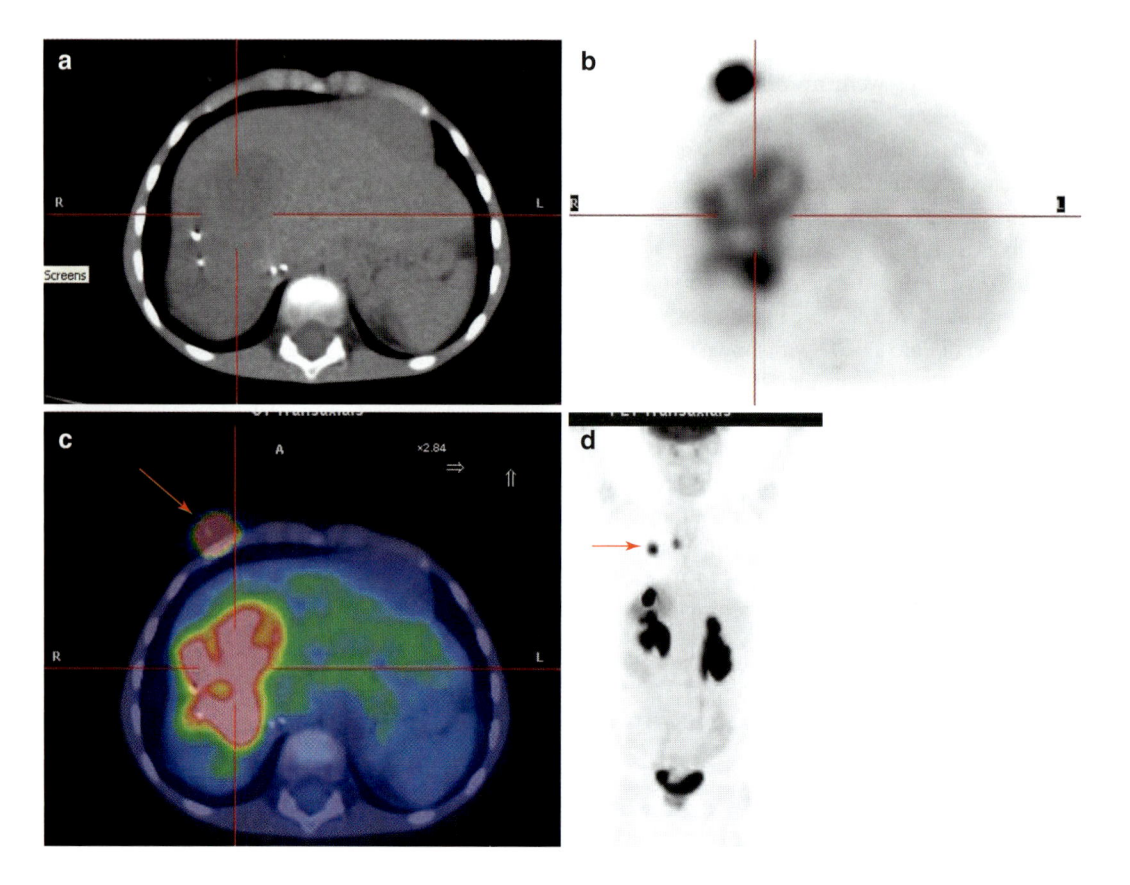

10.4 Carcinoid

Derived from neuroendocrine cells, carcinoid tumors spread throughout the body, especially to the liver (Fig. 10.6), and often produce functional peptide hormones. Approximately 56 % arise in the gastrointestinal tract followed by the lungs (30.1 %), pancreas (2.3 %), reproductive system (1.2 %), biliary tract (1.1 %), and head and neck (0.4 %). Primary hepatic carcinoid tumors (PHCT) are extremely rare [34]. Neither CT, nor MRI is advantageous in the imaging of neuroendocrine tumors (NETs), which are generally better detected by OctreoScan scintigraphy [35]. Recent data indicated that higher quality images obtained with a shorter acquisition protocol are possible with ^{68}Ga-DOTA-NOC PET/CT than with 111In-DTPA-octreotide [36]. ^{18}F-FDG–PET may be useful for identifying NETs characterized by rapid growth or aggressive behavior, with increased tumor uptake of the FDG tracer indicative of a worse prognosis. Although NETs with multiple tumor sites show broad-ranging heterogeneity in tracer uptake, FDG–PET may be able to detect unsuspected distant metastases, contributing to better staging of advanced disease [37].

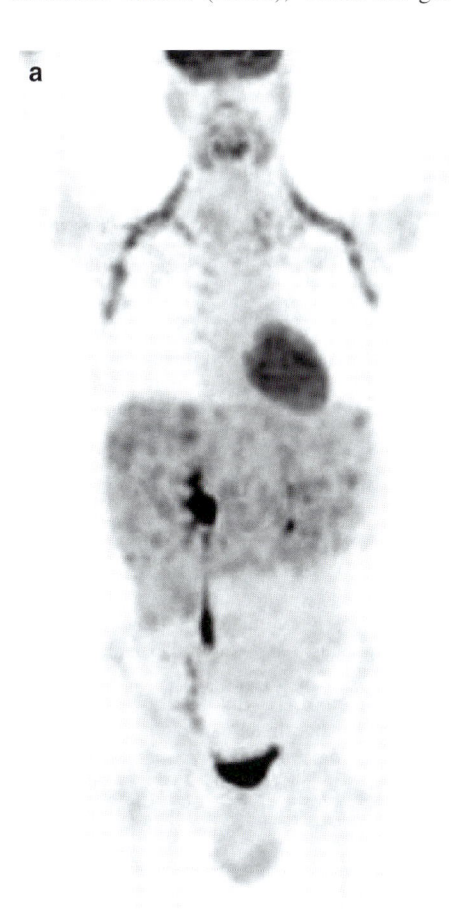

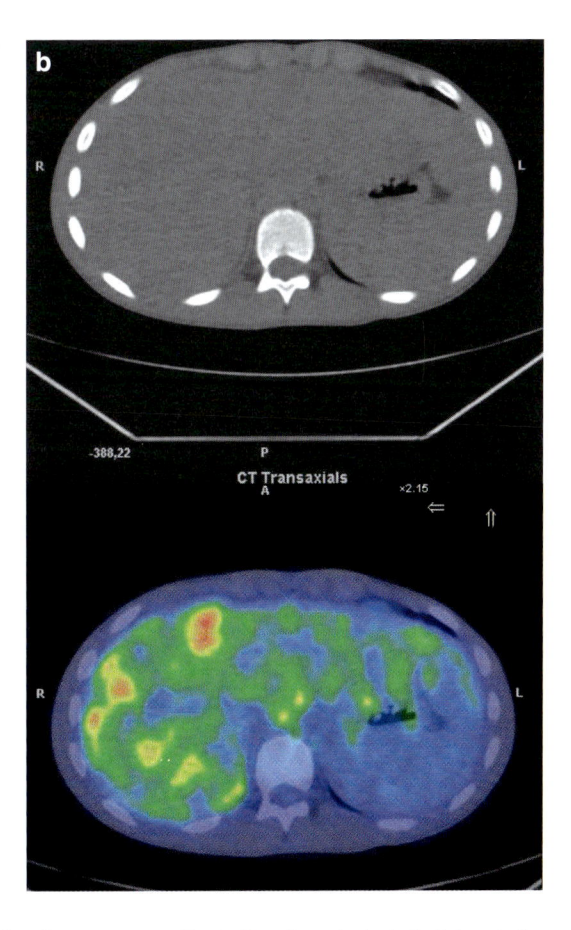

Fig. 10.6 A 7-year-old boy operated on for carcinoid of the terminal ileum. Maximal intensity projection (**a**) and axial and PET/CT fusion images (**b**) show multiple nonhomogeneous ^{18}F-FDG uptake in the right lobe of the liver, corresponding to hepatic metastasis. In (**a**), note the FDG uptake by brown fat in the laterocervical, supraclavicular, and axillary regions

---

Fig. 10.5 (**a–c**) Axial images of the same patient as in Fig. 10.4. The lesion involves almost the entire right lobe of the liver. (**d**) Maximal intensity projection shows two other areas of focal uptake, in the right lung and mediastinum (*red arrow*). On axial images, these areas correspond to tracer stasis in the catheter reservoir of the central venous line (*red arrow* in c)

References

1. Agarwala S (2012) Primary malignant liver tumors in children. Indian J Pediatr 79:793–800
2. Ammann RA, Plaschkes J, Leibundgut K et al (1999) Congenital hepatoblastoma: a distinct entity? Med Pediatr Oncol 32:466–468
3. Herzog CE, Andrassy RJ, Eftekhari F et al (2000) Childhood cancers: hepatoblastoma. Oncologist 5:445–453
4. Litten JB, Tomlinson GE (2008) Liver tumors in children. Oncologist 13:812–820
5. Das CJ, Dhingra S, Gupta AK et al (2009) Imaging of paediatric liver tumours with pathological correlation. Clin Radiol 64:1015–1025
6. Chung EM, Lattin GE Jr, Cube R et al (2011) From the archives of the AFIP: pediatric liver masses: radiologic-pathologic correlation. Part 2. Malignant tumors. Radiographics 31:483–507
7. Zsíros J, Maibach R, Shafford E et al (2010) Successful treatment of childhood high-risk hepatoblastoma with dose-intensive multiagent chemotherapy and surgery: final results of the SIOPEL-3HR study. J Clin Oncol 28:2584–2590
8. Avila LF, Luis AL, Hernandez F et al (2006) Liver transplantation for malignant tumours in children. Eur J Pediatr Surg 16:411–414
9. Perilongo G, Shafford E, Plaschkes J (2000) SIOPEL trials using preoperative chemotherapy in hepatoblastoma. Lancet Oncol 1:94–100
10. Moon SB, Shin HB, Seo JB et al (2011) Hepatoblastoma: 15-year experience and role of surgical treatment. J Korean Surg Soc 81:134–140
11. Abraham H, Dachman MD, Pakter RL et al (1987) Hepatoblastoma: radiologic-pathologic correlation in 50 cases. Radiology 164:15–19
12. King SJ, Babyn PS, Greenberg ML et al (1993) Value of CT in determining the resectability of hepatoblastoma before and after chemotherapy. AJR Am J Roentgenol 160:793–798
13. Miller JH, Greenspan BS (1985) Integrated imaging of hepatic tumors in childhood. Part I: Malignant lesions (primary and metastatic). Radiology 154:83–90
14. Figarola MS, McQuiston SA, Wilson F et al (2005) Recurrent hepatoblastoma with localization by PET-CT. Pediatr Radiol 35:1254–1258
15. Sironi S, Messa C, Cistaro A et al (2004) Recurrent hepatoblastoma in orthotopic transplanted liver: detection with FDG positron emission tomography. AJR Am J Roentgenol 182:1214–1216
16. Philip I, Shun A, McCowage G et al (2005) Positron emission tomography in recurrent hepatoblastoma. Pediatr Surg Int 21:341–345
17. Mody RJ, Pohlen JA, Malde S et al (2006) FDG PET for the study of primary hepatic malignancies in children. Pediatr Blood Cancer 47:51–55
18. Wong KK, Lan LC, Lin SC et al (2004) The use of positron emission tomography in detecting hepatoblastoma recurrence – a cautionary tale. J Pediatr Surg 39:1779–1781
19. Bertagna F, Orlando E, Bosio G et al (2011) Incremental diagnostic value of F-18 FDG PET/CT over MRI in a pediatric patient with suspected hepatoblastoma and histologic diagnosis of focal nodular hyperplasia. Clin Nucl Med 36:305–308
20. Warfel KA, Hull MT (2006) Hepatoblastoma: an ultrastructural and immunohistochemical study. Ultrastruct Pathol 16:451–461
21. Patel C, Kumar R (2007) Positron emission tomography and positron emission tomography – computerized tomography in pediatric patients. J Indian Assoc 12:120–124
22. Exelby PR, Filler RM, Grosfeld JL (1975) Liver tumors in children in the particular reference to hepatoblastoma and hepatocellular carcinoma: American Academy of Pediatrics Surgical Section Survey – 1974. J Pediatr Surg 10:329–337
23. Katzenstein HM, Krailo MD, Malogolowkin MH et al (2003) Fibrolamellar hepatocellular carcinoma in children and adolescents. Cancer 97:2006–2012
24. Donnelly LF, Bisset GS 3rd (1998) Pediatric hepatic imaging. Radiol Clin North Am 36:413–427
25. Finegold MJ, Egler RA, Goss JA et al (2008) Liver tumors: pediatric population. Liver Transpl 14:1545–1556
26. Ni YH, Chang MH, Hsu HY et al (1991) Hepatocellular carcinoma in childhood. Clinical manifestations and prognosis. Cancer 68:1737–1741
27. Czauderna P, Mackinlay G, Perilongo G et al (2002) Hepatocellular carcinoma in children: results of the first prospective study of the International Society of Pediatric Oncology Group. J Clin Oncol 20:2798–2804
28. Jha P, Chawla SC, Tavri S (2009) Pediatric liver tumors – a pictorial review. Eur Radiol 19:209–219
29. Lee JE, Jang JY, Jeong SW et al (2012) Diagnostic value for extrahepatic metastases of hepatocellular carcinoma in positron emission tomography/computed tomography scan. World J Gastroenterol 18:2979–2987
30. Talbot JN, Fartoux L, Balogova S et al (2010) Detection of hepatocellular carcinoma with PET/CT: a prospective comparison of 18F-fluorocholine and 18F-FDG in patients with cirrhosis or chronic liver disease. J Nucl Med 51:1699–1706
31. Dierckx R, Maes A, Peeters M et al (2009) FDG PET for monitoring response to local and locoregional therapy in HCC and liver metastases. Q J Nucl Med Mol Imaging 53:336–342
32. Lee MK, Kwon CG, Hwang KH et al (2009) F-18 FDG PET/CT findings in a case of undifferentiated embryonal sarcoma of the liver with lung and adrenal gland metastasis in a child. Clin Nucl Med 34:107–108
33. Ma L, Liu YP, Geng CZ et al (2008) Undifferentiated embryonal sarcoma of liver in an old female: case report

and review of the literature. World J Gastroenterol 14:7267–7270
34. Maggard MA, O'Connell JB, Ko CY (2004) Updated population-based review of carcinoid tumors. Ann Surg 240:117–122
35. Shi W, Johnston CF, Buchanan KD, Ferguson WR, Laird JD, Crothers JG, McIlrath EM (1998) Localization of neuroendocrine tumours with [111In] DTPA-octreotide scintigraphy (Octreoscan): a comparative study with CT and MR imaging. QJM 91:295–301
36. Krausz Y, Freedman N, Rubinstein R, Lavie E et al (2011) 68Ga-DOTA-NOC PET/CT imaging of neuroendocrine tumors: comparison with ^{111}In-DTPA-octreotide. Mol Imaging Biol 13:583–593
37. Pasquali C, Rubello D, Sperti C et al (1998) Neuroendocrine tumor image: can 18F-fluorodeoxyglucose positron emission tomography detect tumors with poor prognosis and aggressive behavior? World J Surg 22:588–592

Neuroendocrine Tumors

Egesta Lopci and Angelina Cistaro

11.1 Introduction

Neuroendocrine tumors (NETs) are rare neoplasms that arise from the diffuse endocrine system and spread throughout the different organs and tissues of the body. A common characteristic of this group of tumors is the ability of the neoplastic cells to produce, store, and release biogenic amines and hormones [1, 2]. Among children and young adults, NETs comprise a very small percentage of malignant tumors, with an overall incidence of 0.65 per million in Italy and 0.1–0.6 per million in the USA [3–5]. NETs generally include neuroblastoma, pheochromocytoma, paraganglioma, gastroenteropancreatic and lung carcinoids, medullary carcinoma, and islet cell tumors. Less commonly acknowledged NETs are Ewing's sarcoma, benign and malignant schwannomas, neurofibromas, and primary melanomas [3]. The majority of NETs occurring in the pediatric population are sporadic, but they are also seen within inherited syndromes, such as multiple endocrine neoplasia (MEN) type I and II, the Carney complex, neurofibromatosis 1 (NF-1), and von Hippel–Lindau (VHL) disease [3].

With the exception of more aggressive forms of these tumors, NET patients typically have a multiyear anamnesis of symptoms. The majority of these cases involve hormone-releasing tumors whose diagnosis is frequently delayed. In fact, up to 10 % of the newly diagnosed NETs in children and young adults have already metastasized to the liver, bone, etc. [3, 6, 7]. Instrumental imaging is therefore essential in the initial work-up of patients with suspected NETs and is associated with a high probability of true-positive findings [8].

In this chapter, the principal types of NETs seen in children and young adults are discussed. Tumors of particular relevance in the pediatric population, such as neuroblastoma, Ewing's sarcoma, and neurofibromatosis 1, are discussed separately in other chapters of this volume.

E. Lopci, MD
Nuclear Medicine Unit,
Humanitas Cancer Center, IRCCS Humanitas,
Via Manzoni 56, Rozzano (MI) 20089, Italy
e-mail: egesta.lopci@cancercenter.humanitas.it

A. Cistaro, MD (✉)
Department of Nuclear Medicine, Positron Emission Tomography Center IRMET S.p.A., Euromedic Inc., Via Onorato Vigliani 89, Turin 10100, Italy

Institute of Cognitive Sciences and Technologies, National Research Council, Rome, Italy
e-mail: a.cistaro@irmet.com

11.2 Pheochromocytomas and Paragangliomas

These two types of NETs have a common origin, as both derive from chromaffin cells. In pheochromocytomas, these are localized in the adrenal medulla, while in paragangliomas, they are found in the extra-adrenal sympathetic ganglia [1]. Only 10 % of all pheochromocytomas and paragangliomas are seen in children, and almost

80 % of these tumors secrete catecholamines, accounting for the abnormally increased serum or urinary levels of their metabolites and for symptoms such as headache, palpitations, and hypertension [1, 9]. Pheochromocytomas also occur as part of several syndromes, including MEN types IIA and IIB, VHL, and NF-1 [3].

Diagnosis is partially based on laboratory testing, i.e., 24-h urine sampling to detect the excretion of catecholamines, metanephrines, and other metabolites and serum levels of chromogranin A and metanephrines, and partially on morphological and functional imaging. CT and MRI are the initial investigations in clinically suspicious cases especially when looking for primary pheochromocytoma, which in 90 % of patients is found in the adrenal glands. Functional imaging, starting with ^{123}I-MIBG, ^{18}F-DOPA, ^{68}Ga-DOTA peptides, etc., is another important tool in the detection of NETs and in disease staging [1, 10].

In relapsing or advanced pheochromocytomas and paragangliomas, a positive MIBG scan is indicative of the need for additional systemic radiometabolic therapy with ^{131}I-MIBG [11, 12].

11.3 Gastroenteropancreatic (GEP) Carcinoid Tumors

The term "carcinoid" is a rather nonspecific definition applied to some NETs arising from the enterochromaffin or Kulchitsky cells, which are diffusely present in several human epithelia [1, 13]. The GEP tract is the most common site for primary carcinoid in children, with the appendix being the most frequent NET site, as 0.5 % of all post-appendicectomy specimens are carcinoids [6, 14]. According to their site of origin, GEP carcinoids are divided into foregut (stomach, first part of the duodenum, pancreas), midgut (second part of the duodenum, jejunum, ileum, appendix), and hindgut carcinoids (colon, rectum) tumors. In 50–70 % of the cases, large amounts of active hormone or bioamines are released, resulting in the so-called carcinoid syndrome [15]. Typically, these patients present with the carcinoid "triad" (flushing, diarrhea, and cardiac involvement), mostly related to the release of serotonin, tachykinins, and vasoactive peptides [16]. Since the hepatic "filter" tends to neutralize these molecules, the criteria for the onset of a carcinoid syndrome is either an extra-gastrointestinal origin of the primary NET or a GEP carcinoid that has already metastasized to the liver [16]. Other tumors of the GEP tract that are characterized by hormone release are pancreatic NETs (pNETs). They account for almost 30 % of pancreatic tumors in children and young adults [6], with gastrinomas and insulinomas as the more common types [1]. Gastrinomas are responsible for the Zollinger–Ellison syndrome, in which patients typically present with peptic ulcers, malabsorption, and diarrhea. Insulinomas, mostly seen in older children and adults, determines hypoglycemia and must therefore be included in the differential diagnosis along with hyperinsulinemic hypoglycemia and congenital hyperinsulinism [17]. Some pNETs occur in the setting of inherited syndromes, such as MEN and VHL disease, although in these cases, the majority of the tumors are nonfunctional [1].

Instrumental diagnosis in GEP-NET is a valuable adjuvant to clinical suspicion, but it is more useful in the detection of secondary lesions, i.e., in liver and bone, rather than primary tumors, which can be very limited in size or even disappear completely. Functional imaging with different PET radiopharmaceuticals and morphological imaging with MRI and contrast-enhanced CT complement each other and overcome many of the limitations of each technique alone at disease diagnosis and staging.

11.3.1 Liver Carcinoids

This site of neuroendocrine disease is rather controversial. In some series [6, 18], the liver is the second most common site of NET occurrence after the appendix. However, it is unclear whether these tumors are the primary lesion or a metastasis. Functional rather than morphological imaging can be of utmost utility because it offers the unique possibility to visualize the entire body and to detect, when present, a previously unknown primary.

11.3.2 Lung Carcinoids

In the pediatric population, pulmonary NET is the most common cause of primary lung neoplasia, accounting for up to 80 % of cases [18, 19]. The lesions typically present as round or oval masses close to the main bronchus or in the hilus and are thus frequently associated with wheezing, bronchospasm, and atelectasia [6]. Less common is a carcinoid syndrome, unless the tumor is particularly large or has already metastasized to the liver. While detection with morphological imaging is rather easy, the correct diagnosis is possible with functional modalities such as ^{18}F-DOPA PET, ^{68}Ga-DOTA peptides, and other PET and SPECT radiopharmaceuticals.

11.4 PET Imaging in Neuroendocrine Tumors

11.4.1 ^{18}F-Dihydroxyphenylalanine (^{18}F-DOPA)

Dihydroxyphenylalanine is an amino acid naturally present in the human body, as well as an intermediary in the metabolic pathway that leads to catecholamine synthesis (Fig. 11.1) [20]. When labeled with 18-fluoride (^{18}F-DOPA), it yields a positron-emitting compound that has been widely used in clinical practice since the early 1980s [21, 22] to image the basal ganglia [23].

In oncology, ^{18}F-DOPA is mostly employed in imaging tumors arising from neural crest cells and mimicking APUD (amine precursor uptake and decarboxylation) cells in their ability to accumulate and decarboxylate L-DOPA, as a precursor of dopamine [24]. Today, the main application of is in the study of NETs, both primitive and metastatic, including carcinoid (Fig. 11.2),

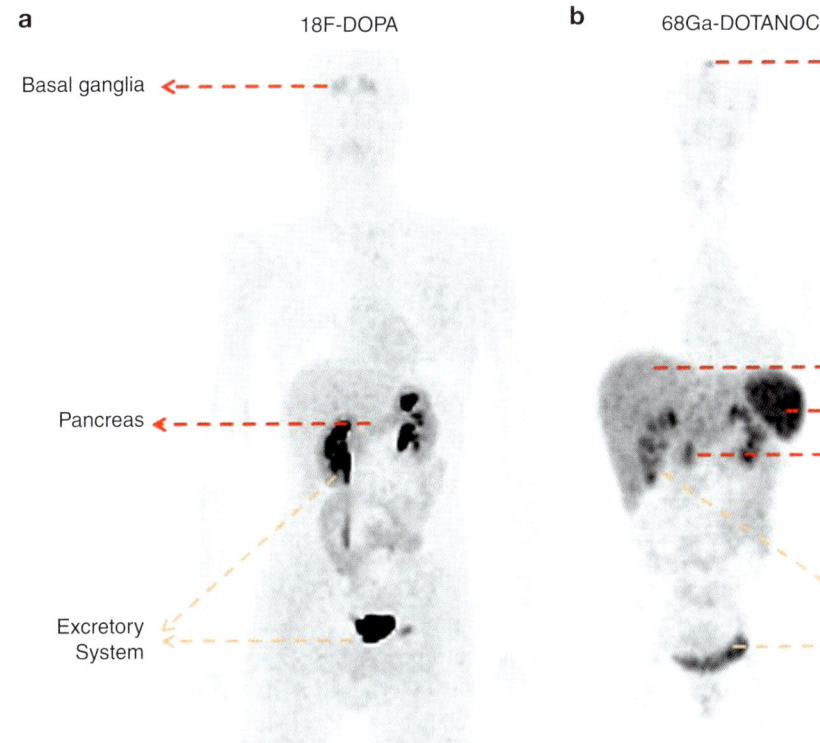

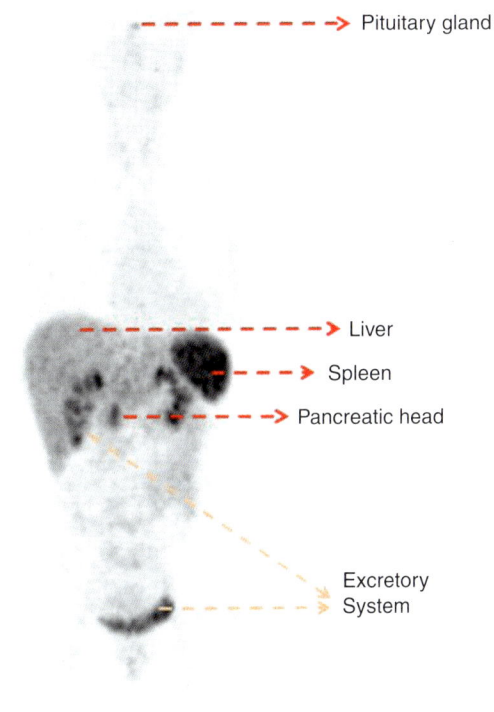

Fig. 11.1 (**a**, **b**) MIP (maximal intensity projection) images showing the physiological distribution of two different PET tracers, respectively, ^{18}F-DOPA and ^{68}Ga-DOTANOC. Along with the normal tissue activity marked by the *arrows*, ^{18}F-DOPA PET reveals tracer stasis in the gallbladder, which is in part masked by the activity of the renal cortex

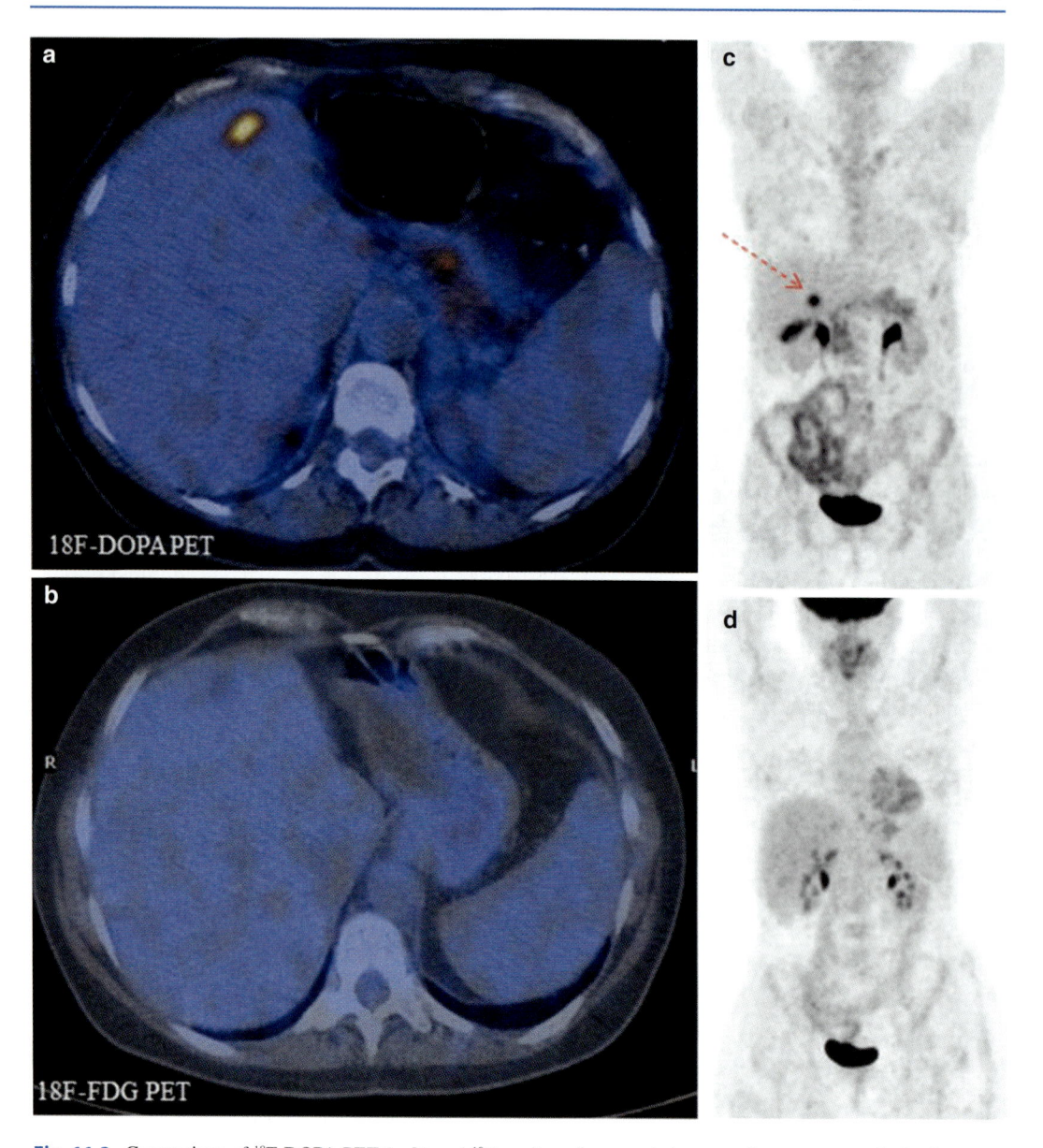

Fig. 11.2 Comparison of ^{18}F-DOPA PET (**a**, **b**) and ^{18}F-FDG–PET (**c**, **d**) scans in a patient with metastatic carcinoid. Note that the ^{18}F-DOPA-avid lesion visible in the liver (**c**, *arrow*) does not show tracer uptake in the corresponding ^{18}F-FDG–PET views (fused axial CT/PET and maximum intensity projections)

GEP tract tumors, glomus tumors, medullary carcinoma of the thyroid, paraganglioma, and pheochromocytoma [25–29].

The diagnostic accuracy of ^{18}F-DOPA PET in these types of neoplasia is very high, surpassing other methods of conventional and anatomic imaging such as CT and MRI, as well as functional scintigraphy with ^{123}I-MIBG and ^{111}In-octreoscan [30–32]

The group of neoplasms best evaluated with ^{18}F-DOPA PET imaging are NETs that excrete large amounts of catecholamines, especially pheochromocytomas (Fig. 11.3), in which imaging sensitivity reaches 90 %, specificity 100 %, and accuracy 92 % [31, 32]. However, while these results are well documented in adults, the experience in children is very limited, although the superimposable behavior of these tumors in

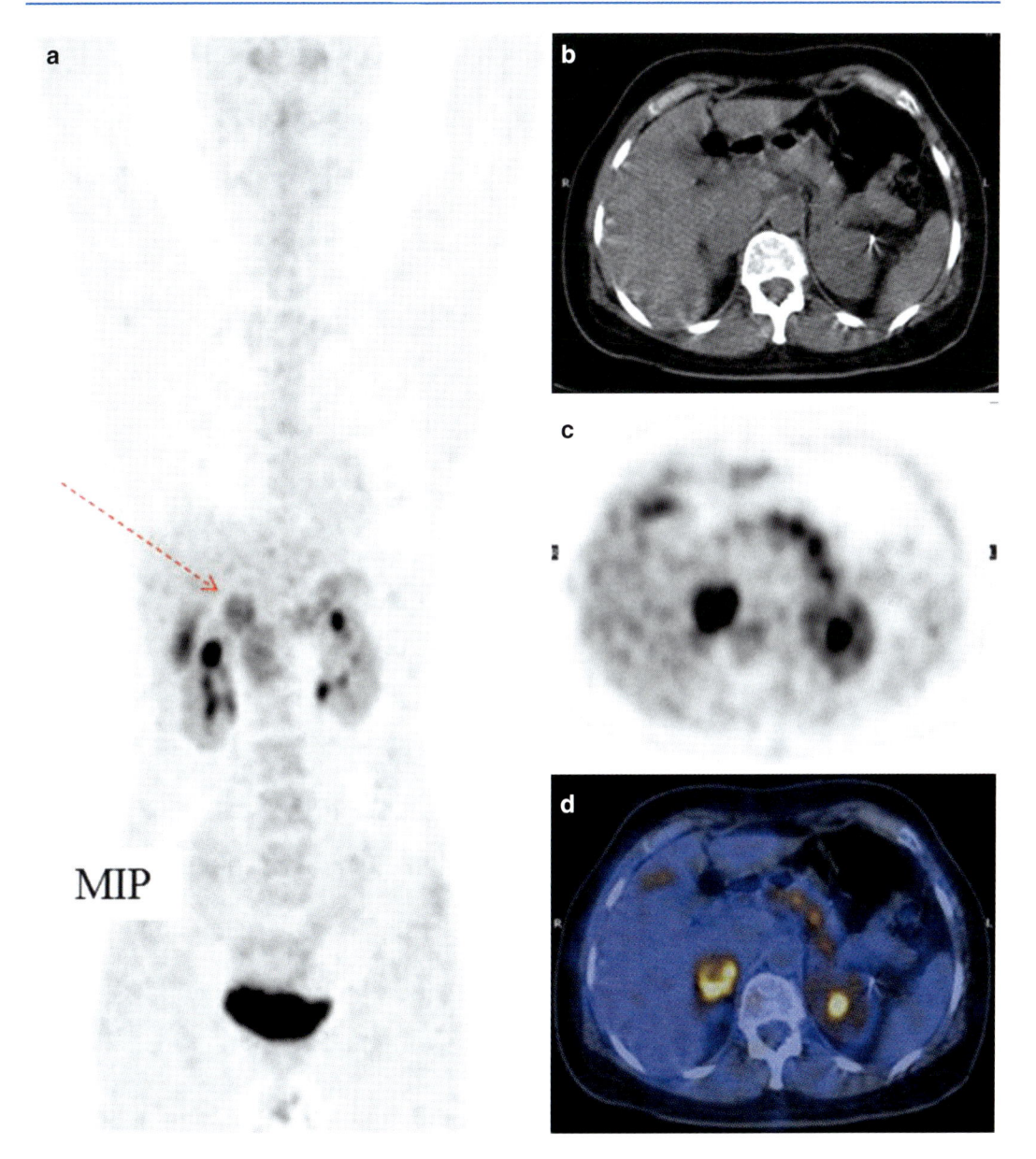

Fig. 11.3 Pheochromocytoma of the right adrenal gland (*arrow*), imaged by means of ^{18}F-DOPA CT/PET. (**a**) Maximum intensity projection, (**b**) CT, (**c**) PET, and (**d**) CT/PET fusion image

patients of all ages supports the applicability of the findings also in the pediatric population.

11.4.2 ^{68}Ga-DOTA Peptides

The group of radiopharmaceuticals comprising ^{68}Ga-DOTA peptides (-NOC, -TOC, -TATE) includes several octreotide analogues, all targeting somatostatin receptors with variable affinity (Fig. 11.1) [33, 34]. The rationale for using radiolabeled octreotide analogues in NET imaging is the finding that in >80 % of the cases, these tumors overexpress somatostatin receptors (SSTRs) [35, 36].

^{68}Ga-DOTA peptides were first investigated for clinical purposes in 2001 [37], immediately followed by the development of several promising PET tracers [38, 39] for use in the diagnosis of primary NETs and in tumor staging (Figs. 11.4 and 11.5) [34, 40, 41]. Compared to other

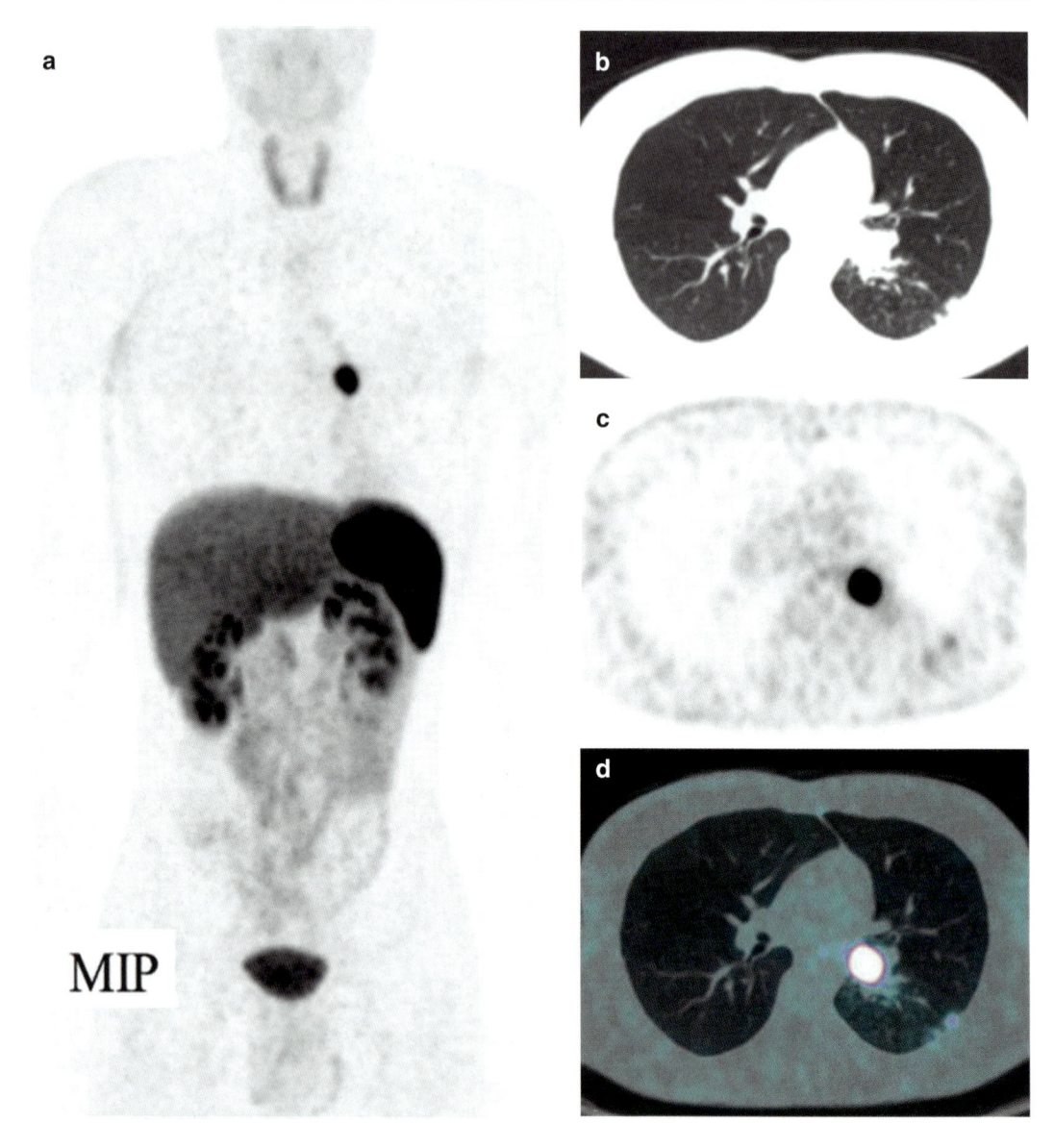

Fig. 11.4 A bronchial carcinoid at the level of the left lung hilus, imaged by means of ^{68}Ga-DOTANOC PET/CT. (**a**) Maximum intensity projection, (**b**) CT, (**c**) PET, and (**d**) CT/PET fusion image

imaging modalities, such as ^{111}In-octreotide or CT, the diagnostic accuracy of PET with ^{68}Ga-DOTA peptides is outstanding, with a 97–100 % sensitivity and 96–100 % specificity [42–46].

At staging or restaging, PET with ^{68}Ga-DOTA peptides has a demonstrated capability to detect unknown metastases in up to 21.4 % of cases, often leading to significant changes in the management of these patients [42, 44, 47]. The ^{68}Ga-DOTA-peptide uptake value (SUV_{max}) correlates with the clinical and pathological characteristics of NETs and is thus a significant prognostic factor in determining patient outcome [48].

Very recently, ^{68}Ga-DOTA peptides were investigated in a pediatric population [49]. Despite the fact that the series was very small and restricted to pheochromocytoma ($n=6$) and

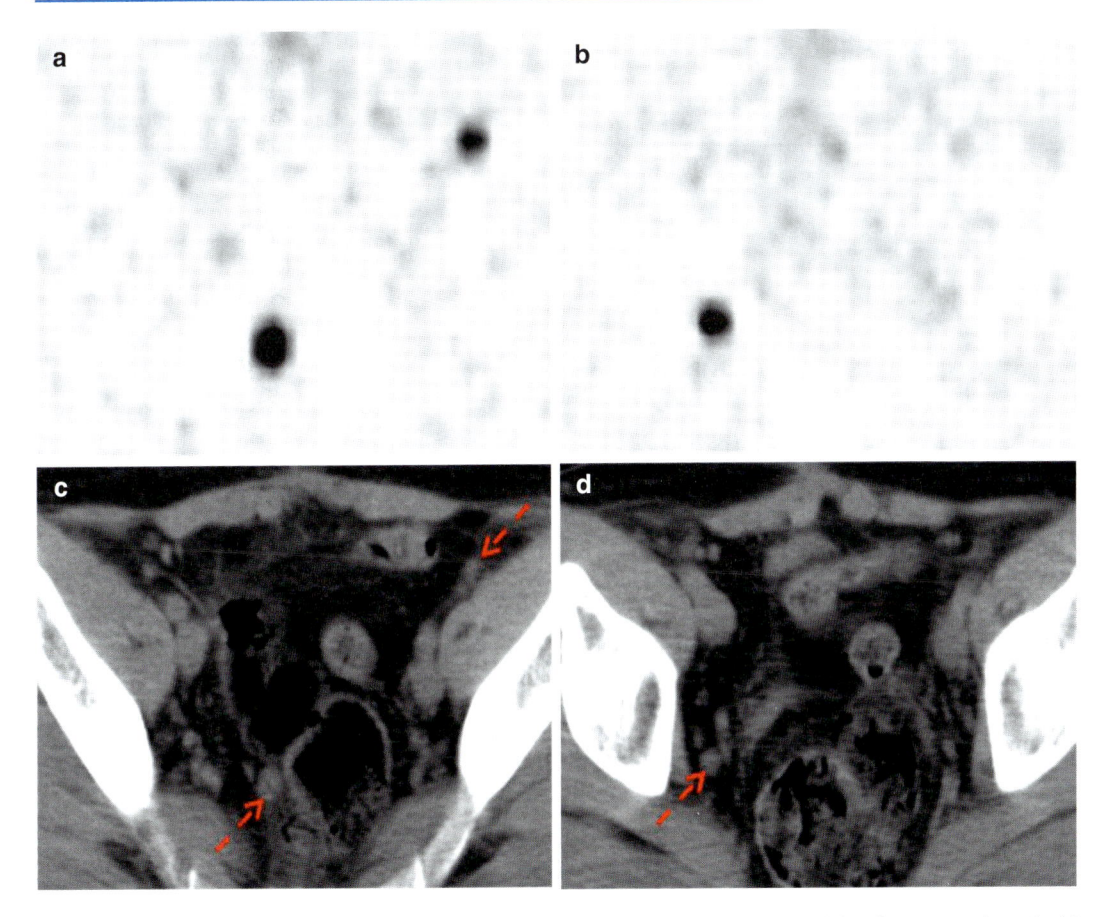

Fig. 11.5 ⁶⁸Ga-DOTANOC PET/CT shows multiple pelvic lymph node metastases deriving from a rectal carcinoid (*red arrows*). (**a, b**) Axial PET images of the pelvis; (**c, d**) corresponding low-dose CT

neuroblastoma ($n=5$) patients, the rather promising results open the way to other applications of radiolabeled DOTA peptides in children, in particular peptide receptor radionuclide therapy (PRRT).

11.4.3 ¹⁸F-Fluorodeoxyglucose

¹⁸F-fluorodeoxyglucose (¹⁸F-FDG) is the tracer of choice in the imaging of most malignant tumors, but its utility in NETs is limited because these tumors exhibit relatively low uptake of ¹⁸F-FDG as the vast majority of NETs are well differentiated [50, 51]. However, since tumor aggressiveness is positively associated with FDG-avidity, ¹⁸F-FDG–PET is advantageous in some types of NETs, i.e., those that are histologically dedifferentiated, or to confirm a poor prognosis [52].

11.4.4 Other PET Tracers

Although not yet used in the pediatric population, other PET tracers may be of clinical relevance when investigating NETs. For example, ¹¹C-hydroxytryptophan (¹¹C-HTP) [53] has been employed in the imaging of islet cell tumors, as has ¹⁸F-fluorodopamine (¹⁸F-FDA) [54] and ¹¹C-hydroxyephedrine (¹¹C-HED) [55], with very good diagnostic capability in pheochromocytoma and paraganglioma. However, one of the major limits of these radiopharmaceuticals is their relatively difficult synthesis and commercial availability, which limit their routine use in clinical practice.

References

1. Howman-Giles R, Shaw PJ, Uren RF, Chung DKV (2007) Neuroblastoma and other neuroendocrine tumors. Semin Nucl Med 37:286–302
2. Wick MR (2000) Neuroendocrine neoplasia. Current concepts. Am J Clin Pathol 113:331–335
3. Sarvida ME, O'Dorisio MS (2011) Neuroendocrine tumors in children: rare or not so rare. Endocrinol Metab Clin North Am 40:65–80
4. Crocetti E, Buiatti E, Amorosi A (1997) Epidemiology of carcinoid tumours in central Italy. Eur J Epidemiol 13:357–359
5. Yao JC, Hassan M, Phan A et al (2008) One hundred years after "carcinoid": epidemiology of and prognostic factors for neuroendocrine tumors in 35,825 cases in the United States. J Clin Oncol 26:3063–3072
6. Khanna G, O'Dorisio SM, Menda Y et al (2008) Gastroenteropancreatic neuroendocrine tumors in children and young adults. Pediatr Radiol 38:251–259
7. Spunt SL, Pratt CB, Rao BN et al (2000) Childhood carcinoid tumors: the St Jude Children's Research Hospital experience. J Pediatr Surg 35:1282–1286
8. Ambrosini V, Campana D, Nanni C et al (2012) Is (68)Ga-DOTA-NOC PET/CT indicated in patients with clinical, biochemical or radiological suspicion of neuroendocrine tumour? Eur J Nucl Med Mol Imaging 39(8):1278–1283
9. Kaltsas GA, Besser GM, Grossman AB (2004) The diagnosis and medical management of advanced neuroendocrine tumors. Endocr Rev 25:458–511
10. Rufini V, Calcagni ML, Baum RP (2006) Imaging of neuroendocrine tumors. Semin Nucl Med 36:228–247
11. Bombardieri E, Giammarile F, Aktolun C et al (2010) 131I/123I-metaiodobenzylguanidine (mIBG) scintigraphy: procedure guidelines for tumour imaging. Eur J Nucl Med Mol Imaging 37(12):2436–2446
12. Giammarile F, Chiti A, Lassman M et al (2008) EANM procedure guidelines for 131I-metaiodobenzylguanidine (131I-mIBG) therapy. Eur J Nucl Med Mol Imaging 35(5):1039–1047
13. Kaplan LM (1998) Endocrine tumors of the gastrointestinal tract and pancreas. In: Isselbacher KJ, Braunwald E, Wilson JD, Martin JB, Fauci AS, Kasper DL (eds) Harrison's principles of internal medicine, 14th edn. McGraw-Hill, New York, pp 584–592
14. Pappo AS, Furman WL (2006) Management of infrequent cancers of childhood. In: Pizzo PA, Poplack DG (eds) Principles and practice of pediatric oncology, 5th edn. Lippincott Williams and Wilkins, Philadelphia, pp 1172–1201
15. Prasad V, Fetscher S, Baum RP (2007) Changing role of somatostatin receptor targeted drugs in NET: nuclear Medicine' view. J Pharm Pharm Sci 10:321s–337s
16. Vinik AI, Renar IP (1995) Neuroendocrine tumors of carcinoid variety. In: De Grool L (ed) Endocrinology, 3rd edn. WB Saunders, Philadelphia, pp 2803–2814
17. Sperling MA (2004) Hypoglycemia. In: Behrman RE, Kliegman RM, Jenson HB (eds) Nelson textbook of pediatrics. Saunders, Philadelphia, pp 505–518
18. Broaddus RR, Herzog CE, Hicks MJ (2003) Neuroendocrine tumors (carcinoid and neuroendocrine carcinoma) presenting at extra-appendiceal sites in childhood and adolescence. Arch Pathol Lab Med 127:1200–1203
19. Hancock BJ, Di Lorenzo M, Youssef S et al (1993) Childhood primary pulmonary neoplasms. J Pediatr Surg 28:1133–1136
20. Jager PL, Chirakal R, Marriot CJ et al (2008) 6-L-18F-fluorodihydroxyphenylalanine PET in neuroendocrine tumors: basic aspects and emerging clinical applications. J Nucl Med 49:573–586
21. Garnett ES, Firnau G, Nahmias C (1983) Dopamine visualized in the basal ganglia of living man. Nature 305:137–138
22. Firnau G, Chiakal R, Garnett ES (1984) Aromatic radiofluorination with 18F fluorine gas: 6-[18F]fluoro-L-dopa. J Nucl Med 25:1228–1233
23. Whal L, Nahmias C (1997) Modeling of fluorine-18-6-fluoro-L-Dopa in humans. J Nucl Med 37(3):432–437
24. Pearce AG (1969) The cytochemistry and ultrastructure of polypeptide hormone-producing cells of the APUD series and the embryologic, physiologic and pathological implications of the concept. J Histochem Cytochem 17:303–313
25. Hoegerle S, Altehoefer C, Ghanem N et al (2001) Whole body 18F-DOPA PET for detection of gastrointestinal carcinoid tumors. Radiology 220:373–380
26. Hoegerle S, Nitzsche E, Altehoefer C et al (2002) Pheochromocytomas: detection with 18F DOPA whole body PET– initial results. Radiology 222(2):507–512
27. Hoegerle S, Ghanem N, Altehoefer C et al (2003) 18F-DOPA positron emission tomography for the detection of glomus tumours. Eur J Nucl Med Mol Imaging 30(5):689–694
28. Gourgiotis L, Sarlis NJ, Reynolds JC et al (2003) Localization of medullary thyroid carcinoma metastasis in a multiple endocrine neoplasia type 2a patient by 6-[18F]-fluorodopamine positron emission tomography. J Clin Endocrinol Metab 88(2):637–641
29. Jacob T, Grahek D, Younsi N et al (2003) Positron emission tomography with [18F]FDOPA and [18F]FDG in the imaging of small cell lung carcinoma: preliminary results. Eur J Nucl Med Mol Imaging 30:1266–1269
30. Becherer A, Szabó M, Karanikas G et al (2004) Imaging of advanced neuroendocrine tumors with (18)F-FDOPA PET. J Nucl Med 45(7):1161–1167
31. Imani F, Agopian VG, Auerbach MS et al (2009) 18F-FDOPA PET and PET/CT accurately localize pheochromocytomas. J Nucl Med 50(4):513–519

32. Fiebrich HB, Brouwers AH, Kerstens MN et al (2009) 6-[F-18]Fluoro-L-dihydroxyphenylalanine positron emission tomography is superior to conventional imaging with (123)I-metaiodobenzylguanidine scintigraphy, computer tomography, and magnetic resonance imaging in localizing tumors causing catecholamine excess. J Clin Endocrinol Metab 94(10):3922–3930
33. Antunes P, Ginj M, Zhang H et al (2007) Are radiogallium-labelled DOTA-conjugated somatostatin analogues superior to those labeled with other radiometals? Eur J Nucl Med Mol Imaging 34:982–993
34. Prasad V, Baum RP (2010) Biodistribution of the Ga-68 labeled somatostatin analogue DOTA-NOC in patients with neuroendocrine tumors: characterization of uptake in normal organs and tumor lesions. Q J Nucl Med Mol Imaging 54(1):61–67
35. Papotti M, Kuma U, Volante M, Pecchiono C, Patel YC (2001) Immunohistochemical detection of somatostatin receptor types 1–5 in medullary carcinoma of the thyroid. Clin Endocrinol 54:641–649
36. Papotti M, Bongiovanni M, Volante M, Allia E, Landolfi S, Helboe L et al (2002) Expression of somatostatin receptor types 1–5 in 81 cases of gastrointestinal and pancreatic endocrine tumors. A correlative immunohistochemical and reverse-transcriptase polymerase chain reaction analysis. Virchows Arch 440(5):461–475
37. Hofmann M et al (2001) Biokinetics and imaging with the somatostatin receptor PET radioligand 68Ga-DOTATOC: preliminary data. Eur J Nucl Med 28:1751–1757
38. Ginj M, Chen J, Walter MA, Eltschinger V, Reubi JC, Maecke HR (2005) Preclinical evaluation of new and highly potent analogues of octreotide for predictive imaging and targeted radiotherapy. Clin Cancer Res 11(3):1136–1145
39. Maecke HR, Hofmann M, Haberkorn U (2005) 68Ga-labeled peptides in tumor imaging. J Nucl Med 46:172S–178S
40. Baum RP et al (2005) Receptor PET/CT imaging of neuroendocrine tumors using the Ga-68 labelled, high affinity somatostatin analogue DOTA-1-NaI3-octreotide (DOTA-NOC): clinical results in 327 patients. Eur J Nucl Med Mol Imaging 32:109s
41. Wild D, Mäcke HR, Waser B, Reubi JC, Ginj M, Rasch H et al (2005) 68Ga-DOTANOC: a first compound for PET imaging with high affinity for somatostatin receptor subtypes 2 and 5. Eur J Nucl Med Mol Imaging 32(6):724
42. Gabriel M et al (2007) 68Ga-DOTA-Tyr3-octreotie PET in neuroendocrine tumours: comparison with somatostatin receptor scintigraphy and CT. J Nucl Med 48:508–518
43. Putzer D, Gabriel M, Henninger B, Kendler D, Uprimny C, Dobrozemsky G et al (2009) Bone metastasis in patients with neuroendocrine tumor: [68Ga] DOTA-Tyr3-octreotide PET in comparison to CT and bone scintigraphy. J Nucl Med 50:1214–1221
44. Ambrosini V, Tomassetti P, Franchi R, Fanti S (2010) Imaging of NETs with PET radiopharmaceuticals. Q J Nucl Med Mol Imaging 54(1):16–23
45. Buchmann I, Henze M, Engelbrecht S et al (2007) Comparison of 68GA-DOTATOC PET and 111In-DTPAOC (Octreoscan) SPECT in patients with neuroendocrine tumours. Eur J Nucl Med Mol Imaging 34:1617–1626
46. Haug A, Auernhammer CJ, Wängler B, Tling R, Schmidt G, Göke B et al (2009) Intraindividual comparison of [68Ga]DOTA-TATE and [18F]DOPA PET in patients with well-differentiated metastatic neuroendocrine tumours. Eur J Nucl Med Mol Imaging 36:765–770
47. Prasad V, Ambrosini V, Hommann M, Hoersch D, Fanti S, Baum RP (2010) Detection of unknown primary neuroendocrine tumours (CUP-NET) using (68)Ga-DOTA-NOC receptor PET/CT. Eur J Nucl Med Mol Imaging 37:67–77
48. Campana D, Ambrosini V, Pezzilli R, Fanti S, Labata AMM, Santini D et al (2010) Standardized uptake values of 68Ga-DOTANOC PET: a promising prognostic tool in neuroendocrine tumors. J Nucl Med 51:353–359
49. Kroiss A, Putzer D, Uprimny C et al (2011) Functional imaging in phaeochromocytoma and neuroblastoma with 68Ga-DOTA-Tyr3-octreotide positron emission tomography and 123I-metaiodobenzylguanidine. Eur J Nucl Med Mol Imaging 38:865–873
50. Adams S, Baum R, Rink T et al (1998) Limited value of fluorine-18 fluorodeoxyglucose positron emission tomography for the imaging of neuroendocrine tumours. Eur J Nucl Med 25(1):79–83
51. Bombardieri E, Maccauro M, De Deckere E et al (2001) Nuclear medicine imaging of neuroendocrine tumours. Ann Oncol 12(Suppl 2):S51–S61
52. Binderup T, Knigge U, Loft A et al (2010) 18F-fluorodeoxyglucose positron emission tomography predicts survival of patients with neuroendocrine tumors. Clin Cancer Res 16(3):978–985
53. Koopmans KP, Neels OC, Kema IP et al (2008) Improved staging of patients with carcinoid and islet cell tumors with [18F]dihydroxy-phenyl-alanine and [11C]5-hydroxy-tryptophan positron emission tomography. J Clin Oncol 26:1489–1495
54. Ilias I, Yu J, Carresquillo JA et al (2003) Superiority of 6-[18F]-fluorodopamine positron emission tomography versus [131I]-metaiodobenzylguanidine scintigraphy in the localization of metastatic pheochromocytoma. J Clin Endocrinol Metab 88: 4083–4087
55. Shulkin BL, Wieland DM, Baro ME et al (1996) PET hydroxyephedrine imaging of neuroblastoma. J Nucl Med 37(1):16–21

Neuroblastoma

12

Egesta Lopci, Umberto Ficola, and Angelina Cistaro

12.1 Introduction

Neuroblastoma (NB) is a malignant neoplasm that originates from neuroectodermal cells of the neural crest. During embryonic life, these cells migrate, eventually giving rise to the sympathetic ganglia and adrenal medulla [1]. In 1864, the German physician Rudolf Virchow was the first to define an abdominal tumor in a child as a "glioma," but only in 1910 did James Homer-Wright realize that the tumor originated from primitive neural cells and therefore referred to it as a "neuroblastoma" [2, 3]. Homer-Wright also noticed the characteristic cellular roundish accumulations visible in samples of bone marrow, which were then called Homer-Wright "pseudorosettes" [3].

NB is the third most frequent pediatric cancer (7–10 % of all neoplasias) after leukemia and tumors of the central nervous system but the most frequent solid tumor in children younger than 5 years [4]. The mean age at diagnosis is around 2 years, with 90 % of the cases diagnosed in children under the age of 6 years; it is rare in adolescents and in adults [5]. In 40 % of the cases, the NB is localized at the level of the adrenal glands, although it can develop anywhere in the sympathetic nervous system: neck (1 %), chest (19 %), elsewhere in the abdomen (30 %), or in the pelvis (1 %) [6, 7].

The degree of malignancy of the tumor is determined by the proportion of cellular and extracellular maturation. The most aggressive and undifferentiated forms of NB occur in young children (average age: 2 years), while the more mature forms, represented by ganglioneuroma, are usually seen in older children [8].

Over the past two decades, there has been considerable progress in understanding the biology of NB and in identifying the chromosomal alterations of NB cells that correlate with prognosis. Amplification of the *MYCN* oncogene was the first molecular NB-specific marker to be identified as a predictor of poor prognosis regardless of the child's age or disease stage. However, MYCN amplification occurs only in 20 % of the cases; hence, additional molecular markers allowing a more exhaustive prognostic stratification are needed [9, 10]. Chromosomal alterations such as 1p and 11q deletions, trisomy, or polysomy also correlate with a poor prognosis [11–13].

Usually, the presenting symptoms reflect disease location and extent. In some cases, NB presents as disseminated disease, without any

E. Lopci, MD
Nuclear Medicine Unit, Humanitas Cancer Center,
IRCCS Humanitas, Via Manzoni 56,
Rozzano (MI) 20089, Italy
e-mail: egesta.lopci@cancercenter.humanitas.it

U. Ficola, MD
Nuclear Medicine Unit, La Maddalena Hospital,
Via San Lorenzo Colli 312, Palermo 90146, Italy
e-mail: ficola@lamaddalena.it

A. Cistaro, MD (✉)
Department of Nuclear Medicine, Positron Emission Tomography Center IRMET S.p.A., Euromedic Inc.,
Via Onorato Vigliani 89, Turin 10100, Italy

Institute of Cognitive Sciences and Technologies,
National Research Council, Rome, Italy
e-mail: a.cistaro@irmet.com

clinical symptoms. Indeed, in 50–60 % of the newly diagnosed patients, the disease is already metastatic [6]. The most common sites of metastases are the bone and bone marrow, often in combination with symptoms related to tumor dissemination such as fever, anorexia, pallor, bone pain, and proptosis [7]. Approximately 30 % of patients have a positive history of pain, whether due to abdominal distension or bone metastases, while 11 % present with problems of weight gain or even weight loss [14]. Other common presenting symptoms are neurological deficits, such as intraspinal tumor growth [14], Horner's syndrome, hypertension, or Kinsbourne syndrome (opsoclonus-myoclonus-ataxia) [6, 15]. In children with advanced disease (stage 4S), there may be skin nodules, called "blueberry spots," or periorbital bruising due to NB metastases. Over 90 % of NB patients have high levels of catecholamines in the serum and urine [15]. Therefore a 24-h urine collection is an important test, both for diagnostic and follow-up purposes [6].

The clinical course is more favorable in children less than 1 year of age and/or with localized disease, while in adolescents and adults relapse tends to be later and is associated with a poor prognosis.

Patients with stage 1 or stage 2 have an excellent prognosis, with 5-year disease-free survival (DFS) rates of 85–90 %, while those with stage 3, stage 4s, and stage 4 have a poor prognosis, with DFS rates of 40–60, 60–70, and 15–25 %, respectively [16–18]. Relapse occurs mostly in the first 2 years after surgery, in the localized forms of the disease, or, in case of metastatic forms, after the end of treatment. In the first postoperative year, attention to symptoms and physical examination are the cornerstones of follow-up, which should also include a complete blood count, urinary catecholamines, and an instrumental examination.

The current standard for staging and restaging NB is metaiodobenzylguanidine (MIBG) scintigraphy [19]. MIBG is an analogue of norepinephrine that is captured by catecholamine-secreting tumors (both primary and metastatic) [6]. For scintigraphy purposes, it is labeled with $^{123}I/^{131}I$ ($^{123}I/^{131}I$-MIBG). In 70–80 % of NB patients, MIBG positivity has a high sensitivity (88 %) and specificity (99 %) in identifying the presence of the disease [20]. Moreover, the method has also been successfully applied in monitoring the response to treatment and in determining the utility of radiometabolic treatment with ^{131}I-MIBG (Figs. 12.1 and 12.2) [52]. However, NB also shows a wide-ranging variability in tracer uptake, which lead to false-negative results in 10 % of the patients. The main reasons for this variability likely include (a) modifications of active transport and tracer entrapment in tumor cells [53, 54], (b) increased levels of catecholamine metabolites [55], (c) the frequent prevalence of necrotic tissue in the primary tumor, (d) pharmacological interferences [20, 55], and (e) the dose-dependent sensitivity of ^{123}I-MIBG [56]. Furthermore, ^{123}I-MIBG scintigraphy is carried out using a gamma camera, with its obvious limits of resolution. It is also a lengthy examination and thus not patient friendly. All of these limits have stimulated a search for other radiopharmaceuticals, specifically, PET tracers.

12 Neuroblastoma

Fig. 12.1 (**a**, **b**) Whole-body ^{123}I-MIBG scan of a patient with stage IV neuroblastoma. The scan was performed before treatment was started

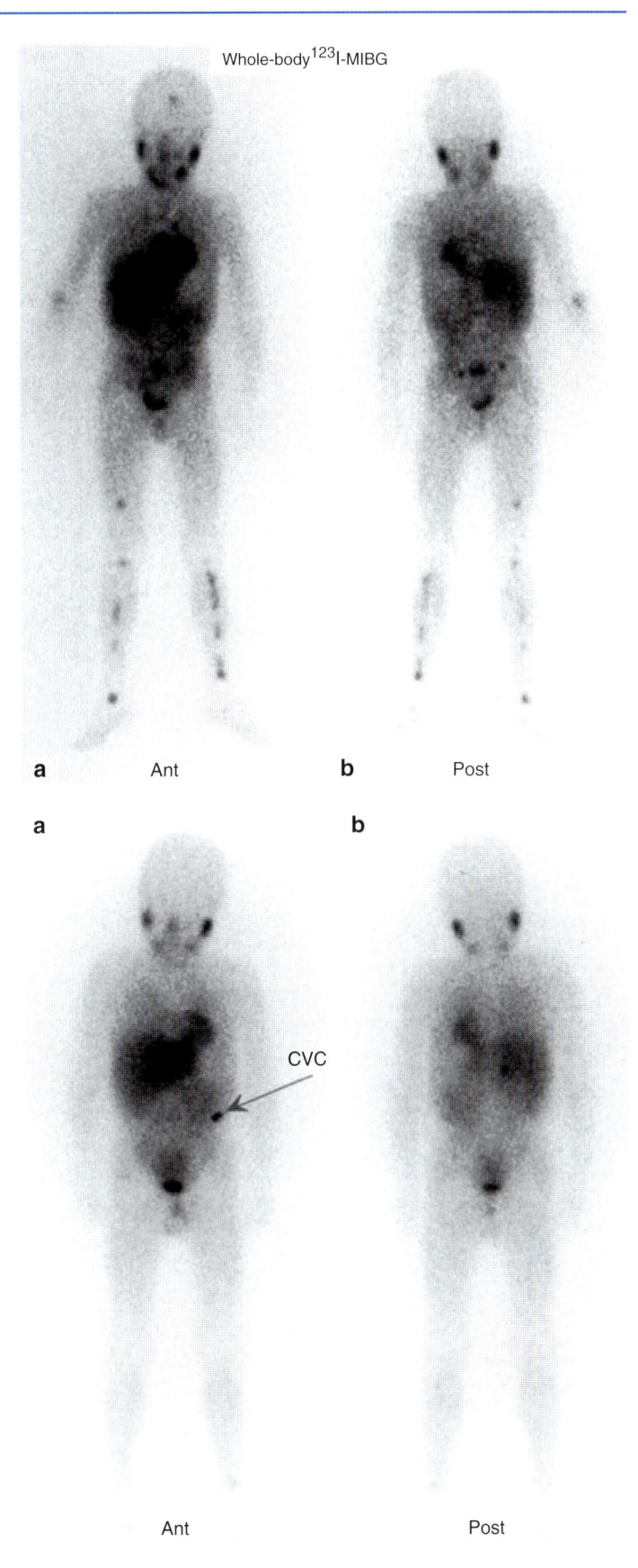

Fig. 12.2 The same patient as in Fig. 12.1. (**a**, **b**) This second whole-body scan was performed to monitor the response to induction therapy. The patient obtained a complete response (CR). Note the residual tracer stasis in the central venous catheter (*CVC*) reservoir (*arrow* in **a**)

12.2 PET Imaging in Neuroblastoma

12.2.1 Fluorodeoxyglucose

The principal PET tracer in oncology is undoubtedly ^{18}F-FDG, and its role in NB has been accordingly investigated [21–27]. Its most frequent use has thus far been in patients with a negative or inconclusive ^{123}I-MIBG scan (Fig. 12.3). In this setting, the superior performance of ^{18}F-FDG–PET has proven, based on a sensitivity and specificity of 78 and 92 %, respectively, whereas for ^{123}I-MIBG scintigraphy, the corresponding values are 50 and 75 % [24].

^{18}F-FDG–PET has also been suggested as a complementary rather than a substitute exam for MIBG scintigraphy in NB staging and treatment monitoring [21–23]. Its diagnostic use to evaluate the response to therapy, especially in patients with high-risk, advanced stage disease, has been assessed [27]. The FDG-avidity of NB tumors increases with their aggressiveness and in those with an unfavorable histology, such that NB detection with ^{18}F-FDG–PET is feasible and may even be superior to MIBG scintigraphy [24]. Further advantages of ^{18}F-FDG–PET are its high resolution, short scanning period, and patient-friendliness. The principal limitations of ^{18}F-FDG as a tracer for NB imaging are its overall low accuracy in the detection of disease in the bone and bone marrow, which are common sites of distant metastasis, the difficult visualization of disease occurring in the skull because of the intense physiological uptake of ^{18}F-FDG in normal brain, and the reduced capability of ^{18}F-FDG–PET to properly assess the response to therapy (Fig. 12.4) [25, 26].

Recently, new indications for this imaging method have been investigated, mainly based on the prognostic role of the FDG-avidity of tumors in patients with high-risk NB under consideration for ^{131}I-MIBG therapy [27]. However, in that study, ^{123}I-MIBG was shown to be superior in the detection of disease extent (Fig. 12.5). Both the SUV_{max} and the FDG-avidity of bone and bone marrow metastases were identified as adverse prognostic factors (Figs. 12.6, 12.7, 12.8, 12.9, 12.10, and 12.11).

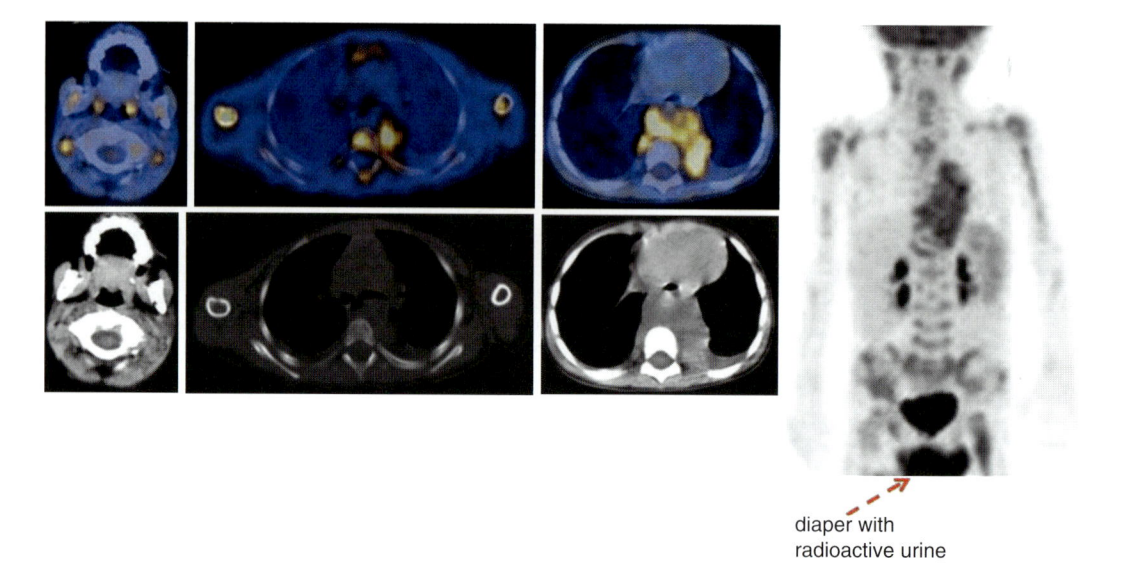

Fig. 12.3 ^{18}F-FDG–PET/CT staging in a patient with stage IV neuroblastoma. Note the large tumor in the chest, associated with massive bone marrow and multiple lymph node involvement

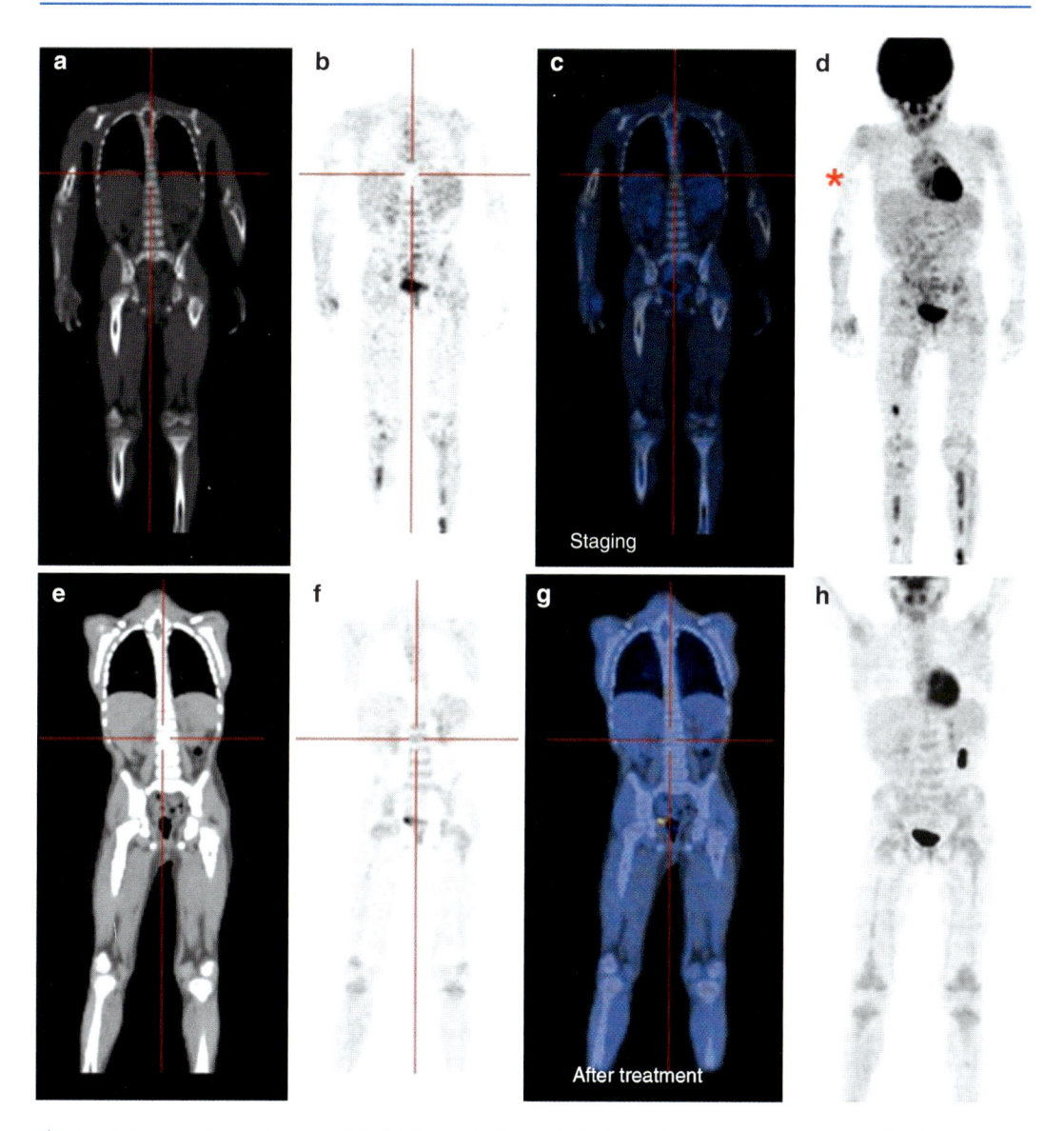

Fig. 12.4 Same patient as in Figs. 12.1, 12.2, and 12.5c, d. (**a–d**) ¹⁸F-FDG–PET/CT staging documents almost all disease sites, except the frontal lesion, which is masked by the intense physiological uptake of tracer in the brain. The *red asterisk*, seen on the MIP image, points to a technical artifact derived from movement during image acquisition. (**e–h**) Corresponding coronal and MIP views obtained with ¹⁸F-FDG–PET after the end of treatment. All previous disease sites now show normal uptake

118 E. Lopci et al.

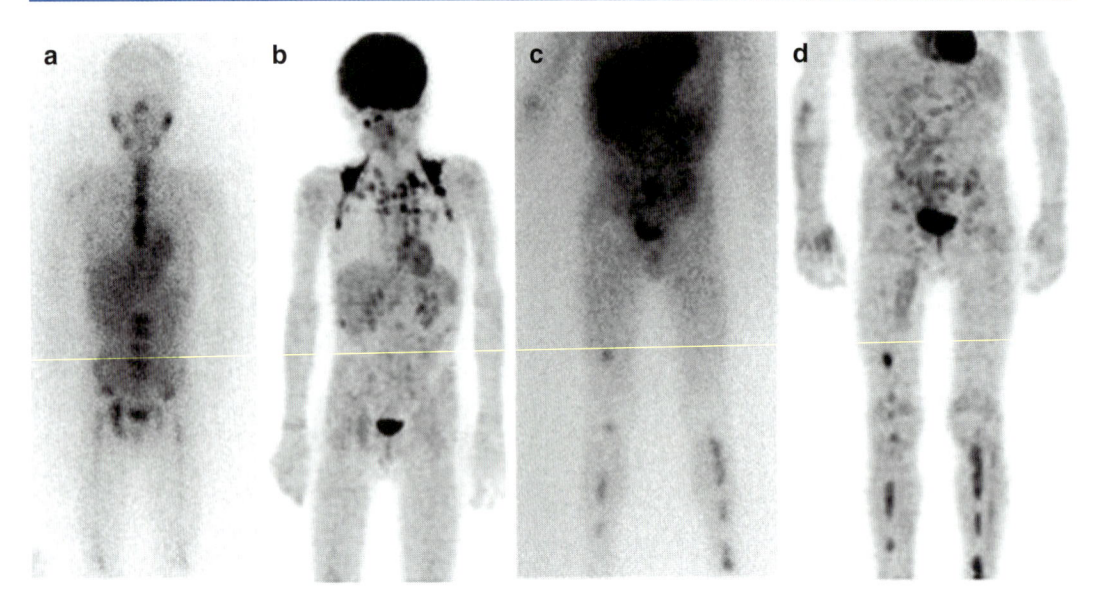

Fig. 12.5 Two different patterns of neuroblastoma detection, by means of ^{123}I-MIBG (**a**, **c**) and ^{18}F-FDG (**c**, **d**). Images (**a**, **b**) were obtained in the same patient. Note the extensive bone marrow involvement visible on the MIBG scan at the level of the spine, pelvic basin, and both femora, which is almost undetectable on the ^{18}F-FDG–PET. Images (**c**, **d**) were obtained from another patient, during staging. Bone and bone marrow involvement of both legs is seen both on the ^{123}I-MIBG scan and on ^{18}F-FDG–PET

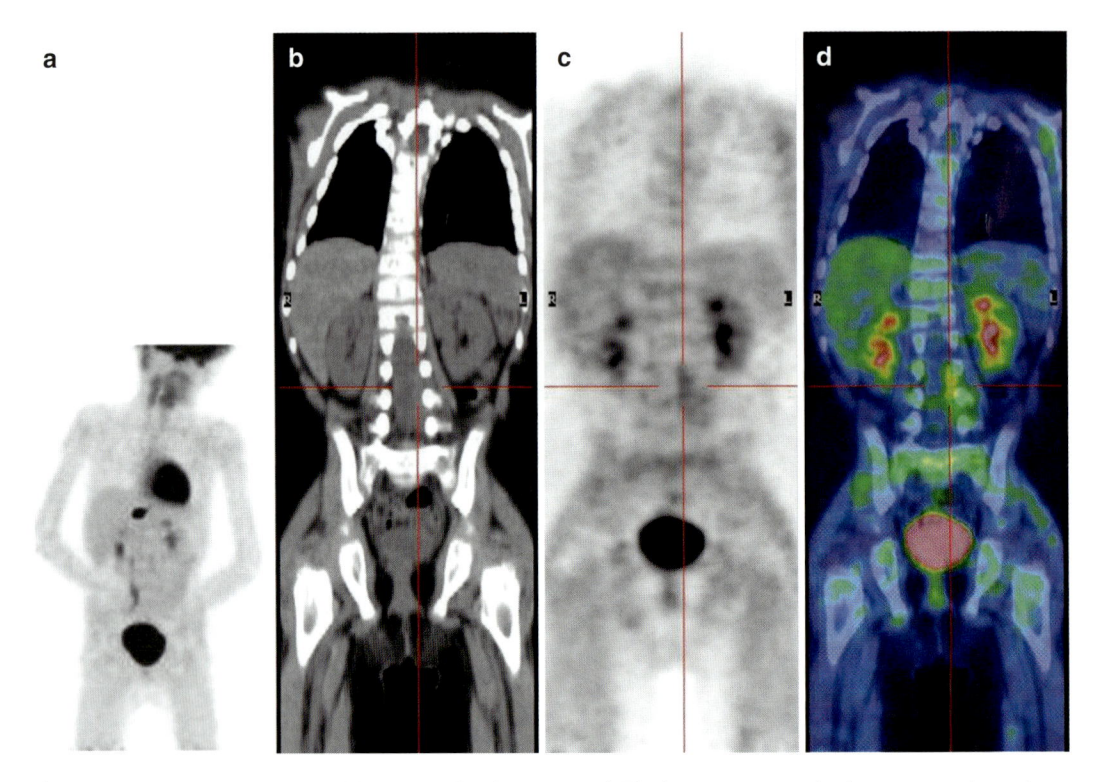

Fig. 12.6 A 5-year-old boy treated 3 years earlier for a thoracic neuroblastoma, stage IV, not amplified, 1p36 deleted. Following the development of pain in his right leg and difficulty walking, he underwent MRI, which showed the presence of epidural tissue in the L3–L5 vertebral canal. The bone marrow aspiration was negative, urinary catecholamines were normal, and ^{123}I-MIBG scintigraphy was negative. (**a**) MIP; (**b**) coronal CT, (**c**) PET, (**d**) PET/CT fusion images show inhomogeneous ^{18}F-FDG uptake in the left L3–L5 vertebral canal

12 Neuroblastoma

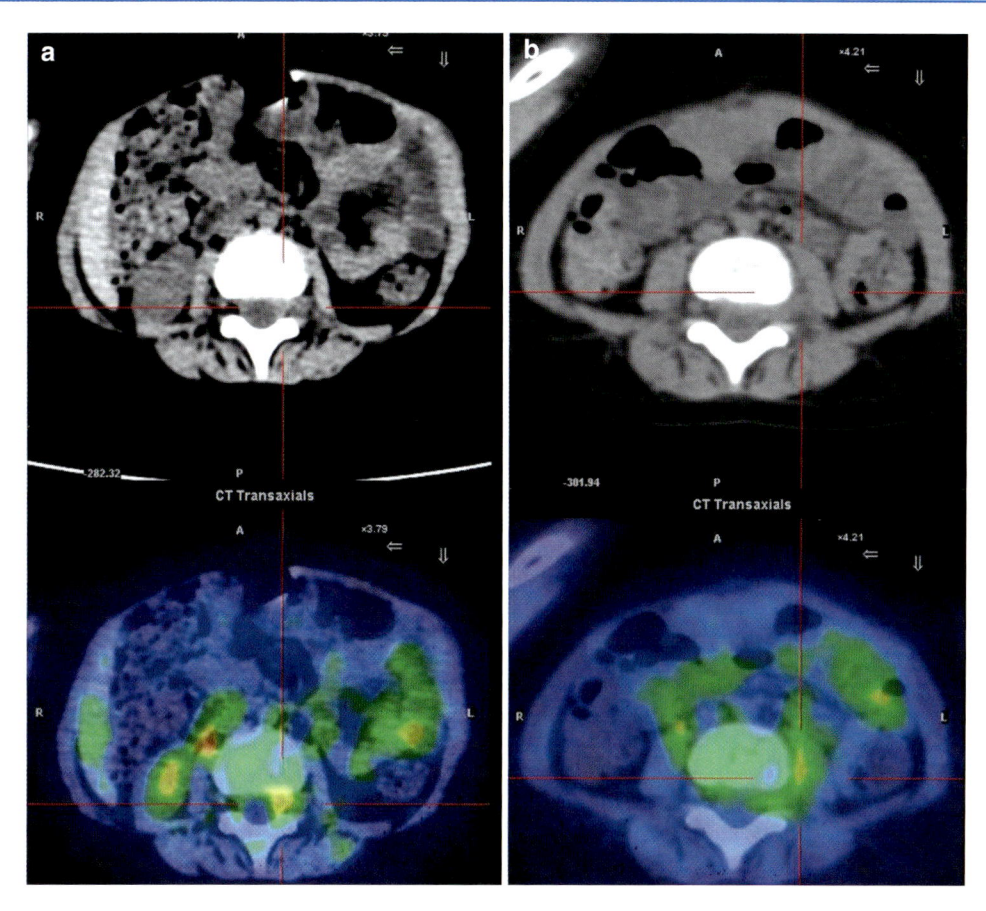

Fig. 12.7 Same patient as in Fig. 12.6. Axial CT and PET/CT fusion images of the intra-canal (**a**) and extra-canal (**b**) lesion. The patient underwent chemotherapy followed by interleukin-2 and isotretinoin treatment

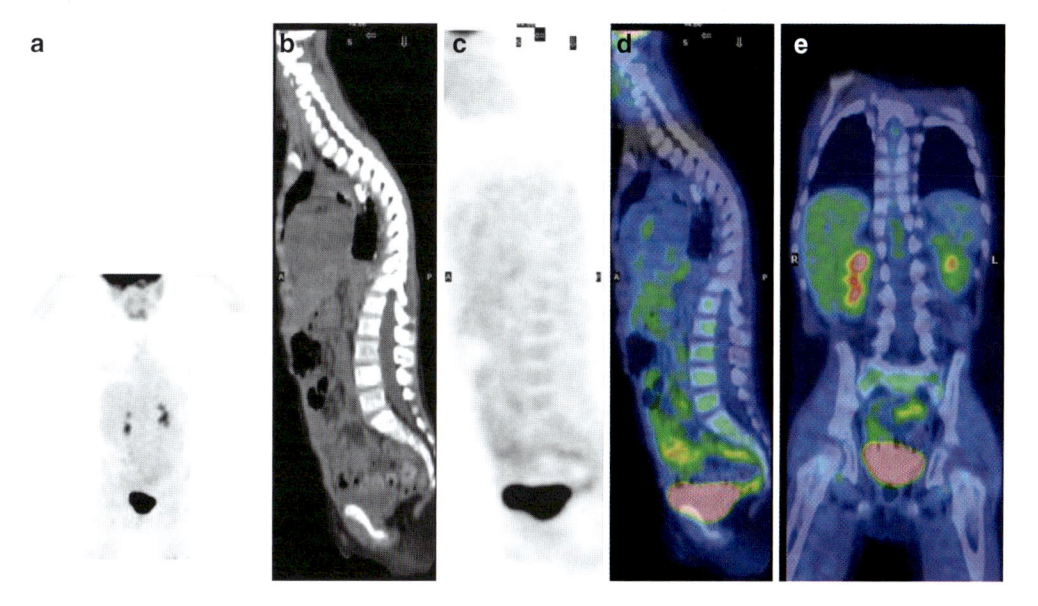

Fig. 12.8 Same patient as in Fig. 12.7, after chemotherapy. (**a**) MIP, sagittal (**b**) CT, (**c**) PET, (**d**) PET/CT, and (**e**) coronal PET/CT fusion images show the complete disappearance of any ^{18}F-FDG uptake. Note the presence of movement artifacts on the MIP and coronal PET images, at the level of the neck–thorax

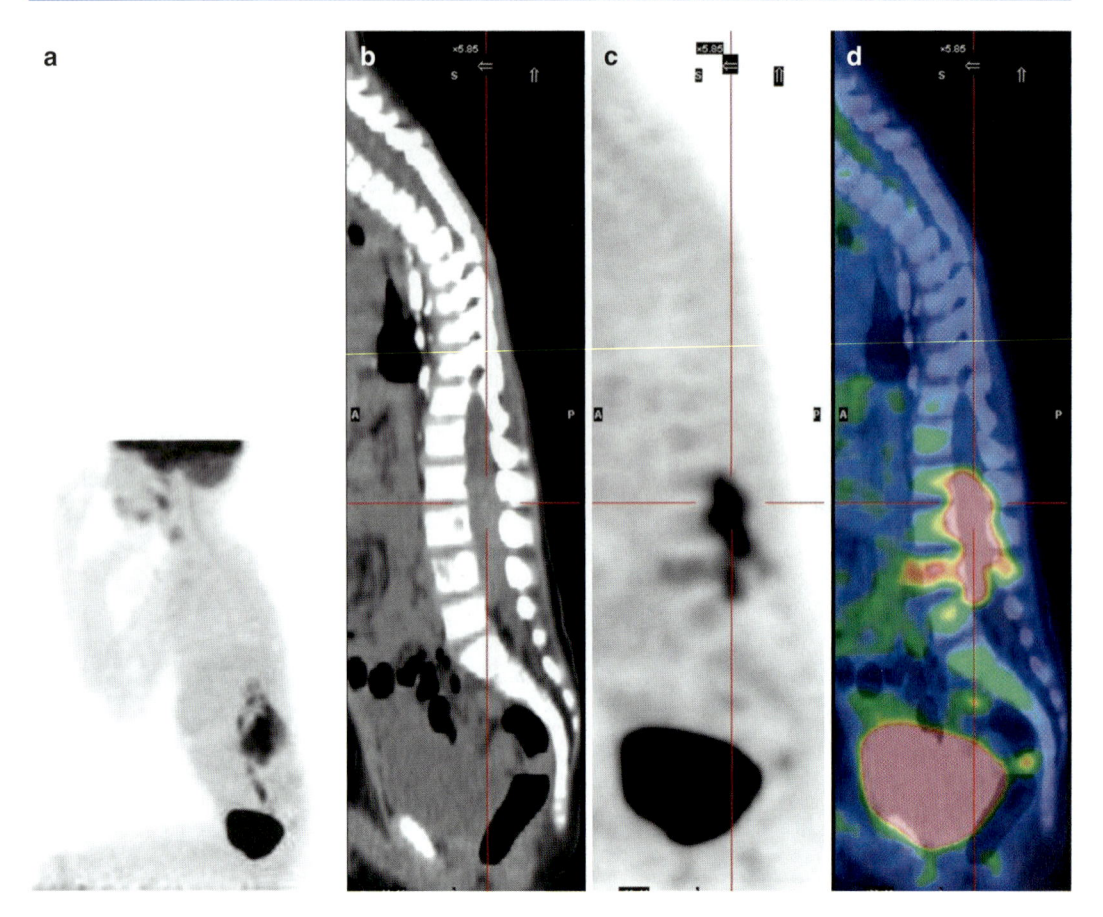

Fig. 12.9 Same patient as above. (**a**) MIP (position chosen to minimize the intense pain reported by the patient), sagittal (**b**) CT, (**c**) PET, and (**d**) PET/CT fusion images 7 months later show important disease relapse. The intensity and extent of ^{18}F-FDG uptake are greater than in the first PET exam, suggesting the aggressiveness of the new tumor

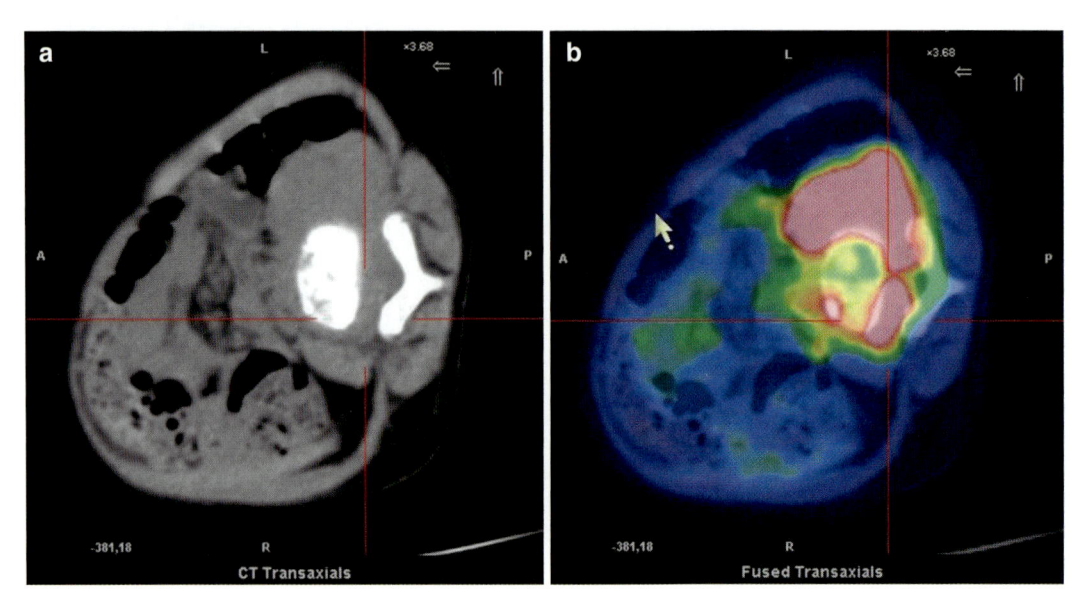

Fig. 12.10 Same patient as above, now in the lateral position. (**a**) CT and (**b**) PET/CT fusion images show intense and extensive uptake at the level of the 4th lumbar vertebra. The lesion involved both the intra- and extra-canal areas. The child died 4 months later

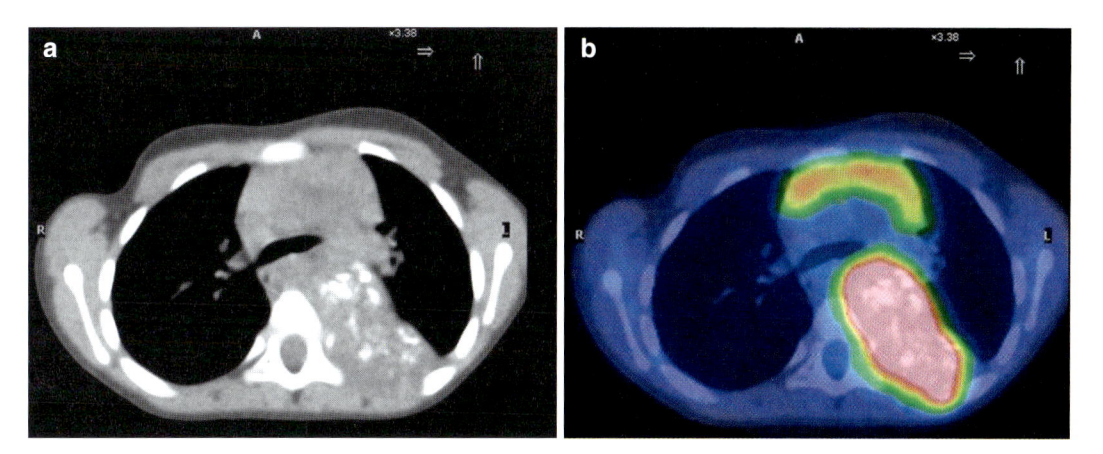

Fig. 12.11 (**a**, **b**) A 4-year-old girl with neuroblastoma underwent a PET/CT study for staging. Note the presence of calcifications in the pathological mass, typical of this type of disease

12.2.2 ^{18}F-DOPA

In NB, the tumors typically produce biologically active hormones such as norepinephrine and several of its precursors, including dihydroxyphenylalanine (DOPA) and dopamine [28, 29]. ^{18}F-dihydroxyphenylalanine (^{18}F-DOPA), the radiolabeled formulation of dihydroxyphenylalanine, is a multivalent molecule widely used in the functional imaging of neuroendocrine tumors and the best PET alternative to ^{123}I-MIBG because of its similar ability to follow catecholamine metabolism, which is increased in NB [30–34]. PET carried out with ^{18}F-DOPA has a better diagnostic accuracy than either ^{123}I-MIBG scintigraphy or conventional imaging modalities, such as CT and MRI, in the study of tumors excreting high levels of catecholamines (Fig. 12.12) [48–51], with a sensitivity vs. these latter methods of 90, 65, and 67 %, respectively [51].

Consequently, several pilot studies have recently investigated the role of ^{18}F-DOPA in NB patients. In a cohort of high-risk patients with primary/relapsed disease ($n=19$), the ^{18}F-DOPA distribution at NB sites was similar to that of ^{123}I-MIBG [35], but the accuracy of ^{18}F-DOPA–PET was higher than that of ^{123}I-MIBG scintigraphy, especially for smaller lesions (<1.5 cm). This difference influenced patient management and treatment decisions in 32 % of the cases.

In a direct comparison with morphological imaging (CT/MRI), ^{18}F-DOPA–PET performed better (Fig. 12.13) [47].

While these findings are encouraging, they require further validation in larger, multicenter, prospective trials.

12.2.3 ^{68}Ga-DOTATOC

As with other neuroendocrine tumors, NB tumors overexpress somatostatin receptors (SSTRs), especially SSTR types 1 and 2 [36, 37]. This observation led to studies of ^{111}In-pentetreotide scintigraphy or somatostatin receptor scintigraphy (SRS) in the assessment of NB [38, 39]; however, neither method was superior to ^{123}I-MIBG. Instead, complementary roles, based on the ability of these methods to provide prognostic information, were recommended, as a positive SRS scan was shown to be a predictor of better outcome in NB patients [38, 39].

Recently, the use of PET tracers such as ^{68}GA-DOTATOC to follow SSTRs in NB has been examined [40]. In a limited cohort comprising pheochromocytoma ($n=6$) and NB ($n=5$) patients, the accuracy of ^{123}I-MIBG scintigraphy and ^{68}GA-DOTATOC PET was investigated. According to a lesion-based analysis, the sensitivity of ^{68}GA-DOTATOC and ^{123}I-MIBG for NB was 97.2 and 90.7 %, respectively.

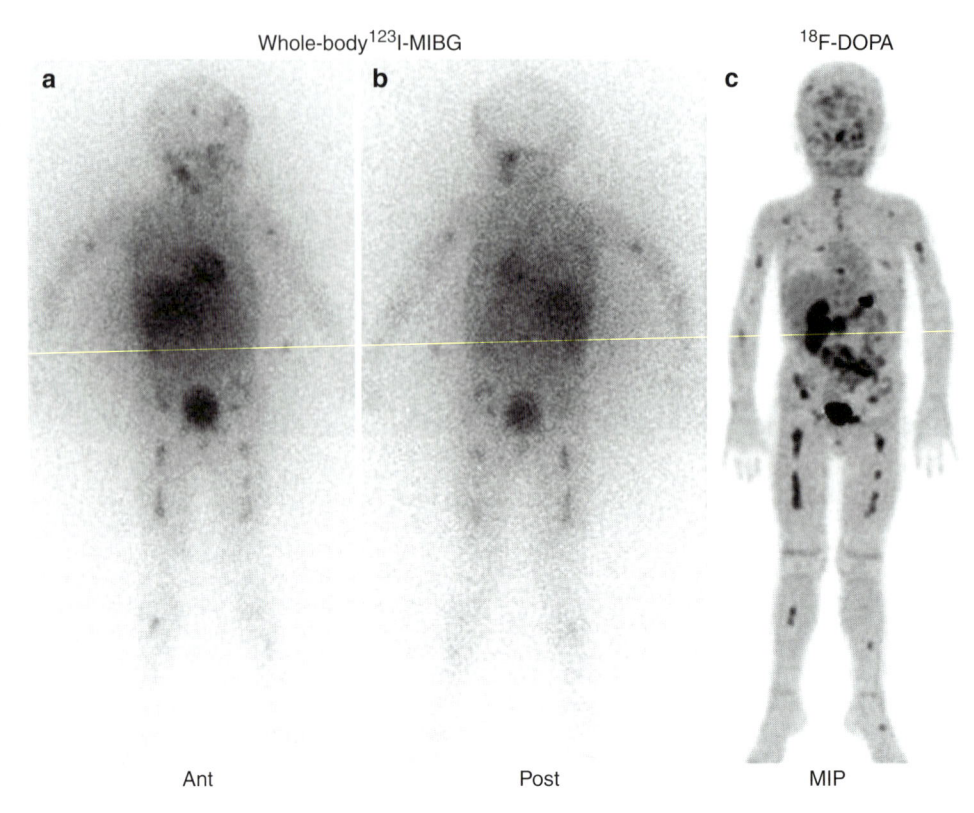

Fig. 12.12 Direct comparison of the whole-body ^{123}I-MIBG scintigraphy (**a**, **b**) and ^{18}F-DOPA–PET scan (**c**) of the same patient as in Fig. 12.3. Note the superimposable pathological distribution of the tracers visible on the two imaging modalities (Courtesy of Arnoldo Piccardo MD, Galliera Hospital, Genoa, Italy)

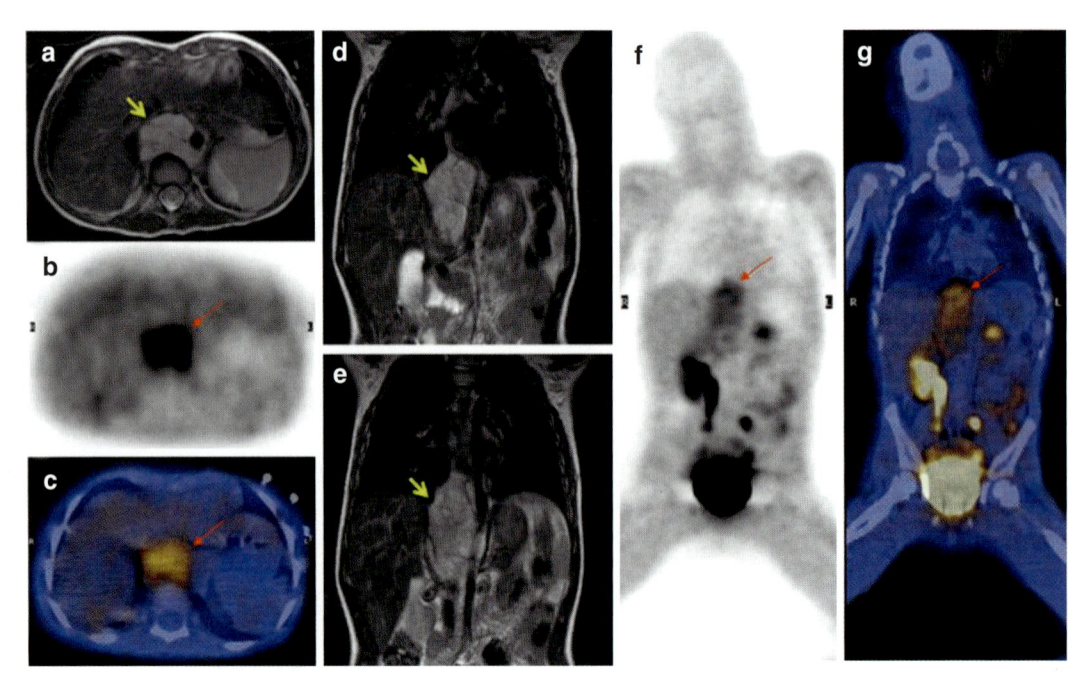

Fig. 12.13 ^{18}F-DOPA–PET/CT and fast spin-echo T2-weighted MRI scans of the same patient, who presented with a thoracic–abdominal neuroblastoma (*arrows*). (**a**, **d**, **e**) Axial and coronal MRI; (**b**, **f**) axial and coronal ^{18}F-DOPA–PET images; (**c**, **g**) fused PET/CT images, axial and coronal views. Note also the important PET tracer retention in the excretory system, namely, the right renal pelvis, proximal ureter, and urinary bladder

Primary NB lesions were better definable in ^{68}GA-DOTATOC PET imaging than in ^{123}I-MIBG scintigraphy, suggesting the advantage of the former especially regarding the peptide receptor radionuclide therapy (PRRT) planning [41]. Undoubtedly, this indication for ^{68}GA-DOTATOC must still be thoroughly assessed in children and the inclusion criteria precisely delineated before this imaging method replaces the already available and safe ^{131}I-MIBG scintigraphy.

12.2.4 ^{124}I-MIBG

We conclude by mentioning the potential introduction of MIBG-labeled with a positron-emitting compound, such as iodine-124. Already used in dosimetry, ^{124}I-MIBG PET may demonstrate the effective "revenge" of a molecule (metaiodobenzylguanidine) that, despite investigations of alternative compounds, has long made an enormous difference in the diagnostic and therapeutic approach to NB patients [42, 43]. A potential disadvantage of ^{124}I-MIBG is the decay scheme of iodine-124, which is rather impure, with the emission of both gamma rays and positrons and thus their coincidence with annihilation photons [44–46]. However, the reported low-quality images obtained in preclinical investigations can be significantly improved in modern PET/CT scanners (Figs. 12.14 and 12.15). The main limitation remains the absence of clinical studies investigating the role ^{124}I-MIBG PET in NB, which makes any statements on its utility mere speculation. Dedicated studies in this direction are therefore welcome.

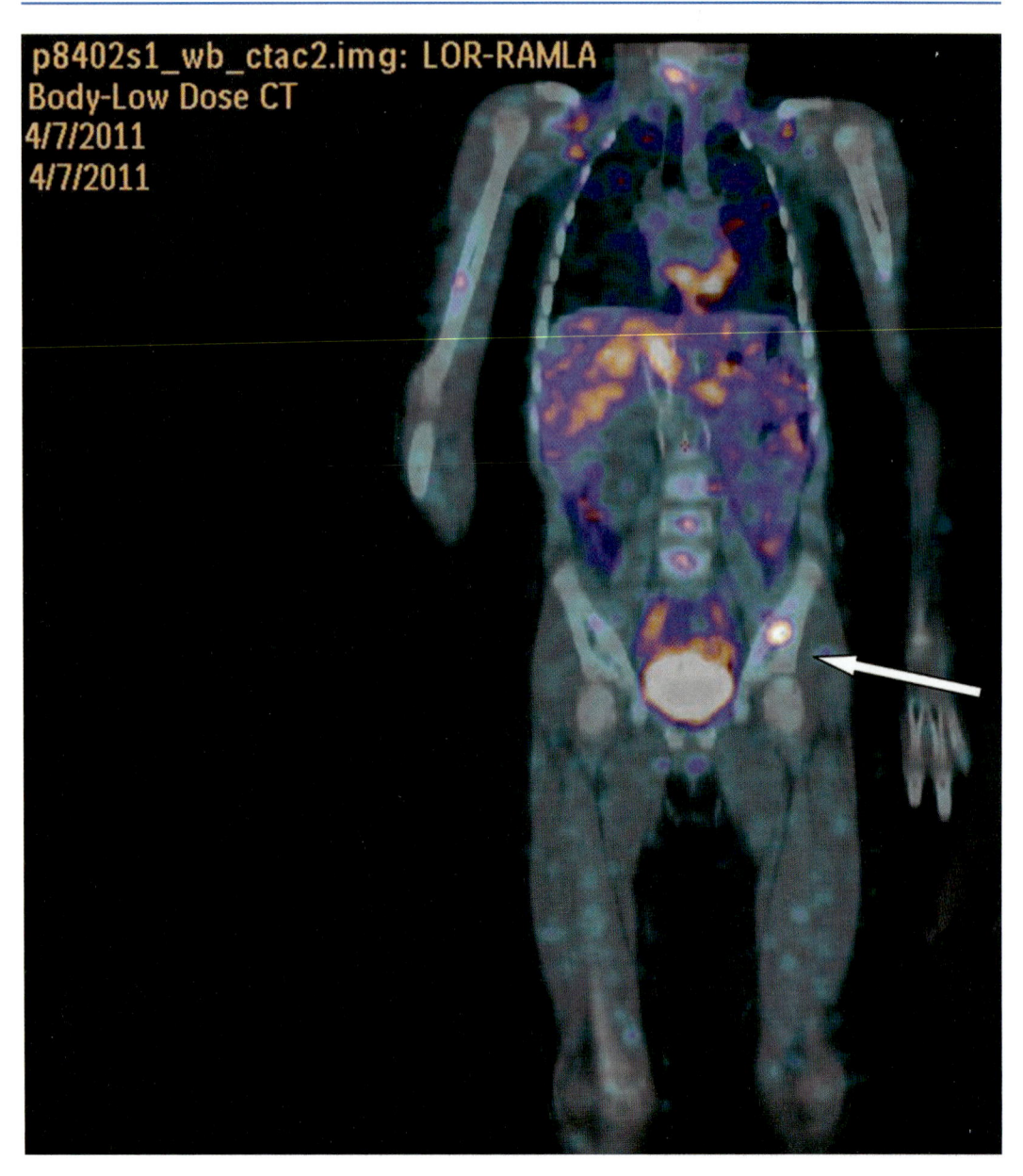

Fig. 12.14 A 7-year-old boy underwent surgery, chemotherapy, radiotherapy, and ^{131}I-MIBG radiometabolic therapy (dose 9,975 MBq) for abdominal neuroblastoma stage IV (bone metastasis). The coronal [124]I-MIBG PET/CT fusion image shows pathological uptake in left iliac (*white arrow*)

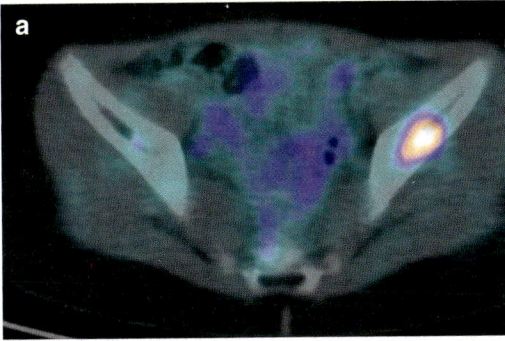

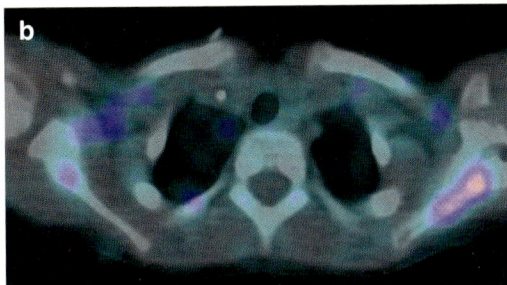

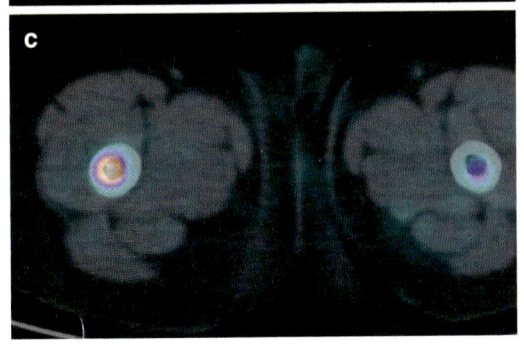

Fig. 12.15 Axial ^{124}I-MIBG PET/CT fusion images show pathological uptake in the left iliac bone (**a**), left shoulder blade (**b**), and right femur (**c**)

References

1. Caron HN, Pearson ADJ (2005) Neuroblastoma. In: Voute PA, Barrett A, Stevens MCG, Caron HN (eds) Cancer in children, 5th edn. Oxford University Press, Oxford, pp 337–352
2. Beckwith JB, Perrin EV (1963) In situ neuroblastomas: a contribution to the natural history of neural crest tumors. Am J Pathol 43(6):1089–1104
3. Rothenberg AB, Berdon WE, D'Angio GJ et al (2009) Neuroblastoma-remembering the three physicians who described it a century ago: James Homer Wright, William Pepper, and Robert Hutchison. Pediatr Radiol 39(2):155–160
4. Conte M, Parodi S, De Bernardi B et al (2006) Neuroblastoma in adolescents: the Italian experience. Cancer 106:1409–1417
5. Tateishi U, Hasegawa T, Makimoto A, Moriyama N (2003) Adult neuroblastoma: radiologic and clinicopathologic features. J Comput Assist Tomogr 27(3):321–326
6. Ley S, Ley-Zaporozhan J, Günther P et al (2011) Neuroblastoma imaging. Rofo 183(3):217–225
7. Lonergan GJ, Schwab CM, Suarez ES et al (2002) Neuroblastoma, ganglioneuroblastoma, and ganglioneuroma: radiologic-pathologic correlation. Radiographics 22:911–934
8. Papaioannou G, McHugh K (2005) Neuroblastoma in childhood: review and radiological findings. Cancer Imaging 5:116–127
9. Look AT, Hayes FA, Shuster JJ et al (1991) Clinical relevance of tumor cell ploidy and N-myc gene amplification in childhood neuroblastoma. A pediatric Oncology Group Study. J Clin Oncol 9:581–591
10. Tonini GP, Boni L, Pession A et al (1997) MYCN oncogene amplification in neuroblastoma is associated with worse prognosis, except in stage 4s: the Italian experience with 295 children. J Clin Oncol 15:85–93
11. Caron H, van Sluis P, Buschman R et al (1996) Allelic loss of chromosome 1p as a predictor of unfavorable outcome in patients with neuroblastoma. N Engl J Med 334:225–230
12. Bown N, Cotterill S, Lastowska M et al (1999) Gain of chromosome arm 17q and adverse outcome in patients with neuroblastoma. N Eng J Med 340:1954–1961
13. Asgharzadeh S, Pique-Regi R, Sposto R et al (2006) Prognostic significance of gene expression profiles of metastatic neuroblastomas lacking MYCN gene amplification. J Natl Cancer Inst 98:1193–1203
14. Berthold F, Simon T (2005) Clinical presentation of neuroblastoma. In: Cheung NK, Cohn SL (eds) Neuroblastoma. Springer, New York, pp 63–85
15. Strenger V, Kerbl R, Dornbusch HJ et al (2007) Diagnostic and prognostic impact of urinary catecholamines in neuroblastoma patients. Pediatr Blood Cancer 48:504–509
16. Schmidt ML, Lukens JN, Seeger RC et al (2000) Biologic factors determine prognosis in infants with stage IV neuroblastoma: a prospective Children's Cancer Group study. J Clin Oncol 18:1260–1268
17. Perez CA, Matthay KK, Atkinson JB et al (2000) Biologic variables in the outcome of stage I and II neuroblastoma treated with surgery as primary therapy: a Children's Cancer Group study. J Clin Oncol 18:18–26
18. Ceschel S, Casotto V, Valsecchi MG et al (2006) Survival after relapse in children with solid tumors: a follow-up study from the Italian off-therapy registry. Pediatr Blood Cancer 47(5):560–566
19. Goo HW (2010) Whole-body MRI of neuroblastoma. Eur J Radiol 75(3):306–314
20. Biasotti S, Garaventa A, Villavecchia GP et al (2000) False-negative metaiodobenzylguanidine scintigraphy at diagnosis of neuroblastoma. Med Pediatr Oncol 35:153–155

21. Shulkin BL, Hutchinson RJ, Castle VP, Yanik GA, Shapiro B, Sisson JC (1996) Neuroblastoma: positron emission tomography with 2-[fluorine-18]-fluoro-2-deoxy-D-glucose compared with metaiodobenzylguanidine scintigraphy. Radiology 199:743–750
22. Kushner BH, Yeung HW, Larson SM, Kramer K, Cheung NK (2001) Extending positron emission tomography scan utility to high-risk neuroblastoma: fluorine-18 fluorodeoxyglucose positron emission tomography as sole imaging modality in follow-up of patients. J Clin Oncol 219:3397–3405
23. Kushner BH (2004) Neuroblastoma: a disease requiring a multitude of imaging studies. J Nucl Med 45:1172–1188
24. Melzer HI, Coppenrath E, Schmid I, Albert MH, von Schweinitz D, Tudball C et al (2011) (123)I-MIBG scintigraphy/SPECT versus (18)F-FDG PET in paediatric neuroblastoma. Eur J Nucl Med Mol Imaging 38:1648–1658
25. Taggart DR, Han MM, Quach A, Groshen S, Ye W, Villablanca JG et al (2009) Comparison of iodine-123 metaiodobenzylguanidine (MIBG) scan and [18F] fluorodeoxyglucose positron emission tomography to evaluate response after iodine-131 MIBG therapy for relapsed neuroblastoma. J Clin Oncol 27:5343–5349
26. Sharp SE, Shulkin BL, Gelfand MJ, Salisbury S, Furman WL (2009) 123I-MIBG scintigraphy and 18F-FDG PET in neuroblastoma. J Nucl Med 50:1237–1243
27. Papathanasiou ND, Gaze MN, Sullivan K, Aldridge M, Waddington W, Almuhaideb A, Bomanji JB (2011) 18F-FDG PET/CT and 123I-metaiodobenzylguanidine imaging in high-risk neuroblastoma: diagnostic comparison and survival analysis. J Nucl Med 52:519–525
28. LaBrosse EH et al (1976) Catecholamine metabolism in neuroblastoma. J Natl Cancer Inst 57(3):633–638
29. Brodeur GM (1991) Neuroblastoma and other peripheral neuroectodermal tumors. In: Fernbach DJ, Vietti TJ (eds) Clinical pediatric oncology, 4th edn. CV Mosby, St. Louis, p 337
30. Hoegerle S, Altehoefer C, Ghanem N et al (2001) 18F-DOPA positron emission tomography for tumour detection in patients with medullary thyroid carcinoma and elevated calcitonin levels. Eur J Nucl Med Mol Imaging 28(1):64–71
31. Becherer A, Szabó M, Karanikas G et al (2004) Imaging of advanced neuroendocrine tumors with (18)F-FDOPA PET. J Nucl Med 45(7):1161–1167
32. Koopmans KP, de Vries EG, Kema IP et al (2006) Staging of carcinoid tumours with 18FDOPA PET: a prospective, diagnostic accuracy study. Lancet Oncol 7(9):728–734
33. Jager PL, Chirakal R, Marriott CJ et al (2008) 6-L-18F-fluorodihydroxyphenylalanine PET in neuroendocrine tumors: basic aspects and emerging clinical applications. J Nucl Med 49(4):573–586
34. Minn H, Kauhanen S, Seppänen M, Nuutila P (2009) 18F-FDOPA: a multiple-target molecule. J Nucl Med 50(12):1915–1918
35. Piccardo A, Lopci E, Conte M, Garaventa A, Foppiani L, Altrinetti V et al (2012) Comparison of (18)F-DOPA PET/CT and (123)I-MIBG scintigraphy in stage 3 and 4 neuroblastoma: a pilot study. Eur J Nucl Med Mol Imaging 39:57–61
36. O'Dorisio MS, Chen F, O'Dorisio TM et al (1994) Characterization of somatostatin receptors on human neuroblastoma tumors. Cell Growth Differ 5:1–8
37. Albers AR, O'Dorisio MS, Balster DA et al (2000) Somatostatin receptor gene expression in neuroblastoma. Regul Pept 88:61–73
38. Kropp J, Hofmann M, Bihl H (1997) Comparison of MIBG and pentetreotide scintigraphy in children with neuroblastoma. Is the expression of somatostatin receptors a prognostic factor? Anticancer Res 17(3B):1583–1588
39. Shalaby-Rana E, Majd M, Andrich MP, Movassaghi N (1997) In-111 pentetreotide scintigraphy in patients with neuroblastoma. Comparison with I-131 MIBG, N-MYC oncogene amplification, and patient outcome. Clin Nucl Med 22(5):315–319
40. Kroiss A, Putzer D, Uprimny C, Decristoforo C, Gabriel M, Santner W et al (2011) Functional imaging in phaeochromocytoma and neuroblastoma with 68Ga-DOTA-Tyr 3-octreotide positron emission tomography and 123I-metaiodobenzylguanidine. Eur J Nucl Med Mol Imaging 38:865–873
41. Gains JE, Bomanji JB, Fersht NL, Sullivan T, D'Souza D, Sullivan KP et al (2011) 177Lu-DOTATATE molecular radiotherapy for childhood neuroblastoma. J Nucl Med 52:1041–1047
42. Lopci E, Chiti A, Castellani MR, Pepe G, Antunovic L, Fanti S et al (2011) Matched pairs dosimetry: 124I/131I metaiodobenzylguanidine and 124I/131I and 86Y/90Y antibodies. Eur J Nucl Med Mol Imaging 38:S28–S40
43. Lee CL, Wahnishe H, Sayre GA, Cho HM, Kim HJ, Hernandez- Pampaloni M et al (2010) Radiation dose estimation using preclinical imaging with 124I-metaiodobenzylguanidine (MIBG) PET. Med Phys 37(9):4861–4866
44. Herzog H, Tellmann L, Scholten B, Coenen HH, Qaim SM (2007) PET imaging problems with the non-standard positron emitters yttrium-86 and iodine-124. Q J Nucl Med Mol Imaging 52:159–165
45. Mariani G, Bruselli L, Duatti A (2008) Is PET always an advantage versus planar and SPECT imaging? Eur J Nucl Med Mol Imaging 35:1560–1565
46. Pentlow KS, Graham MC, Lambrecht RM, Cheung NKV, Larson SM (1991) Quantitative imaging of I-124 using positron emission tomography with applications to radioimmunodiagnosis and radioimmunotherapy. Med Phys 18(3):357–366
47. Lopci E, Piccardo A, Nanni C, Altrinetti V, Garaventa A, Pession A, Cistaro A, Chiti A, Villavecchia G, Fanti S (2012) F18-DOPA PET/CT in neuroblastoma: comparison with conventional imaging with CT/MR. Clin Nucl Med 37:e73–e78
48. Fottner C, Helisch A, Anlauf M et al (2010) 6-18F-Fluoro-L-dihydroxyphenylalanine positron emission

tomography is superior to 123i-metaiodobenzylguanidine scintigraphy in the detection of extrarenal and hereditary pheochromocytomas and paragangliomas: correlation with vesicular monoamine transporter expression. J Clin Endocrinol Metab 95(6):2800–2810
49. Timmers HJ, Chen CC, Carrasquillo JA et al (2009) Comparison of 18F-fluoro-LDOPA, 18F-fluorodeoxyglucose, and 18F-fluorodopamine PET and 123I-MIBG scintigraphy in the localization of pheochromocytoma and paraganglioma. J Clin Endocrinol Metab 94(12):4757–4767
50. Fiebrich HB, Brouwers AH, Kerstens MN et al (2009) 6-[F-18]fluoro-l-dihydroxyphenylalanine positron emission tomography is superior to conventional imaging with 123i-metaiodobenzylguanidine scintigraphy, computer tomography, and magnetic resonance imaging in localizing tumors causing catecholamine excess. J Clin Endocrinol Metab 94:3922–3930
51. Kauhanen S, Seppanen M, Ovaska J et al (2009) The clinical value of [18F]fluoro-dihydroxyphenylalanine positron emission tomography in primary diagnosis, staging, and restaging of neuroendocrine tumors. Endocr Relat Cancer 16:255–265
52. Giammarile F, Chiti A, Lassman M et al (2008) EANM procedure guidelines for 131I-metaiodobenzylguanidine (131I-mIBG) therapy. Eur J Nucl Med Mol Imaging 35(5):1039–1047
53. Moyenes JSE, Babich JW, Carter R, Meller ST, Agrawal M, McElwain TJ (1989) Quantitative study of radioiodinated metaiodobenzylguanidine uptake in children with neuroblastoma: correlation with tumor histopathology. J Nucl Med 30(4):474–480
54. Lebtahi Hadj-Djilani N, Lebtahi NE, Bischof Delaloye A, Laurini R, Beck D (1995) Diagnosis and follow-up of neuroblastoma by means of iodine-123 metaiodobenzylguanidine scintigraphy and bone scan, and the influence of histology. Eur J Nucl Med 22:322–329
55. Khafagi FA, Shapiro B, Fig LM, Mallette S, Sisson JC (1989) Labetalol reduces iodine-131 uptake by pheochromocytoma and normal tissues. J Nucl Med 30:481–489
56. Giammarile F, Lumbroso J, Ricard M, Aubert B, Hartmann O, Schlumberger M et al (1995) Radioiodinated metaiodobenzylguanidine in neuroblastoma: influence of high dose on tumour site detection. Eur J Nucl Med 22:1180–1183

Part III

Other Tumors

Pediatric Nasopharyngeal Carcinoma

Silvia Morbelli

13.1 Introduction

Nasopharyngeal carcinoma (NPC) is a malignancy of epidermoid origin. It differs from other head and neck carcinomas by its unique histological, epidemiological, and biological characteristics [1]. Even if NPC is a rare malignant tumor in childhood, in pediatric patients, it is one of the most frequent neoplasms in the nasopharyngeal and respiratory tracts [2]. Histologically, NPC is nearly always an undifferentiated carcinoma or lymphoepithelioma. Its pathogenesis is closely related to a preceding infection with Epstein–Barr virus (EBV) [3]. NPC that develops in childhood is characterized by not only the advanced clinical stage at onset but also the better chances of survival of these patients. Several studies, both in adult and in children, demonstrated the ability of combined therapy (neoadjuvant chemotherapy and radiotherapy or concomitant chemoradiotherapy) to significantly improve the prognosis of NPC patients [3].

Clinical Case

A 13-year-old HIV-positive boy underwent neck ultrasound for a nodular neck swelling. Echography revealed bilateral multiple cervical lymph nodes up to 2 cm, with the subsequent cervical lymph node biopsy showing total effacement by poorly differentiated large cells, suggesting a poorly differentiated NPC. The diagnosis was confirmed by means of endoscopic evaluation. The patients were then submitted to MRI and contrast-enhanced (ce)-CT scan for staging and to a whole-body ^{18}F-FDG–PET/CT scan for staging and radiotherapy planning. The PET/CT scan for radiotherapy planning was performed using the same rigid bed and restraint aids used in radiotherapy treatment. The ce-CT confirmed the presence of a right-side nasopharyngeal mass and multiple bilateral enlarged necrotic cervical lymph nodes. It also revealed an unexpected metastatic lesion in the right posterior parietal pleura. These findings were confirmed by ^{18}F-FDG–PET/CT (Fig. 13.1).

S. Morbelli, MD
Nuclear Medicine Unit, IRCCS AOU San Martino – IST, Largo R. Benzi 10, Genoa 16132, Italy
e-mail: silviadaniela.morbelli@hsanmartino.it

Clinical Case (continued)

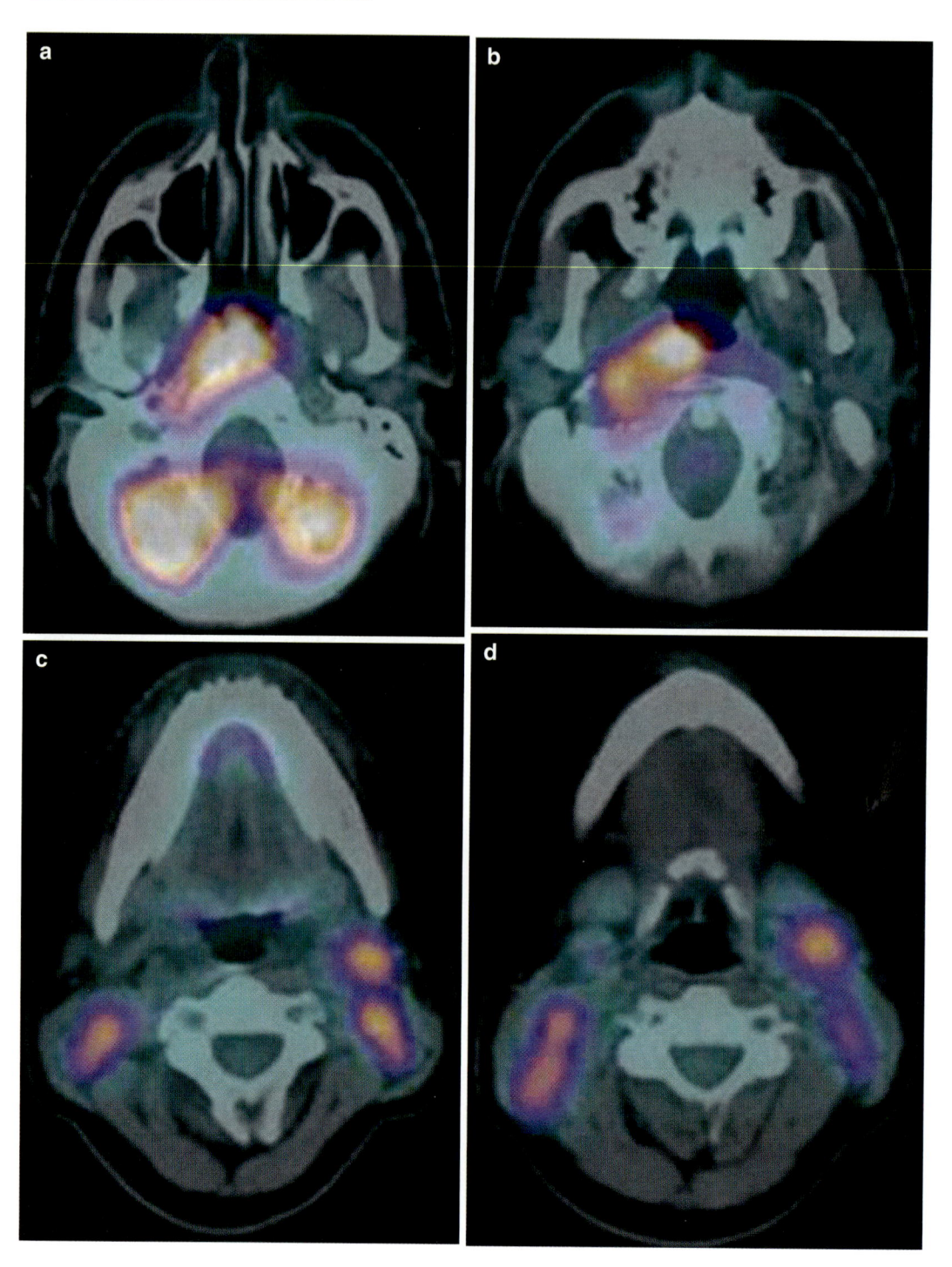

Fig. 13.1 Baseline ¹⁸F-FDG–PET/CT scan shows intense uptake in the nasopharyngeal primary lesion (**a**, **b**, **f**) as well as in multiple bilateral enlarged cervical lymph nodes (**c**, **d**) and in a metastatic right pleural lesion (**e**, **g**)

13 Pediatric Nasopharyngeal Carcinoma

Clinical Case (continued)

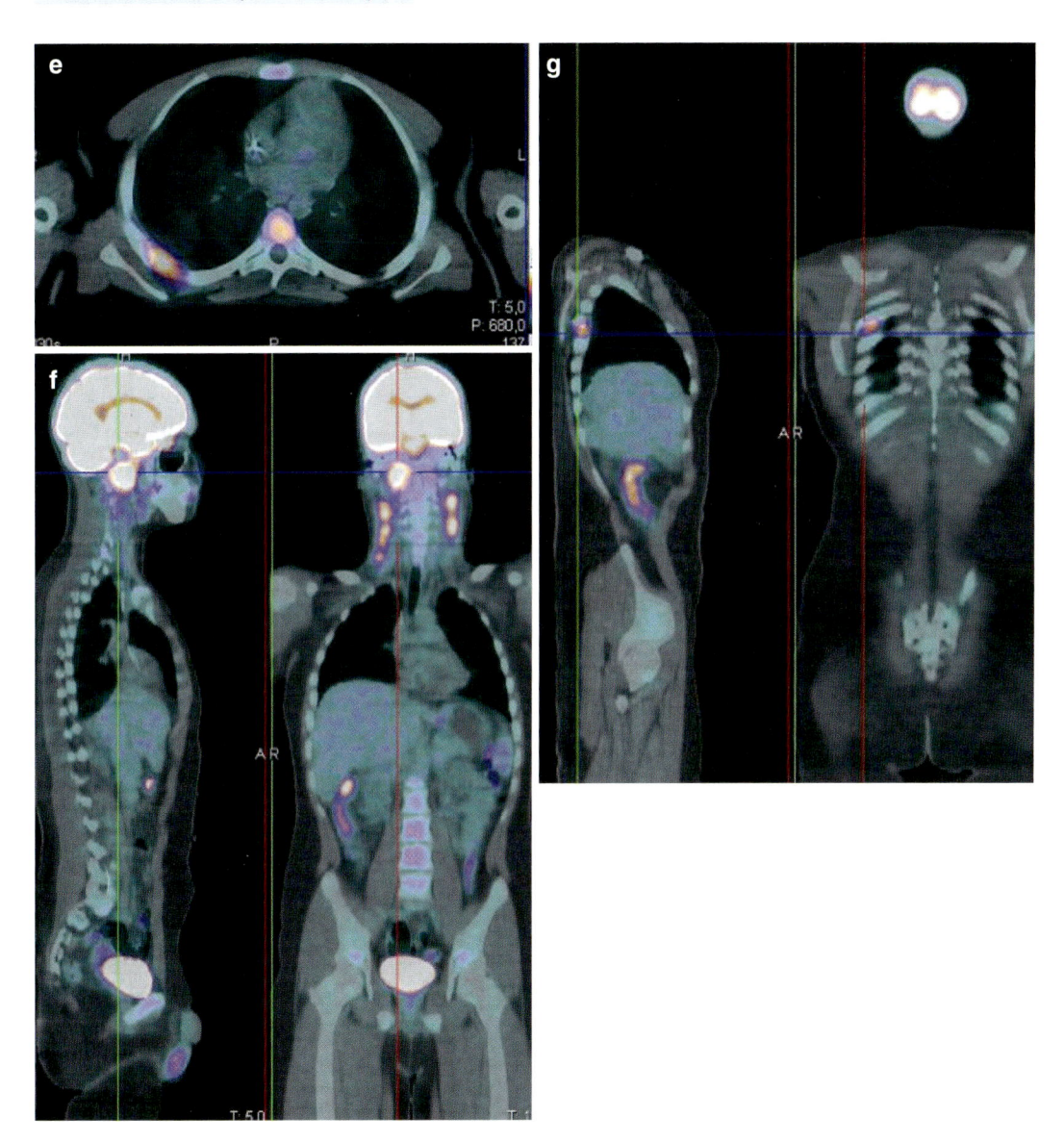

Fig. 13.1 (continued)

The patient then underwent two cycles of chemotherapy (cisplatin and fluorouracil). His early response to chemotherapy was evaluated with ce-CT and ^{18}F-FDG–PET/CT. Both examinations highlighted the positive response to chemotherapy. However, whereas several cervical lymph nodes >10 mm (arrow in Fig. 13.2) and persistent posterior right pleural thickening were still evident on the ce-CT, ^{18}F-FDG–PET/CT showed a complete metabolic response (Fig. 13.2).

Clinical Case (continued)

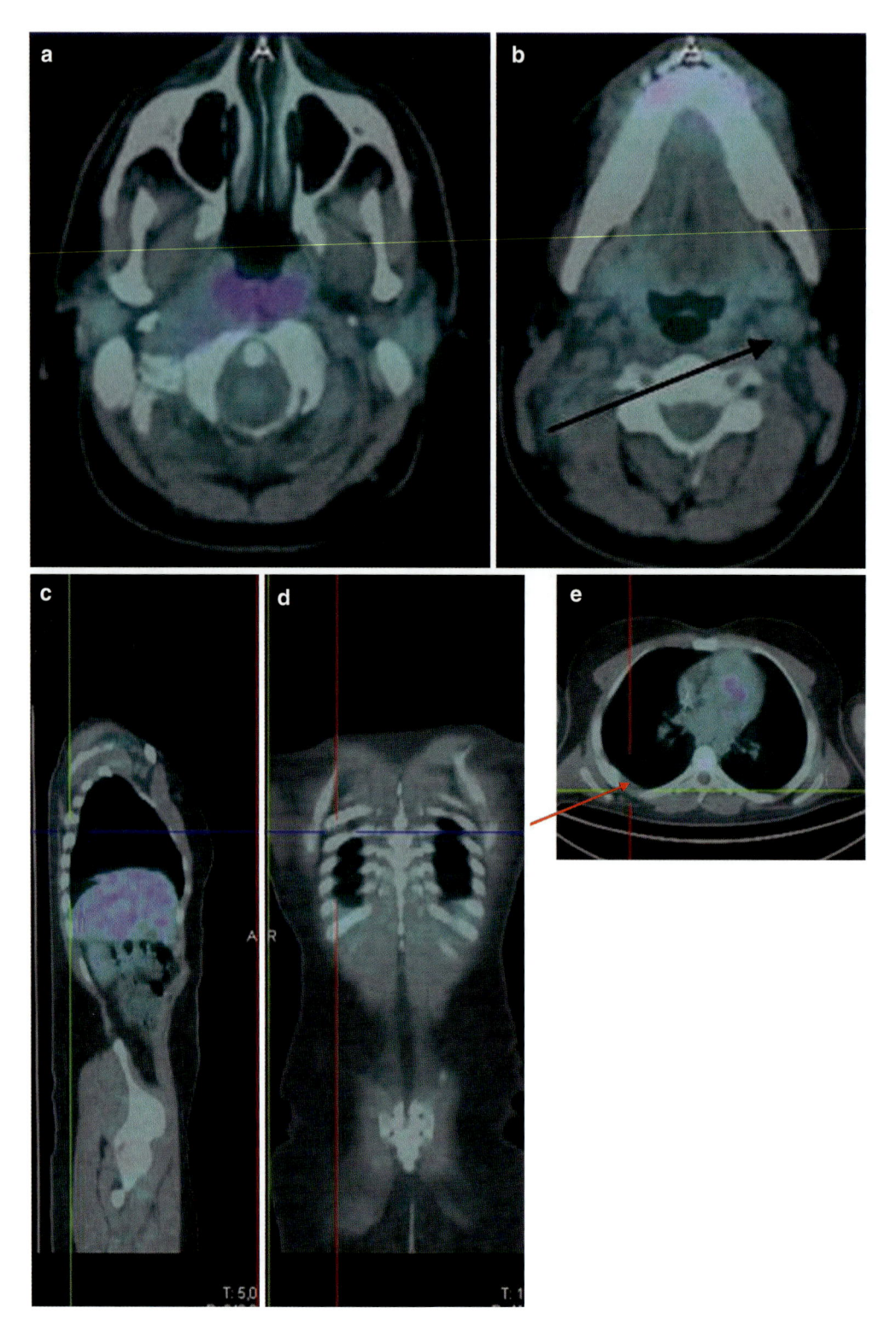

Fig. 13.2 ¹⁸F-FDG–PET/CT performed after two cycles of chemotherapy shows a complete metabolic response of the all pathological uptakes (**a–e**). On the opposite, enlarged cervical lymph nodes (*black arrow* in **b**) and posterior right pleural thickening were still evident on the coregistered CT images (*red arrow* in **e**)

Teaching Points

In children with NPC, an ^{18}F-FDG–PET-based metabolic response after chemotherapy has a high sensitivity and specificity in evaluating the treatment response and may result in the improved management of patients with advanced disease [4].

References

1. Sultan I, Casanova M, Ferrari A, Rihani R, Rodriguez-Galindo C (2010) Differential features of nasopharyngeal carcinoma in children and adults: a SEER study. Pediatr Blood Cancer 55(2): 279–284
2. Casanova M, Bisogno G, Gandola L, Cecchetto G, Di Cataldo A, Basso E, Rare Tumors in Pediatric Age Group et al (2012) A prospective protocol for nasopharyngeal carcinoma in children and adolescents: the Italian Rare Tumors in Pediatric Age (TREP) project. Cancer 118(10):2718–2725
3. Mertens R, Granzen B, Lassay L, Bucsky P, Hundgen M, Stetter G, Heimann G, Weiss C, Hess CF, Gademann G (2005) Treatment of nasopharyngeal carcinoma in children and adolescents: definitive results of a multicenter study (NPC-91-GPOH). Cancer 104(5):1083–1089
4. Chan SC, Yen TC, Ng SH, Lin CY, Wang HM, Liao CT, Fan KH, Chang JT (2006) Differential roles of 18F-FDG PET in patients with locoregional advanced nasopharyngeal carcinoma after primary curative therapy: response evaluation and impact on management. J Nucl Med 47(9):1447–1454

Poorly Differentiated Thyroid Carcinoma

14

Somali Gavane and Heiko Schoder

14.1 Introduction

Thyroid cancer, although uncommon in childhood, represents the most common pediatric endocrine neoplasia [1]. Poorly differentiated thyroid cancers are very rare [2]. Currently, whole-body PET/CT is approved for use in assessing suspected recurrence of well-differentiated thyroid cancer in patients with radioiodine-negative scans and detectable thyroglobulin (Tg) levels [3]. Evidence is emerging on the advantages of PET/CT imaging in other histological types of thyroid malignancy, such as Hürthle cell, medullary, and the anaplastic variants. Due to its aggressive growth and subsequent significantly elevated glucose utilization, several case reports have shown FDG-PET/CT's ability to detect both primary and metastatic anaplastic thyroid cancer [4].

Clinical Case

Lung abnormalities were detected as an incidental ultrasound finding in a 17-year-old girl who was asymptomatic for pulmonary disease. The left lobe measured 6.5×3.2×3.7 cm. Three solid thyroid nodules with scattered calcification were noted, the largest one measuring 3.3×2.0×2.8 cm. No suspicious adenopathy was reported. Serum calcitonin levels were low.

After a second evaluation, fine-needle aspiration was performed. During that time, a nodule in the left thyroid doubled in size and another, dominant nodule measured 4.9×3.3×4.3 cm. A prominent level 4 lymph node measuring 1.5 cm was detected in the posterior left jugular vein. Another lymph node (2.3 cm) was noted on the right side. Fine-needle aspiration of the three thyroid nodules on the left side indicated poorly differentiated carcinoma.

The patient underwent thyroidectomy, bilateral central neck dissection, and left modified dissection. Pathology reported poorly differentiated carcinoma, insular in origin, with extensive necrosis, focal extrathyroidal extension, and vascular invasion. Three out of six parathyroid lymph nodes were positive for metastasis, with extracapsular extension. On left neck dissection, one of the five lymph nodes was positive for metastasis. The postoperative course was complicated by bilateral vocal cord paralysis, requiring tracheostomy, and hypoparathyroidism. Postoperative thyroglobulin (Tg) was 0.3 ng/ml, TgAb 25.6, and parathyroid hormone <4 (Fig. 14.1).

She received radioimmunotherapy (^{131}I, activity: 155.23 mCi). The post-therapy ^{131}I scan did not show uptake in the lateral neck, lungs, or bones. The synthroid dose was adjusted to keep TSH suppressed to close to 0.1 ng/ml.

After 4 months, the patient developed two masses in the left neck, which on MRI measured

S. Gavane, MD (✉) • H. Schoder, MD
Nuclear Medicine Department,
Memorial Sloan-Kettering Cancer Center,
1275 York Avenue, New York, NY 10065, USA
e-mail: gavanes@mskcc.org; schoderh@mskcc.org

5 × 3.8 and 3.0 × 2.3 cm (Fig. 14.2). Thyroglobulin increased until 27 ng/ml.

The patient's disease was considered radioimmunotherapy refractory and PET positive (Fig. 14.2). She underwent surgery and was subsequently treated with 175 mcg of synthroid. Her most recent TSH value was 0.03 ng/ml, T4 1.59 ng/ml, and thyroglobulin 0.2 ng/ml, and antibodies were undetectable.

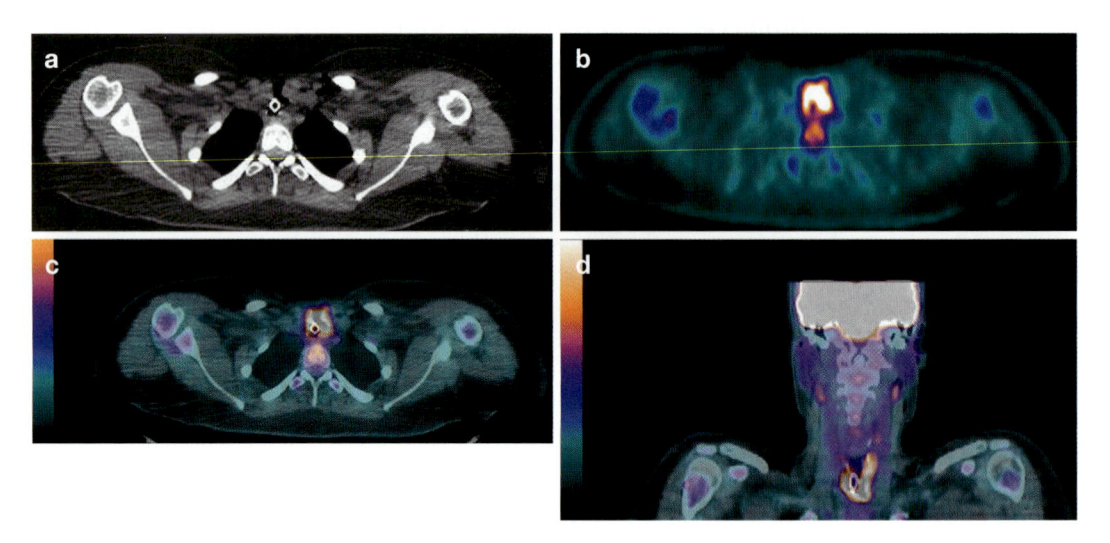

Fig. 14.1 (**a–d**) The patient underwent PET/CT, which showed hypermetabolic soft tissue at the tracheostomy site. This was more likely an infectious/inflammatory change than malignancy. Otherwise, there were no suspicious hypermetabolic lesions

14 Poorly Differentiated Thyroid Carcinoma

Clinical Case (continued)

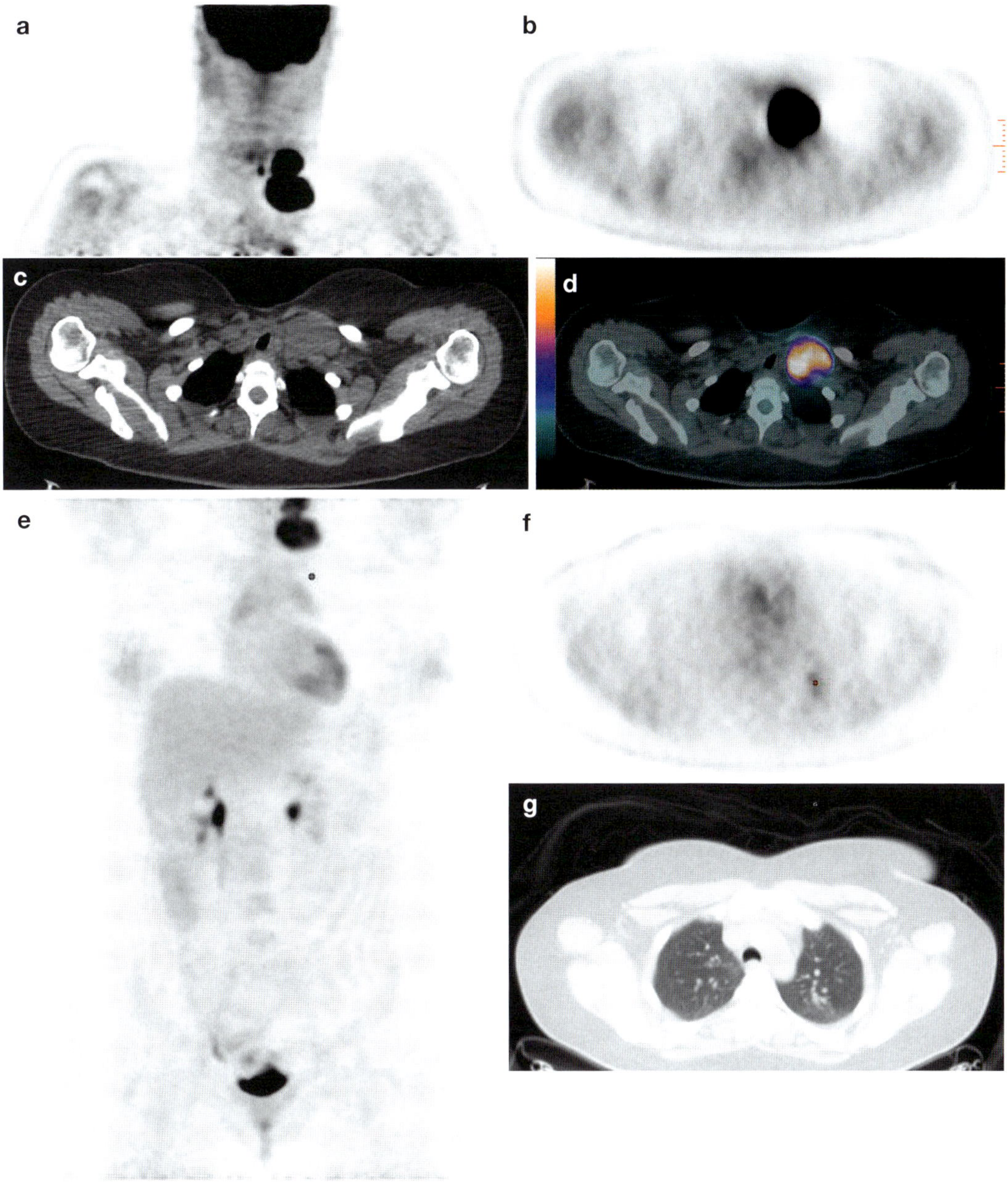

Fig. 14.2 (**a–d**) The PET/CT study showed a new, hypermetabolic bilobed mass in the left neck that was suspicious for relapse malignancy (SUV$_{max}$ 12.0) and (**e–h**) mild FDG uptake associated with a left upper lobe nodule seen on CT, possibly malignancy or inflammatory change

Clinical Case (continued)

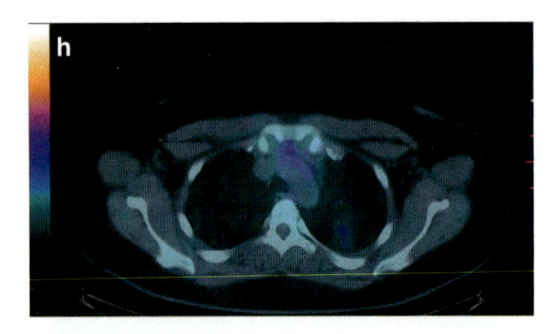

Fig. 14.2 (continued)

References

1. Luster M, Lassmann M, Freudenberg LS, Reiners C (2007) Thyroid cancer in childhood: management strategy, including dosimetry and long-term results. Hormones (Athens) 6(4):269–278
2. Mosci C, Iagaru A (2011) PET/CT imaging of thyroid cancer. Clin Nucl Med 36(12):e180–e185
3. Juweid M, O'Dorisio T, Milhem M (2008) Diagnosis of poorly differentiated thyroid cancer with radioiodine scanning after thyrotropin alfa stimulation. N Engl J Med 359:1295–1297
4. Nguyen BD, Ram PC (2007) PETCT staging and post-therapeutic monitoring of anaplastic thyroid carcinoma. Clin Nucl Med 32:145–149

Phylloid Tumor of the Breast

15

Mariapaola Cucinotta and Angelina Cistaro

Phylloid tumor, formerly called cystosarcoma phylloides, is a very unusual neoplasia. It accounts for <0.5 % of all breast neoplasms and approximately 2.5 % of fibro-epithelial tumors [1–3]. Like fibroadenoma, it histologically comprises two components, in which connective tissue predominates [3–5]. Hodges et al. studied the genome of a synchronous fibroadenoma and a phylloid tumor placed in the same breast mass and found that both neoplasms had an allelic loss at D7S522. However, in the phylloid tumor but not in the fibroadenoma, allelic losses also occurred at TP53 and D22S264. These latter mutations were suggested to be involved in the progression of fibroadenoma to phylloid tumor [5].

Phylloid neoplasias may be benign, borderline, or malignant [3]. They are generally seen in adult women and only rarely in girls (Fig. 15.1). In the study of Bässler and Zahner, 133 tumors occurred in the female and only 1 in the male breast [6]. In 1998, Blanckaert et al. described a case in an 11-year-old child, in whom the tumor presented as a painless, voluminous (6-cm diameter), and rapidly growing mass [4]. Among the clinical characteristics of phylloid tumor is a high local recurrence rate, independent of the tumor's degree of malignancy [1, 2]. Consequently, surgical therapy, either conservative or radical depending not only on the tumor grade and growth rate but also on the size of the neoplasm and the breast, should always consist of a complete resection, with tumor-free margins [1, 2, 6].

M. Cucinotta, MD
Nuclear Medicine Unit, Department of Radiological Sciences, Policlinico Gaetano Martino Hospital, University of Messina, Via Consolare Valeria, 1, Messina 98125, Italy
e-mail: mariapaola.cucinotta@gmail.com

A. Cistaro, MD (✉)
Department of Nuclear Medicine, Positron Emission Tomography Center IRMET S.p.A., Euromedic Inc., Via Onorato Vigliani 89, Turin 10100, Italy

Institute of Cognitive Sciences and Technologies, National Research Council, Rome, Italy
e-mail: a.cistaro@irmet.com

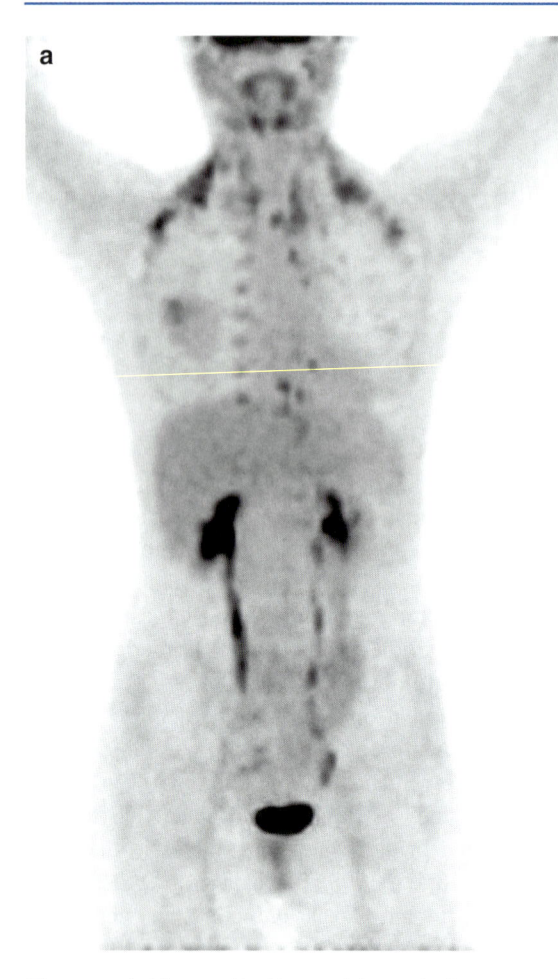

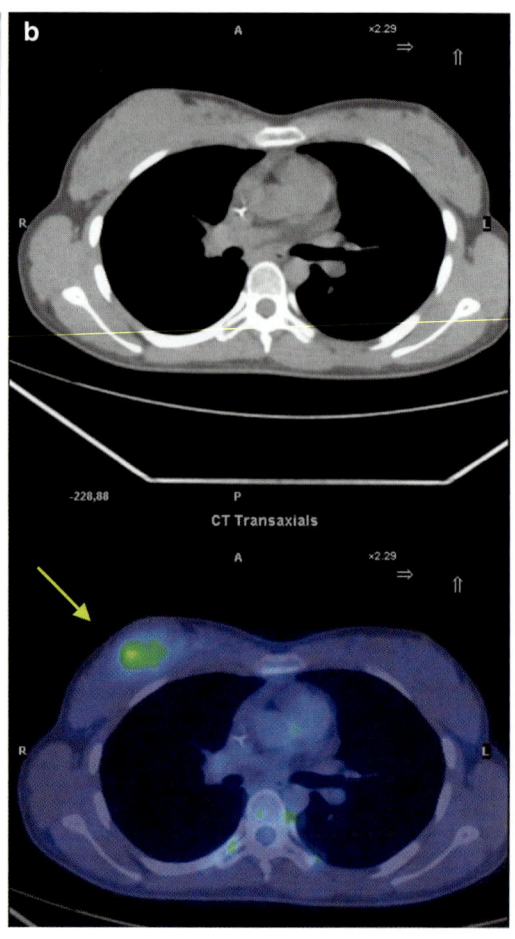

Fig. 15.1 A 14-year-old girl treated for Hodgkin's lymphoma. Maximum intensity projection (**a**) and axial CT and PET/CT fusion images (**b**) show moderately intense FDG uptake in the right breast, corresponding to phylloid tumor (*yellow arrow* in **b**)

References

1. Abdallah A, Saklaoui O, Stückle C, Sommerer F, Hatzmann W, Audretsch W, Wesemann A, Zink M, Skoljarev L, Papadopoulos S (2009) Case reports of operative management of very large, benign phylloid tumors – is a safety margin necessary? Gynakol Geburtshilfliche Rundsch 49:320–325
2. Finocchi L, Covarelli P, Rulli A, Servoli A, Noya G (2008) Bilateral phylloid cystosarcoma of the breast: a case report and review of the literature. Chir Ital 60:867–872
3. Norat F, Dreant N, Riah Y, Lebreton E (2009) Extraordinary case of malignant phylloid tumor of the breast: surgical reconstruction treatment. Ann Ital Chir 80:475–478
4. Blanckaert D, Lecourt O, Loeuille GA, Six J, Laurent JC (1998) Phyllodes tumor of the breast in an 11-year-old child. Pediatrie 43:405–408
5. Hodges KB, Abdul-Karim FW, Wang M, Lopez-Beltran A, Montironi R, Easley S, Zhang S, Wang N, MacLennan GT, Cheng L (2009) Evidence for transformation of fibroadenoma of the breast to malignant phyllodes tumor. Appl Immunohistochem Mol Morphol 17:345–350
6. Bässler R, Zahner J (1989) Recurrences and metastases of cystosarcoma phylloides (phylloid tumor, WHO). On the 150th birthday of a controversial diagnostic concept. Geburtshilfe Frauenheilkd 49:1–10

Wilms' Tumor

Natale Quartuccio

Wilms' tumor (WT), also called nephroblastoma, is the most common renal cancer in childhood, accounting for 90 % of all renal cancers in children and 6 % of all pediatric cancers [1]. WT arises from a mutation of the *WT1* gene on chromosome 11 (locus 11p13). The WT1 protein is a transcription factor that plays a role in the embryonic development of the kidneys and gonads. However, the genetics underlying WT expression seems to be multifactorial, and other mutations, on chromosomes 1, 12, and 8, have been recognized [2].

Several imaging techniques are currently available for the staging and follow-up of WT, including abdominal ultrasound [3], chest radiograph [4], CT [5], and MRI [6]. Both ^{18}F–FDG–PET/CT and diffusion-weighted imaging (DWI) with MRI have been proposed as tools to obtain additional information on WTs, in the staging of these tumors, in the assessment of treatment response, and in surgical and radiotherapy planning (Figs. 16.1 and 16.2) [6, 7].

Multimodality treatment for WT includes chemotherapy, surgery, and radiotherapy, with 5-year survival rates >80 % reported [8].

N. Quartuccio, MD
Nuclear Medicine Unit, Department of Biomedical
Sciences and Morphological and Functional Images,
University of Messina, Via Consolare Valeria 1,
Messina 98125, Italy
e-mail: natale.quartuccio84@hotmail.it

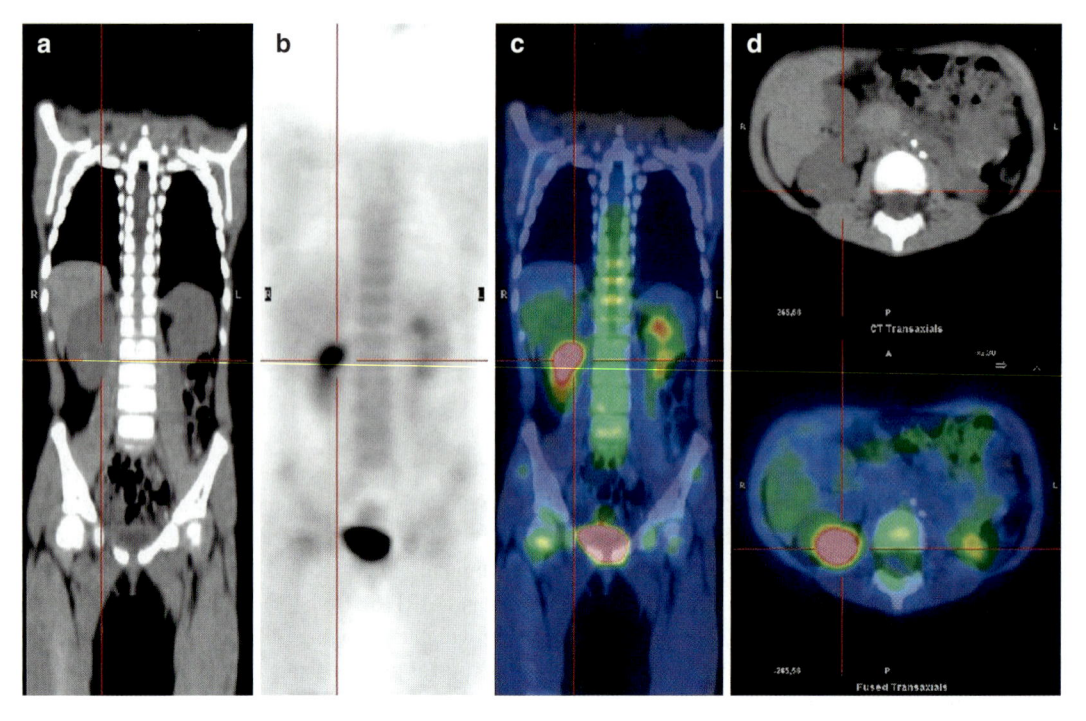

Fig. 16.1 A 3-year-old girl treated for Wilms' tumor. Coronal (**a–c**) CT, PET, and PET/CT fusion images together with an axial (**d**) CT and PET/CT fusion image show an ^{18}F-FDG-avid lesion at the upper pole of the right kidney, corresponding to disease recurrence

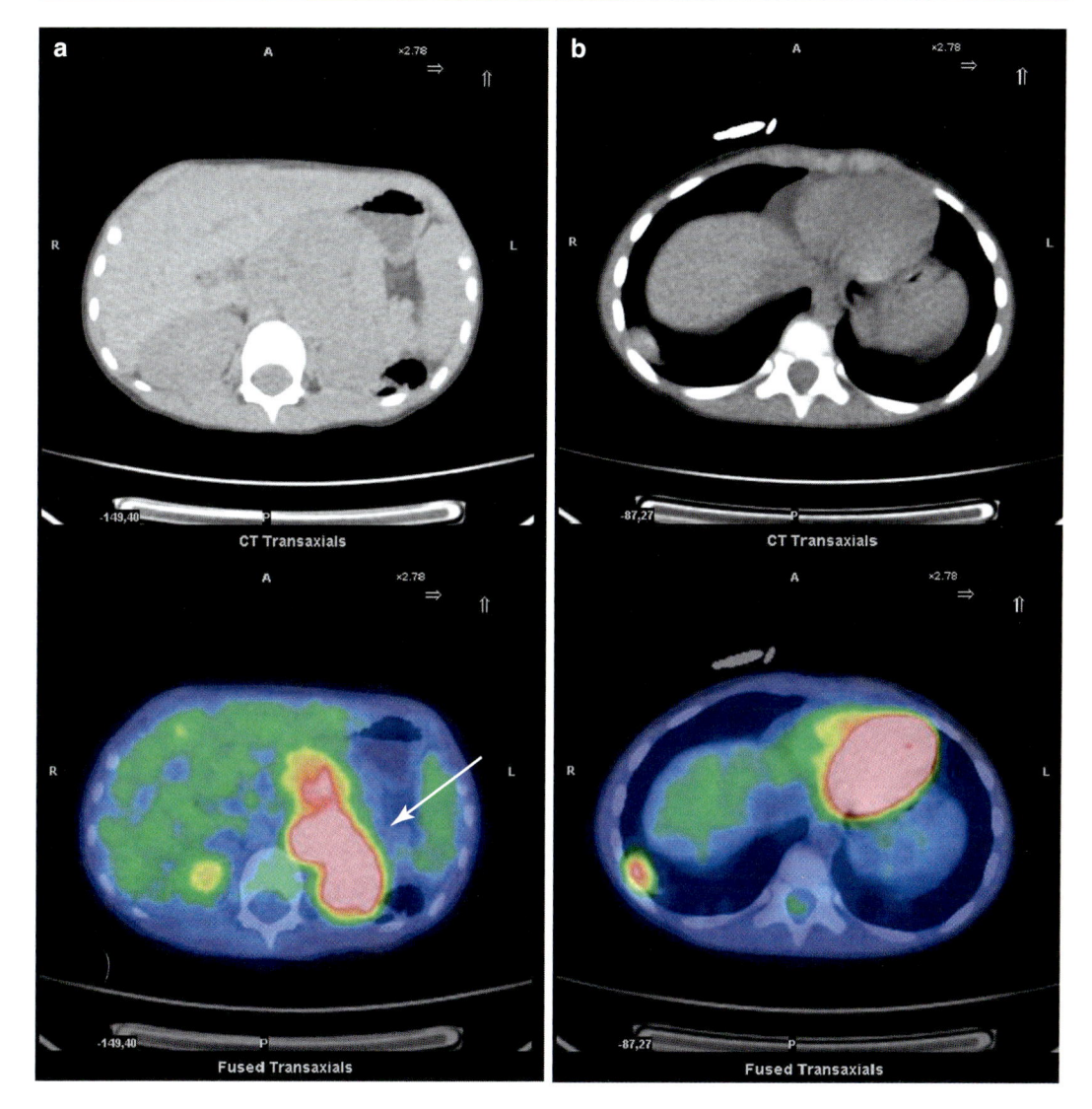

Fig. 16.2 A 3-year-old boy treated for Wilms' tumor. Axial CT of the abdomen (**a**) and chest (**b**) and PET/CT fusion images show the extensive pathological involvement of the left kidney region (*white arrow* in **a**) and another accumulation in the basal segment of the lower right lung lobe

References

1. Smets AM, de Kraker J (2010) Malignant tumours of the kidney: imaging strategy. Pediatr Radiol 40:1010–1018
2. Charles AK, Vujanic GM, Berry PJ (1998) Renal tumours of childhood. Histopathology 32:293–309
3. Israels T, Moreira C, Scanlan T et al (2013) SIOP PODC: clinical guidelines for the management of children with Wilms tumour in a low income setting. Pediatr Blood Cancer 60:5–11
4. Wootton-Gorges SL, Albano EA, Riggs JM et al (2000) Chest radiography versus chest CT in the evaluation for pulmonary metastases in patients with Wilms' tumor: a retrospective review. Pediatr Radiol 30:533–539
5. Grundy PE, Green DM, Dirks AC et al (2012) Clinical significance of pulmonary nodules detected by CT and Not CXR in patients treated for favorable histology Wilms tumor on national Wilms tumor studies-4 and -5: a report from the Children's Oncology Group. Pediatr Blood Cancer 59:631–635
6. Owens CM, Brisse HJ, Olsen ØE et al (2008) Bilateral disease and new trends in Wilms tumour. Pediatr Radiol 38:30–39
7. Moinul Hossain AK, Shulkin BL, Gelfand MJ et al (2010) FDG positron emission tomography/computed tomography studies of Wilms' tumor. Eur J Nucl Med Mol Imaging 37:1300–1308
8. Levitt G (2012) Renal tumours: long-term outcome. Pediatr Nephrol 7:911–916

Adrenal Gland Cancers

17

Natale Quartuccio and Angelina Cistaro

Adrenal gland cancers refer to a heterogeneous group of neoplasms involving the cortex and adrenal medulla [1]. They include adenoma, myelolipoma, pheochromocytoma, metastases, adrenocortical carcinoma, neuroblastoma, and lymphoma [2]. Exact statistics on their incidences are not available [3]. Neuroblastoma is the most common extracranial solid tumor of childhood and accounts for 8 % of all cancers in the pediatric population [1, 4]. Adrenocortical carcinoma and pheochromocytoma, by contrast, are very rarely seen in children [5, 6]. Adrenal masses are currently evaluated by means of CT and MRI, which are of high sensitivity (>90 %) but low specificity [7]. The primary role of FDG-PET is to differentiate benign from malignant adrenal neoplasms [1] and to monitor the response to therapy (Figs. 17.1, 17.2, and 17.3) [8].

N. Quartuccio, MD
Nuclear Medicine Unit, Department of Biomedical Sciences and Morphological and Functional Images, University of Messina, Via Consolare Valeria 1, Messina 98125, Italy
e-mail: natale.quartuccio84@hotmail.it

A. Cistaro, MD (✉)
Department of Nuclear Medicine, Positron Emission Tomography Center IRMET S.p.A., Euromedic Inc., Via Onorato Vigliani 89, Turin 10100, Italy

Institute of Cognitive Sciences and Technologies, National Research Council, Rome, Italy
e-mail: a.cistaro@irmet.com

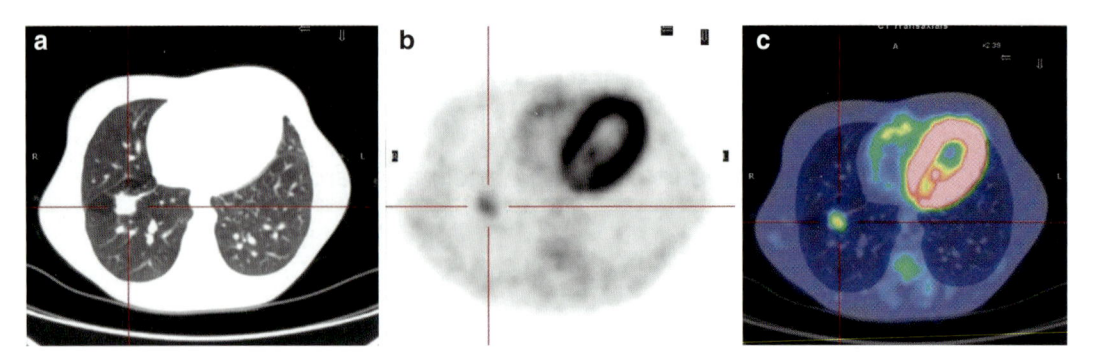

Fig. 17.1 A 9-year-old boy treated for adrenal gland carcinoma. Axial CT with lung window (**a**), PET (**b**), and PET/CT fusion (**c**) images show nonhomogeneous FDG uptake in the right lung, corresponding to a metastasis

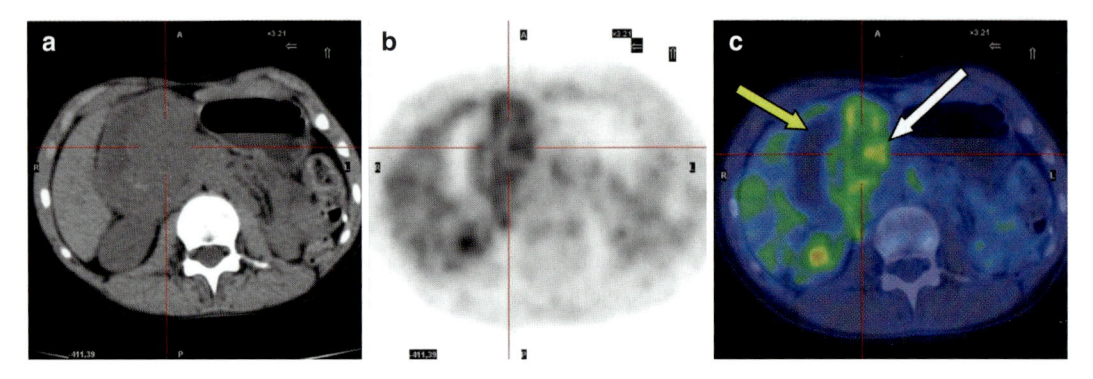

Fig. 17.2 Same patient during treatment with imatinib for disease relapse in the abdomen. Axial CT with abdominal window (**a**), PET (**b**), and PET/CT fusion (**c**) images show extensive nonhomogeneous FDG fixation in the (*right*) abdomen (*white arrow* in **c**). The area without FDG metabolism corresponds to the necrotic component of the lesion (*yellow arrow* in **c**)

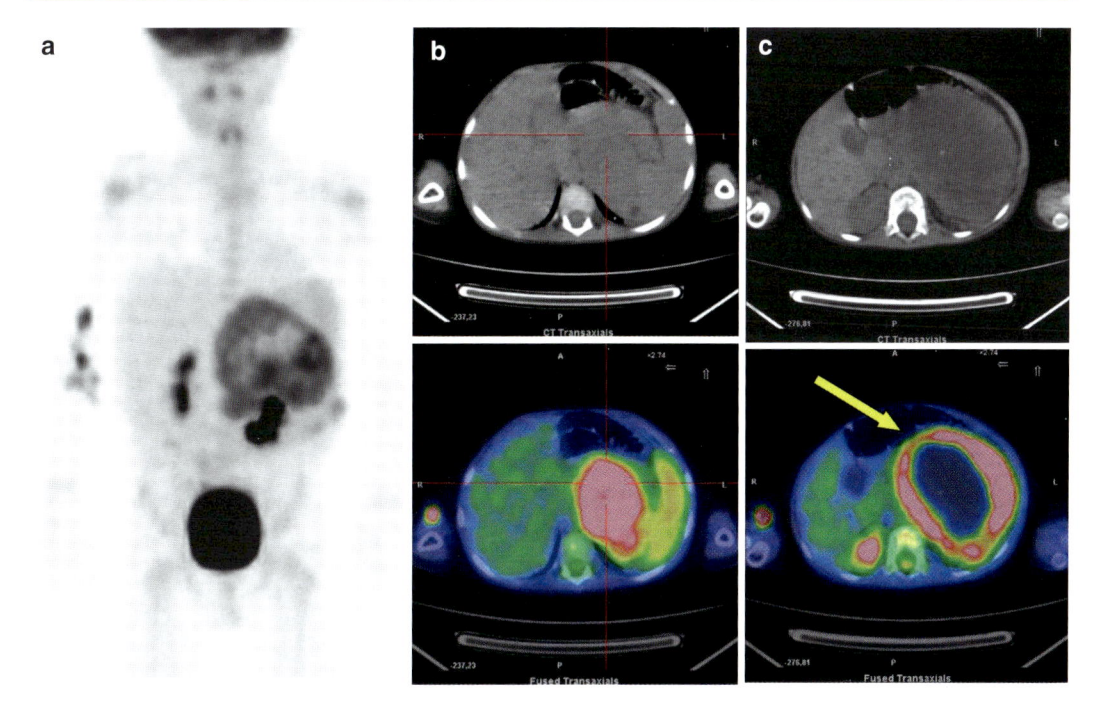

Fig. 17.3 A 3-year-old boy with adrenal gland carcinoma. Maximum intensity projection (**a**) and CT and PET/CT fusion images (**b, c**) show different aspects of the abdominal lesion. Note the broad, non-metabolizing central area, corresponding to necrosis (*yellow arrow* in **c**)

References

1. McHugh K (2007) Renal and adrenal tumours in children. Cancer Imaging 7:41–51
2. Low G, Dhliwayo H, Lomas DJ (2013) Adrenal neoplasms. Clin Radiol 67:988–1000
3. Cancer.Net Editorial Board (2013) Adrenal gland tumor – statistics. Cancer.net http://www.cancer.net/cancer-types/adrenal-gland-tumor/statistics. Accessed 30 Jun 2013
4. Weinstein JL, Katzenstein HM, Cohn SL (2003) Advances in the diagnosis and treatment of neuroblastoma. Oncologist 8:278–292
5. Chen QL, Su Z, Li YH et al (2011) Clinical characteristics of adrenocortical tumors in children. J Pediatr Endocrinol Metab 24:535–541
6. Waguespack SG, Rich T, Grubbs E et al (2010) A current review of the etiology, diagnosis, and treatment of pediatric pheochromocytoma and paraganglioma. J Clin Endocrinol Metab 95:2023–2037
7. Imani F, Agopian VG, Auerbach MS et al (2009) 18F-FDOPA PET and PET/CT accurately localize pheochromocytomas. J Nucl Med 50:513–519
8. Samuel AM (2010) PET/CT in pediatric oncology. Indian J Cancer 47:360–370

Ovarian Teratomas

Angelina Cistaro

Ovarian teratoma, also called dermoid cyst of the ovary, is a bizarre, usually benign tumor in the ovary that typically contains a diversity of tissues, including hair, teeth, and bone. Collectively, teratomas constitute half of all pediatric ovarian neoplasms, and 1 % of these are malignant immature teratomas (Figs. 18.1 and 18.2) [1]. The long-term survival of patients with mature teratomas is good, whereas in those with immature teratomas, long-term survival following surgery only is related to tumor grade and especially to the contribution of neural elements.

A. Cistaro MD
Department of Nuclear Medicine,
Positron Emission Tomography Center IRMET
S.p.A., Euromedic Inc., Via Onorato Vigliani 89,
Turin 10100, Italy

Institute of Cognitive Sciences and Technologies,
National Research Council, Rome, Italy
e-mail: a.cistaro@irmet.com

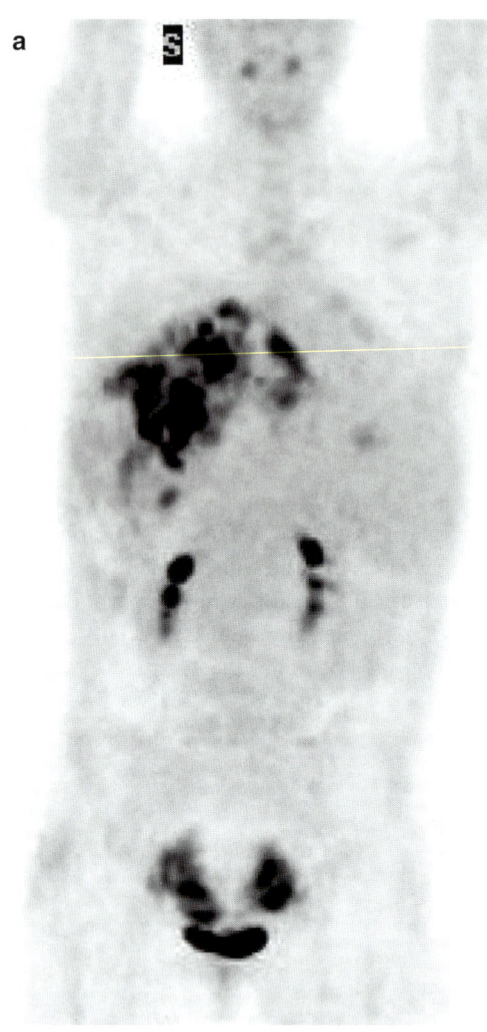

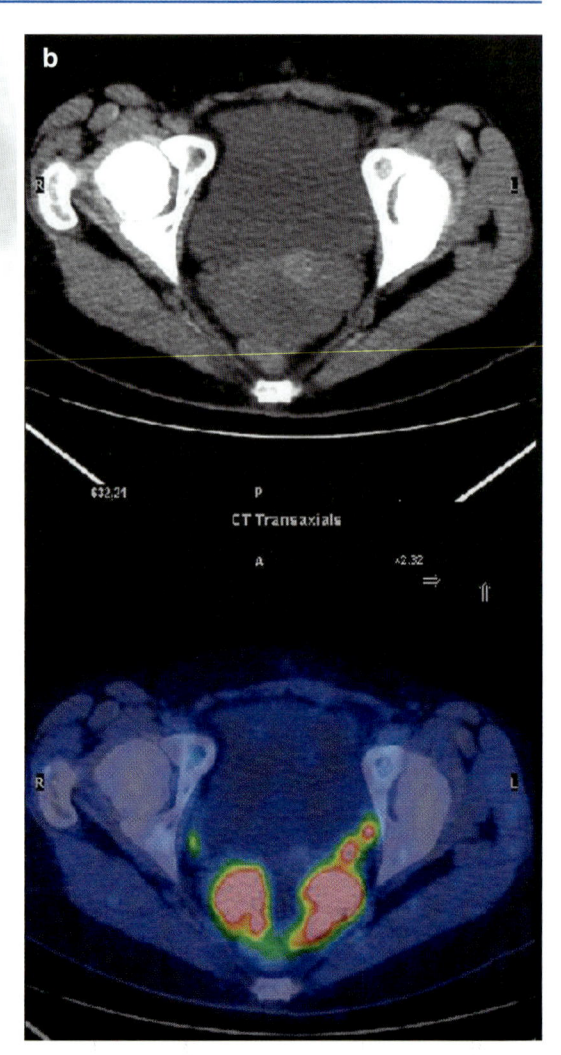

Fig. 18.1 A 12-year-old girl with a positive biopsy for malignant ovarian teratoma. Maximum intensity projection (**a**) shows diffuse pathological FDG uptakes in the pelvis and upper abdomen. Axial abdominal window CT and PET/CT fusion images (**b**) show the FDG-avid lesions in the pelvis

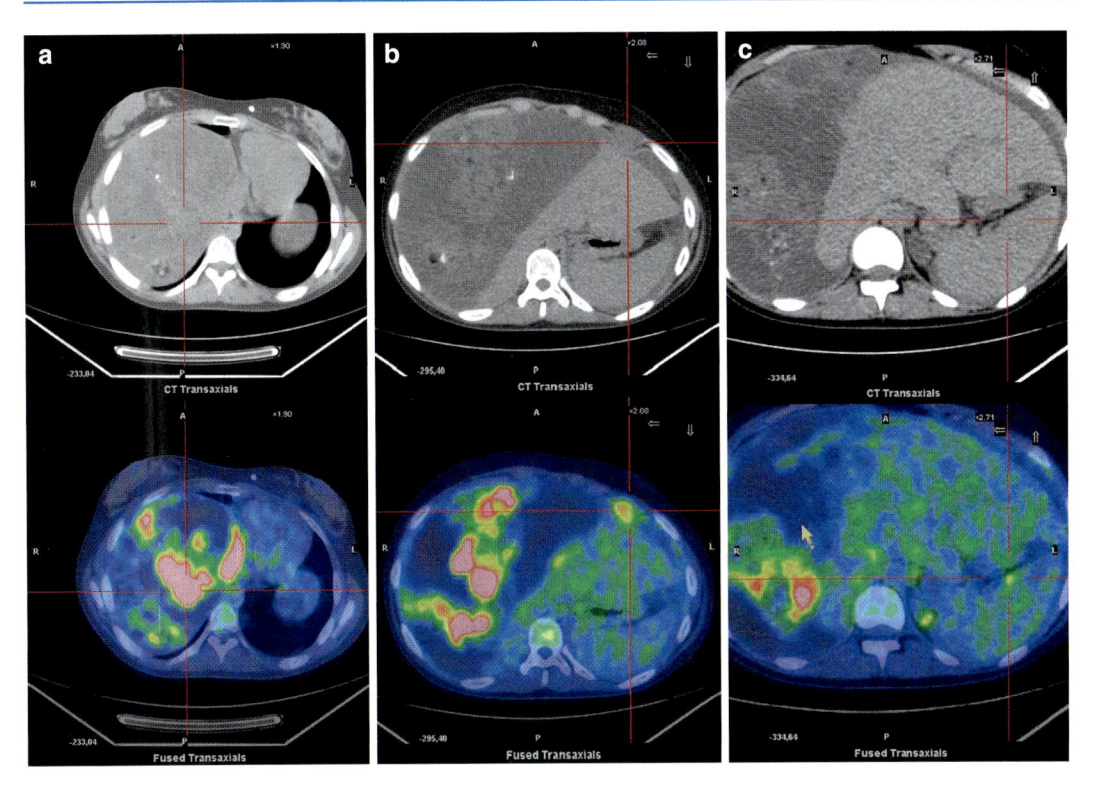

Fig. 18.2 Same patient. (**a–c**) Axial abdominal window CT and PET/CT fusion images show diffuse subglissonian (**a**), peritoneal (**b**), and peri-splenic (**c**) FDG-avid lesions

Teaching Point
In patients with suspected malignant teratoma, ^{18}F-FDG–PET/CT may help in the accurate diagnosis and staging, similar to its use in other malignant diseases, allowing a more aggressive multimodality treatment [2, 3].

References
1. Azizkhan RG, Caty MG (1996) Teratomas in childhood. Curr Opin Pediatr 8(3):287–292
2. Balink H, Apperloo MJ, Collins J (2012) Assessment of ovarian teratoma and lymphadenopathy by 18F-FDG PET/CT. Clin Nucl Med 37(8):804–806
3. Miyasaka N, Kubota T (2011) Unusually intense 18F-fluorodeoxyglucose (FDG) uptake by a mature ovarian teratoma: a pitfall of FDG positron emission tomography. J Obstet Gynaecol Res 37(6):623–628

Part IV

Neurology

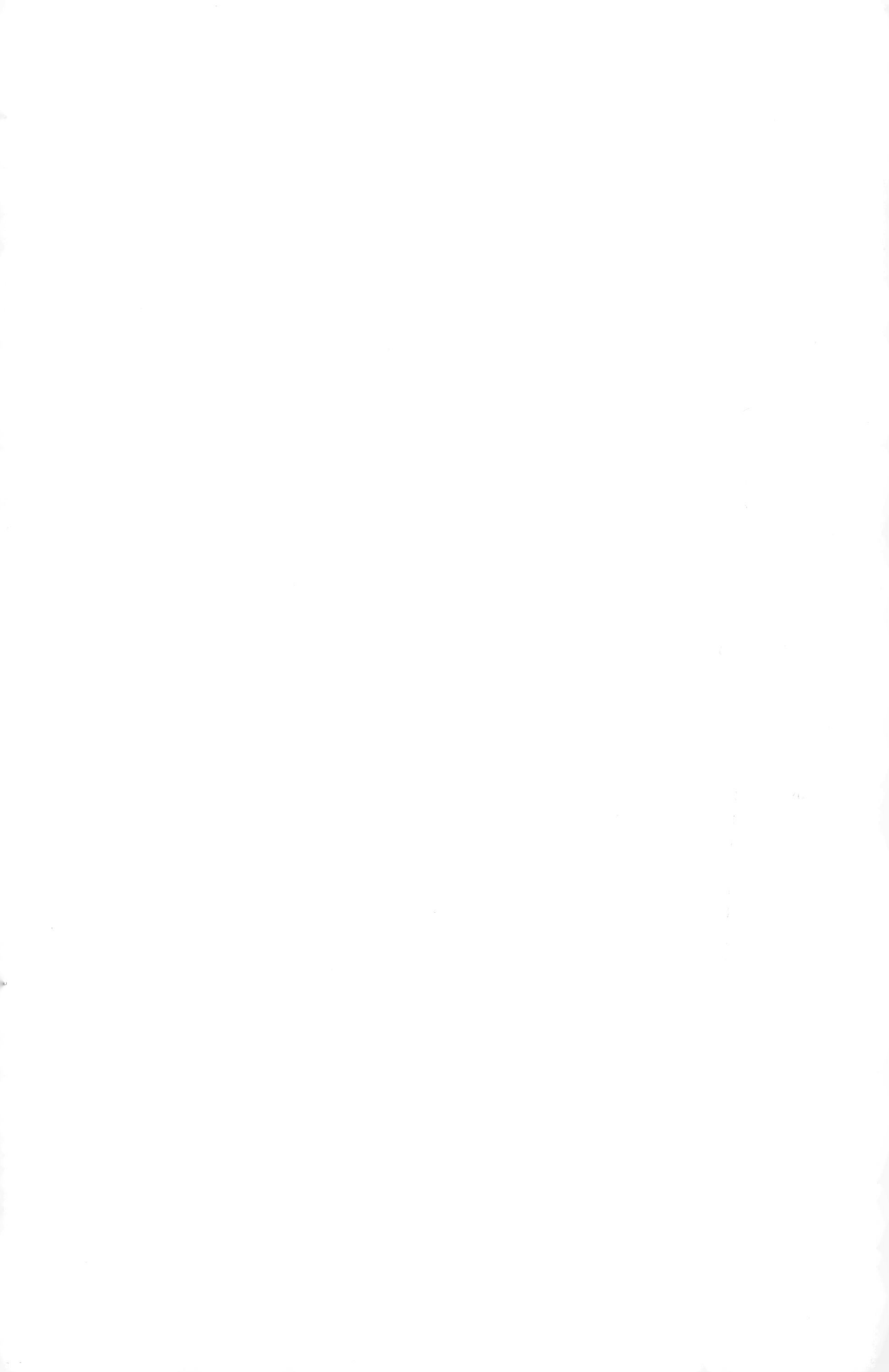

Role of Amino Acid PET Tracers in Pediatric Brain Tumors

19

Arnoldo Piccardo and Giovanni Morana

Brain tumors are the most common solid neoplasm in children, accounting for 20–25 % of all primary pediatric malignancies. Despite the steady and considerable improvement in the prognosis of pediatric patients with brain tumors, current therapies still carry a high risk of side effects, especially for the very young [1]. Central nervous system (CNS) tumors remain the principal cause of cancer mortality in children [2].

Childhood brain tumors display a high pathological heterogeneity regarding the type of tumor, the overall incidence, and the outcome, all of which vary with patient age. Whereas most brain tumors in adults are gliomas (≈70 % malignant anaplastic astrocytoma and glioblastoma), a significant portion of pediatric brain tumors consist of medulloblastoma, pilocytic astrocytomas, ependymomas, and craniopharyngioma [3, 4]. Supratentorial tumors are more common in the first 2 years of life and again in adolescents, whereas infratentorial neoplasms are frequently seen in children between 3 and 11 years of age.

Another major difference from the adult population is the known prevalence of primitive intra-axial tumors, whereas extra-axial and secondary neoplasms are distinctly uncommon [5].

The treatment of children with CNS tumors is challenging and requires an integrated multidisciplinary approach that brings together different disciplines, including neurosurgery, neuro-oncology, diagnostic imaging, neuropathology, and radiation medicine. Surgical resection is the first-line treatment option and is a significant prognostic factor in the management of several pediatric CNS tumors. When complete surgical removal is not possible, biopsy or partial debulking is an alternative, followed by adjuvant therapy consisting of either radiotherapy, chemotherapy, or both. For malignant brain tumors (e.g., medulloblastoma, malignant glioma) and some lower-grade tumors, adjuvant therapy is administered even if a complete resection is achieved because of concerns about residual microscopic disease. Thus, surgery in combination with chemotherapy and/or radiotherapy is the mainstay of treatment for many pediatric brain tumors [6–8].

Advances in neurosurgical techniques, radiotherapy planning, and novel chemotherapeutics have paralleled the increasing demand for noninvasive diagnostic techniques. In this respect, diagnostic imaging plays a key role in determining the most appropriate treatment strategy and then in following its efficacy. Conventional MRI with gadolinium-based contrast agents is the current imaging modality of choice and provides excellent anatomic and morphological imaging

A. Piccardo, MD (✉)
Nuclear Medicine Department, E.O. Ospedali Galliera,
Mura delle Cappuccine 14, Genoa 16128, Italy
e-mail: arnoldo.piccardo@galliera.it

G. Morana, MD
Unit of Pediatric Neuroradiology,
Department of Radiology,
G. Gaslini Children's Research Hospital,
Largo G. Gaslini 5, Genoa 16147, Italy
e-mail: giovannimorana@ospedale-gaslini.ge.it

of brain tumors. However, it suffers from certain limitations in distinguishing tumor from tumor-like pathology and in defining tumor type and grade, nor does it always allow the precise delineation of tumor margins. It also does not readily differentiate between true tumor and treatment-induced changes, such as "pseudoprogression" or "pseudoresponse," especially in the early phase of treatment monitoring. Furthermore, conventional MRI does not provide information about the biological activity of the disease, thus limiting its clinical usefulness in therapeutic decision-making [9–13]. There is an urgent need for novel imaging biomarkers that allow a more precise evaluation of brain tumors, including tumor diagnosis but also treatment planning, response to treatment assessment, and posttreatment surveillance.

Very little research has been published regarding the role of PET in pediatric neuro-oncology. Recent studies have suggested that ^{18}F-FDG–PET is useful in the evaluation of brain tumors in children [14] as it complements MRI and can identify sites of metabolically active disease. However, there are also important limitations of ^{18}F-FDG–PET imaging. Because of the high rate of physiological glucose metabolism in normal brain tissue, the detection of tumors with weak FDG uptake, such as low-grade tumors and, in some cases, recurrent high-grade tumors, is difficult. ^{18}F-FDG uptake in low-grade tumors is usually similar to that in normal white matter, while uptake in high-grade tumors may be less than or similar to that in normal gray matter, thus decreasing the sensitivity of lesion detection. Overall, the principal role of ^{18}F-FDG–PET thus far is in prognosis determination. In fact, an association between tumor tracer uptake and patient outcome has been reported [14–17].

A growing body of evidence suggests that PET carried out with amino acid tracers increases the diagnostic accuracy of brain tumor evaluation. Increased radiolabeled amino acid uptake in brain tumors correlates with their increased use of amino acids for energy, protein synthesis, and cell division, associated with the overexpression of amino acid transporter systems, and provides an estimate of tumor growth and vitality. Amino acid analogues such as ^{11}C-methionine and ^{18}F-DOPA has advantages over ^{18}F-FDG in the metabolic imaging of brain tumors because of the high uptake of these alternate tracers in tumor tissue and their low uptake in normal brain tissue. In addition, as these tracers are taken up by active transport mechanisms, neither the visualization nor the characterization of brain tumors depends on the status of the blood–brain barrier, such that the labeled amino acids are taken up by enhancing as well as non-enhancing tumors. The impact of ^{11}C-methionine PET in adults is well established and has been shown to improve the clinical management of patients with gliomas. Specifically, ^{11}C-methionine PET yields important clinical information on newly diagnosed tumors (high diagnostic accuracy and determination of tumor extent in high- and low-grade gliomas), directly influencing biopsy planning, surgical treatment, and radiotherapy planning [18]. This approach can also be used to assess tumor response after radiotherapy or chemotherapy and in this setting is better than other imaging modalities [18].

In pediatric brain tumors, few data on the role ^{11}C-methionine PET are currently available. A recently published study [19] focusing on children with incidental brain lesions showed that ^{11}C-methionine PET had a much higher sensitivity and specificity than MRI in the detection of tumor tissue and malignant tumors. According to the authors, ^{11}C-methionine PET can have a significant impact on the surgical treatment of these patients. In particular, a more conservative approach is possible for new brain lesions without tracer uptake vs. more aggressive treatment of those exhibiting intense ^{11}C-methionine uptake [19].

A number of second-generation amino acid tracers labeled with radioisotopes of longer half-life are under active development. Among these, ^{18}F-DOPA has shown promise as a tracer for brain tumor imaging, with a high sensitivity for gliomas (96 %) and providing excellent visualization of low- and high-grade lesions (Figs. 19.1, 19.2, 19.3, and 19.4) [17]. ^{18}F-DOPA is an amino acid PET tracer similar to other ^{18}F-labeled radiopharmaceuticals, such as O-(2-[^{18}F]fluoroethyl)-L-tyrosine, L-3-[^{18}F]-fluoromethyltyrosine, or ^{11}C-methionine [20]. ^{18}F-DOPA uptake in brain tumors is essentially

19 Role of Amino Acid PET Tracers in Pediatric Brain Tumors

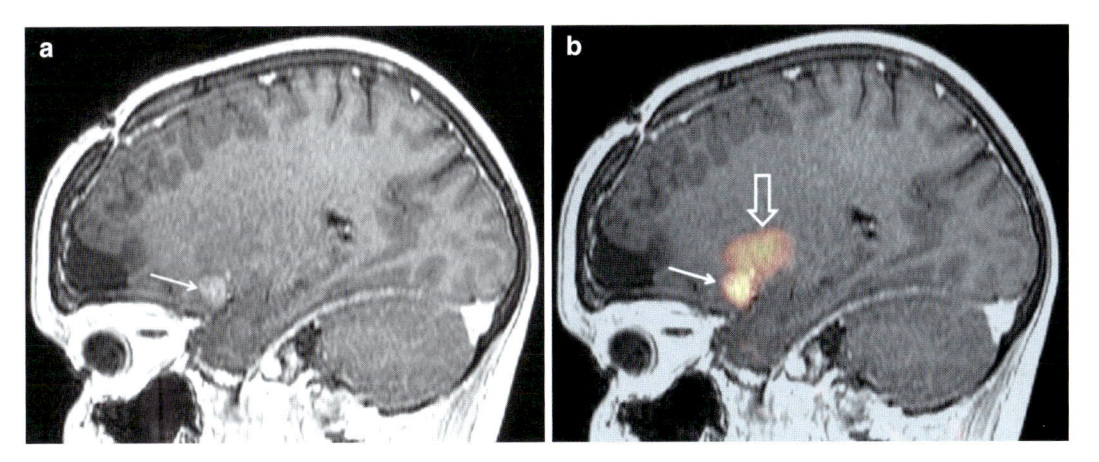

Fig. 19.1 Recurrent ganglioglioma in an 8-year-old girl. (**a**) Sagittal Gd-enhanced T1-weighted image; (**b**) ^{18}F-DOPA–PET/MRI fusion image. There is a focal, rounded, contrast-enhancing lesion in the inferior frontal gyrus (*thin arrow* in **a**) with elevated ^{18}F-DOPA activity (*thin arrow* in **b**). Normal tracer uptake in the adjacent striatum (*open arrow* in **b**) is seen as well

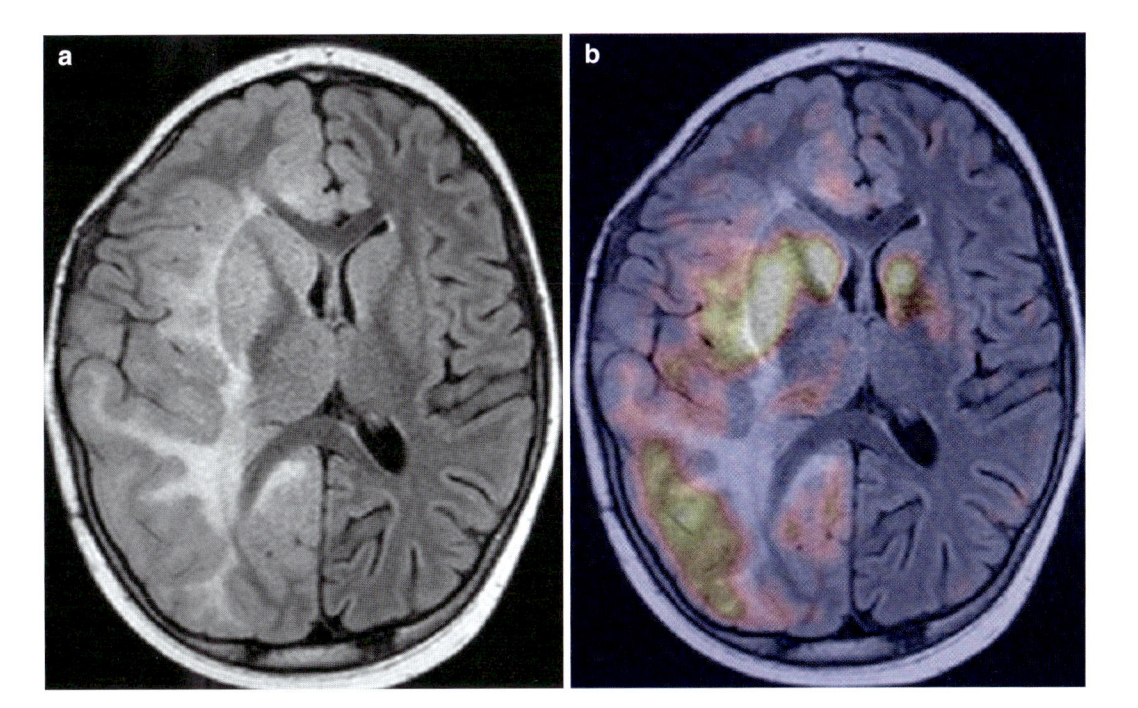

Fig. 19.2 Gliomatosis cerebri in a 10-year-old boy. (**a**) Axial fluid attenuated inversion recovery (FLAIR) image; (**b**) ^{18}F-DOPA–PET/MRI fusion image. There is an extensive diffusely infiltrating lesion involving the right cerebral hemisphere (**a**) with heterogeneous, increased tracer uptake (**b**)

the same as that of ^{11}C-methionine [21, 22], which to date is the most frequently used radiolabeled amino acid in brain tumors. Becherer et al. compared these two different amino acid PET tracers in adults and found that ^{18}F-DOPA and ^{11}C-methionine images matched in all cases, showing all lesions as hot spots with higher uptake than in the contralateral aspect of the

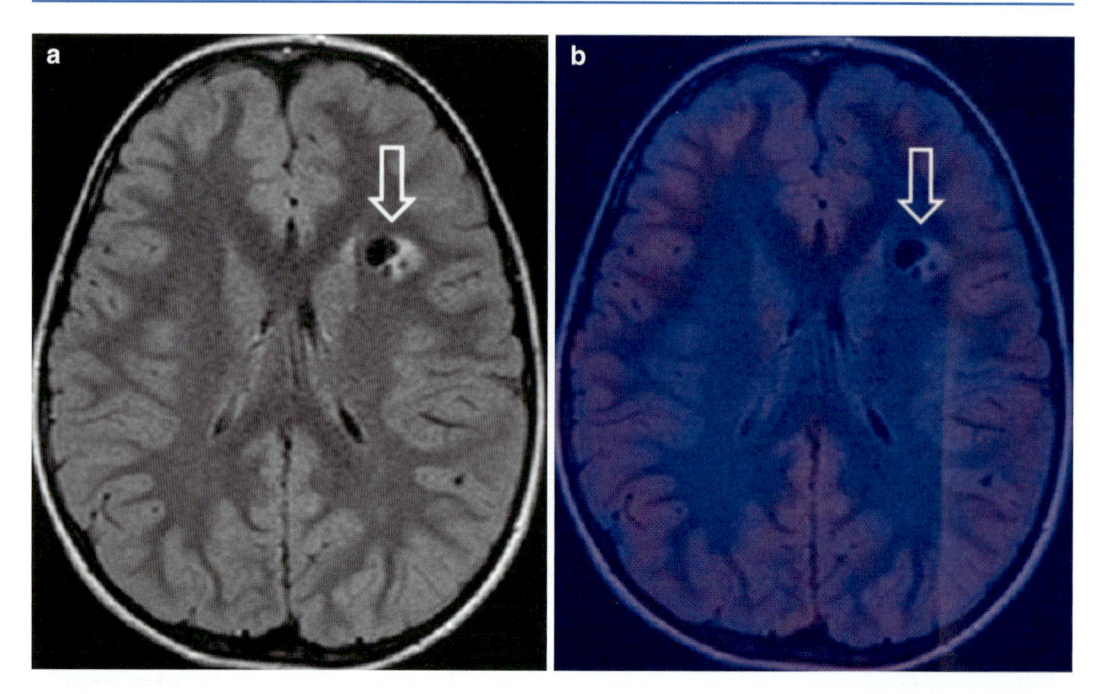

Fig. 19.3 Suspected brain tumor on MRI in a 12-year-old boy. (**a**) Axial FLAIR image shows a focal lesion within the left frontal white matter (*open arrow*) suspicious for a brain tumor. (**b**) ^{18}F-DOPA–PET/MRI fusion image shows a lack of tracer uptake (*open arrow*). No neoplastic tissue was demonstrated after stereotactic biopsy

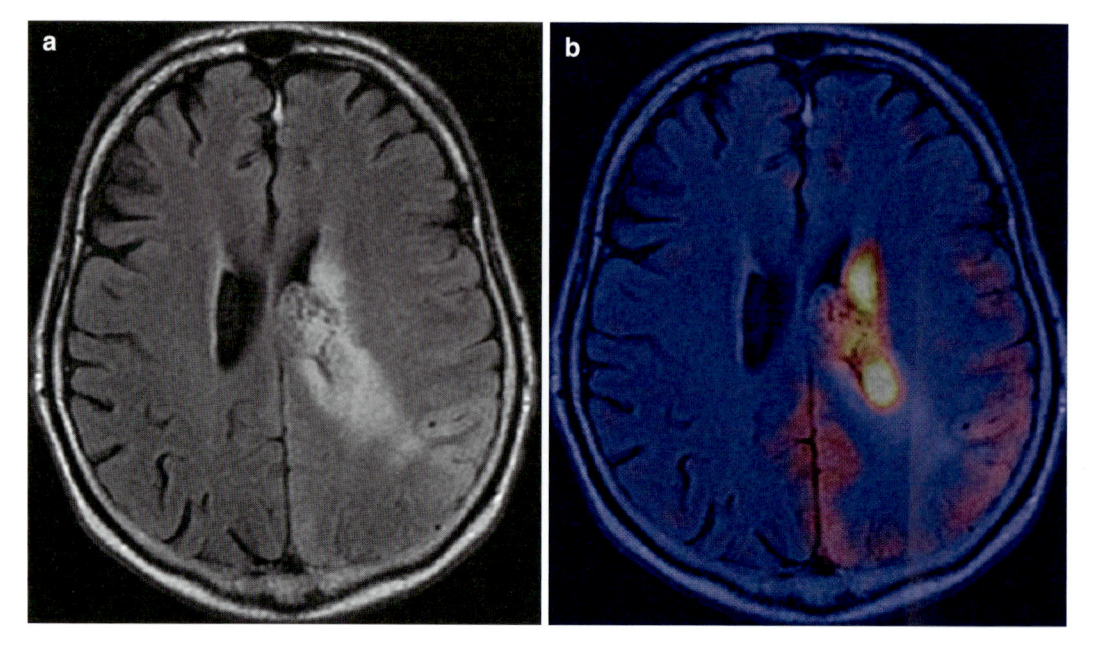

Fig. 19.4 Anaplastic astrocytoma in a 17-year-old boy. (**a**) Axial FLAIR image shows a periventricular expansive/infiltrating lesion with involvement of the left parietal cortex. (**b**) ^{18}F-DOPA–PET/MRI fusion image shows heterogeneous, increased traced uptake

healthy brain [22]. The major advantage of ^{18}F-DOPA over ^{11}C-methionine is its longer half-life, which enables its widespread use without the need for an on-site cyclotron [23]. In children, the use of ^{18}F-DOPA to image catecholamine-producing tumors and in congenital hyperinsulinism is well established; however, the diagnostic impact of this tracer in pediatric brain tumors is thus far largely unexplored [24–27]. Only two children (one with pilocytic astrocytoma and another with ependymoma) have been evaluated with ^{18}F-DOPA by Tripathi et al. in 2009 [28].

We recently studied a pediatric patient with malignant transformation of ganglioglioma treated with bevacizumab and were able demonstrate the significant contribution of combined multimodal MRI and ^{18}F-DOPA–PET in the early diagnosis of tumor "pseudoresponse" and non-enhancing tumor progression [29]. Anti-angiogenic agents, especially those targeting vascular endothelial growth factor, such as bevacizumab, are increasingly used in pediatric patients with high-grade tumors. Previous studies in adults demonstrated that the differentiation between brain tumor response and tumor progression following treatment with bevacizumab poses a complex diagnostic challenge. This monoclonal antibody produces a dramatic decrease in the contrast enhancement of the lesion on conventional MRI, a phenomenon called "pseudoresponse." The prefix "pseudo" refers to the fact that the imaging change reflects restoration of the blood–brain barrier rather than a true tumor response. Despite this stably reduced or absent contrast enhancement, patients can develop neurological worsening, with an increase of T2/FLAIR MRI abnormalities on follow-up studies, in keeping with a pattern of non-enhancing but progressive disease. Since an objective criterion for non-enhancing tumor progression is currently unfeasible, these patients must be closely and repeatedly followed until a confident disease evaluation is possible, as this will significantly influence decision-making regarding treatment continuation or discontinuation.

Our results suggest that ^{18}F-DOPA–PET imaging in patients treated with anti-angiogenesis agents deserves further investigation to evaluate the potentially promising role of this novel imaging modality [29]. Overall, on the basis of our preliminary experience in pediatric patients with brain tumors, the results obtained with ^{18}F-DOPA confirm previous data from adults [30] in terms of the impact of this tracer on patient management and/or treatment decisions. Further investigations with larger series are thus also needed to validate the use of amino acid PET tracers in improving diagnostic accuracy, monitoring dynamic changes within brain tumors during therapy, and establishing whether (and if so, how and when) these radiolabeled amino acids should become a critical part of the clinical management of pediatric patients with brain tumors. Correlation with MRI data is mandatory for an accurate interpretation of PET results and thus a close collaboration between neuroradiologists and nuclear medicine physicians. Greater efforts within the diagnostic imaging community should be directed at improving the integration of information obtained by different imaging modalities in order to overcome their respective limitations. The result will be a more robust tool in the crucial evaluation of pediatric brain tumors.

Teaching Point

Amino acid PET tracers have an important role in adult brain tumors, influencing treatment management. The overall diagnostic accuracy of these tracers for brain tumor evaluation is higher than that of ^{18}F-FDG [17]. Tumor detection and grading, biopsy, radiotherapy planning, posttreatment monitoring, and the evaluation of recurrent disease are among the most important applications [18]. Although few data are available on the role and impact of these newly developed tracers in pediatric brain tumors, ^{11}C-methionine and ^{18}F-DOPA have thus far shown great promise based on their ability to add useful diagnostic information to clinical and conventional MRI data. To further increase their diagnostic role, a correlation between the results obtained with these tracers and MRI findings is mandatory.

References

1. Muller S, Chang S (2009) Pediatric brain tumors: current treatment strategies and future therapeutics approaches. Neurotherapeutics 6:570–586
2. Young H, Baum R, Cremerius U et al (1999) Measurement of clinical and subclinical tumour response using [18F]-fluorodeoxyglucose and positron emission tomography: review and 1999 EORTC recommendations. European Organization for Research and Treatment of Cancer (EORTC) PET Study Group. Eur J Cancer 35:1773–1782
3. Pötter R, Czech TH, Dieckmann I et al (1998) Tumors of the central nervous system. In: Voute PA, Kalifa C, Barrett A (eds) Cancer in children. Clinical management, 4th edn. Oxford University Press, New York, pp 170–193
4. Panigrahy A, Blüml S (2009) Neuroimaging of pediatric brain tumors: from basic to advanced magnetic resonance imaging (MRI). J Child Neurol 24:1343–1365
5. Tortori-Donati P, Rossi A, Biancheri R et al (2005) Brain Tumors. In: Tortori-Donati P (ed) Pediatric neuroradiology. Springer, Berlin
6. Pollack IF (2011) Multidisciplinary management of childhood brain tumors: a review of outcomes, recent advances, and challenges. J Neurosurg Pediatr 8:135–148
7. Kalifa C, Grill J (2005) The therapy of infantile malignant brain tumors: current status? J Neurooncol 75:279–285
8. Sonderkaer S, Schmiegelow M, Carstensen H et al (2003) Long-term neurological outcome of childhood brain tumors treated by surgery only. J Clin Oncol 21:1347–1351
9. Gerstner ER, Sorensen AG, Jain RK, Batchelor TT (2008) Advances in neuroimaging techniques for the evaluation of tumor growth, vascular permeability, and angiogenesis in gliomas. Curr Opin Neurol 21:728–735
10. Gerstner ER, Batchelor TT (2010) Imaging and response criteria in gliomas. Curr Opin Oncol 22:598–603
11. Chen W, Silverman DH (2008) Advances in evaluation of primary brain tumors. Semin Nucl Med 38:240–250
12. Heiss WD, Raab P, Lanfermann H (2011) Multimodality assessment of brain tumors and tumor recurrence. J Nucl Med 52:1585–1600
13. Dhermain FG, Hau P, Lanfermann H, Jacobs AH et al (2010) Advanced MRI and PET imaging for assessment of treatment response in patients with gliomas. Lancet Neurol 9:906–920
14. Zukotynski KA, Fahey FH, Kocak M, Alavi A, Wong TZ, Treves ST et al (2011) Evaluation of 18F-FDG PET and MRI associations in pediatric diffuse intrinsic brain stem glioma: a report from the Pediatric Brain Tumor Consortium. J Nucl Med 52:188–195
15. Pirotte B, Lubansu A, Massager N, Wikler D, Goldman S, Levivier M (2007) Results of positron emission tomography guidance and reassessment of the utility of and indications for stereotactic biopsy in children with infiltrative brainstem tumors. J Neurosurg 107(5 suppl):392–399
16. Williams G, Fahey F, Treves ST et al (2008) Exploratory evaluation of two-dimensional and three-dimensional methods of 18F-FDG PET quantification in pediatric anaplastic astrocytoma: a report from the Pediatric Brain Tumor Consortium (PBTC). Eur J Nucl Med Mol Imaging 35:1651–1658
17. Chen W, Silverman DH, Delaloye S et al (2006) 18F-FDOPA PET imaging of brain tumors: comparison study with 18F-FDG PET and evaluation of diagnostic accuracy. J Nucl Med 47:904–911
18. Singhal T, Narayanan TK, Jain V, Mukherjee J, Mantil J (2008) 11C-L-methionine positron emission tomography in the clinical management of cerebral gliomas. Mol Imaging Biol 10(1):1–18
19. Pirotte BJ, Lubansu A, Massager N et al (2010) Clinical interest of integrating positron emission tomography imaging in the workup of 55 children with incidentally diagnosed brain lesions. J Neurosurg Pediatr 5:479–485
20. Calabria F, Chiaravalloti A, Di Pietro B, Grasso C, Schillaci O (2012) Molecular imaging of brain tumors with 18F-DOPA PET and PET/CT. Nucl Med Commun 33:563–570
21. Fueger BJ, Czernin J, Cloughesy T, Silverman DH, Geist CL, Walter MA, Schiepers C, Nghiemphu P, Lai A, Phelps ME, Chen W (2010) Correlation of 6-18F-fluoro-L-dopa PET uptake with proliferation and tumor grade in newly diagnosed and recurrent gliomas. J Nucl Med 51:1532–1538
22. Becherer A, Karanikas G, Szabó M, Zettinig G, Asenbaum S, Marosi C et al (2003) Brain tumour imaging with PET: a comparison between [18F]fluorodopa and [11C]methionine. Eur J Nucl Med Mol Imaging 30:1561–1567
23. Jager PL, Vaalburg W, Pruim J, de Vries EG, Langen KJ, Piers DA (2001) Radiolabeled amino acids: basic aspects and clinical applications in oncology. J Nucl Med 42:432–445
24. Fiebrich HB, Brouwers AH, Kerstens MN, Pijl ME, Kema IP, de Jong J et al (2009) 6-[F-18] FluoroLdihydroxyphenylalanine positron emission tomography is superior to conventional imaging with (123)I metaiodobenzylguanidine scintigraphy, computer tomography, and magnetic resonance imaging in localizing tumors causing catecholamine excess. J Clin Endocrinol Metab 94(10):3922–3930
25. Piccardo A, Lopci E, Conte M, Garaventa A, Foppiani L, Altrinetti V, Nanni C, Bianchi P, Cistaro A, Sorrentino S, Cabria M, Pession A, Puntoni M, Villavecchia G, Fanti S (2012) Comparison of (18) F-dopa PET/CT and (123)I-MIBG scintigraphy in stage 3 and 4 neuroblastoma: a pilot study. Eur J Nucl Med Mol Imaging 39:57–61
26. Lopci E, Piccardo A, Nanni C, Altrinetti V, Garaventa A, Pession A et al (2012) 18F-DOPA PET/CT in neuroblastoma: comparison of conventional imaging with CT/MR. Clin Nucl Med 37:e73–e78

27. Ribeiro MJ, De Lonlay P, Delzescaux T, Boddaert N, Jaubert F, Bourgeois S et al (2005) Characterization of hyperinsulinism in infancy assessed with PET and 18F-fluoro-L-DOPA. J Nucl Med 46(4):560–566
28. Tripathi M, Sharma R, D'Souza M et al (2009) Comparative evaluation of F-18 FDOPA, F-18 FDG, and F-18 FLT-PET/CT for metabolic imaging of low grade gliomas. Clin Nucl Med 34:878–883
29. Morana G, Piccardo A, Garrè ML, Nozza P, Consales A, Rossi A (2013) Multimodal MRI and 18F-DOPA PET in early characterization of pseudoresponse and nonenhancing tumor progression in a pediatric patient with malignant transformation of ganglioglioma treated with bevacizumab. J Clin Oncol 31:e1–e5
30. Walter F, Cloughesy T, Walter MA, Lai A, Nghiemphu P, Wagle N, Fueger B, Satyamurthy N, Phelps ME, Czernin J (2012) Impact of 3,4-dihydroxy-6-18F-fluoro-L-phenylalanine PET/CT on managing patients with brain tumors: the referring physician's perspective. J Nucl Med 53:393–398

20

^{18}F-FDG in the Imaging of Brain Tumors

Angelina Cistaro, Piercarlo Fania, and Maria Consuelo Valentini

^{18}F-FDG PET in the evaluation of patients suspected of having a brain tumor include grading, localization for biopsy, differentiation of radiation necrosis from tumor recurrence, therapeutic monitoring, and assessment for malignant transformation of low-grade glioma.

^{18}F-FDG-PET imaging of brain tumors presents unique challenges because of the high background glucose metabolism of normal gray matter structures. Coregistration of the MRI or CT and FDG-PET images is essential for accurate evaluation of brain tumors. Together with delayed imaging acquisition, it improves the accuracy of interpretation and would be performed routinely.

A. Cistaro, MD (✉)
Department of Nuclear Medicine, Positron Emission Tomography Center IRMET S.p.A., Euromedic Inc., Via Onorato Vigliani 89, Turin 10100, Italy

Institute of Cognitive Sciences and Technologies, National Research Council, Rome, Italy
e-mail: a.cistaro@irmet.com

P. Fania
Brain Tumors Project, San Paolo IMI Foundation for Neuroradiology Department, CTO Hospital, Via Zuretti 29, Turin 10126, Italy
e-mail: piercarlo.fania_pf@hotmail.it

M.C. Valentini, PhD
Neuroradiology InterDepartment,
CTO – M.Adelaide-OIRM – S.Anna Hospitals and San Giovanni Battista Hospital, Via Zuretti 29, Turin 10126, Italy
e-mail: consuelovalentini@yahoo.it

Metabolic Characterization of Brain Lesions

Case 1

In 1993, the distinct pathological entity known as dysembryoplastic neuroepithelial tumor (DNET) was entered into the WHO classification of brain tumors as a grade I tumor of neuroepithelial origin [1–3]. On neuroimaging, DNETs are cortical lesions with little mass effect and a predilection for the temporal lobes (Figs. 20.1 and 20.2). On computed tomography, DNETs are typically well-demarcated, hypodense, cortical lesions that in some cases cause a deformation of the overlying skull. Magnetic resonance images often show a solid and cystic mass, with the cystic portions appearing slightly more intense than cerebrospinal fluid.

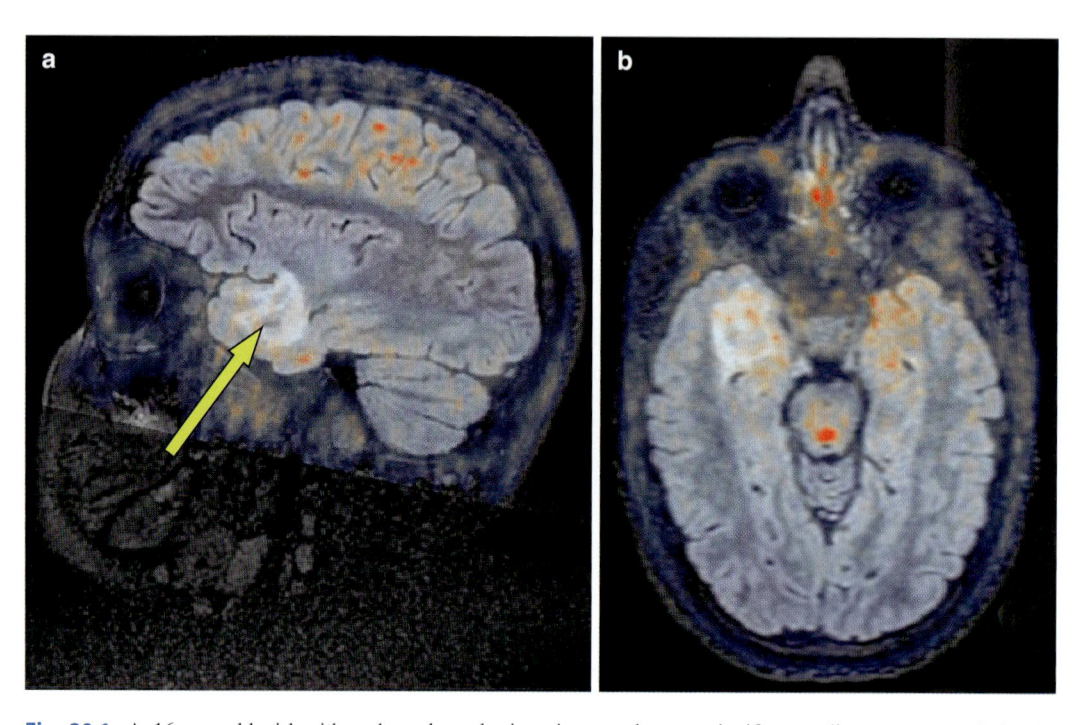

Fig. 20.1 A 16-year-old girl with a dysembryoplastic neuroepithelial tumor (DNET) and partial seizures. Sagittal (**a**) and axial (**b**) ^{18}F-DOPA–PET/MRI fusion images show no significant radiotracer accumulation by the right temporal lesion (*yellow arrow* in **a**)

Case 1 (continued)

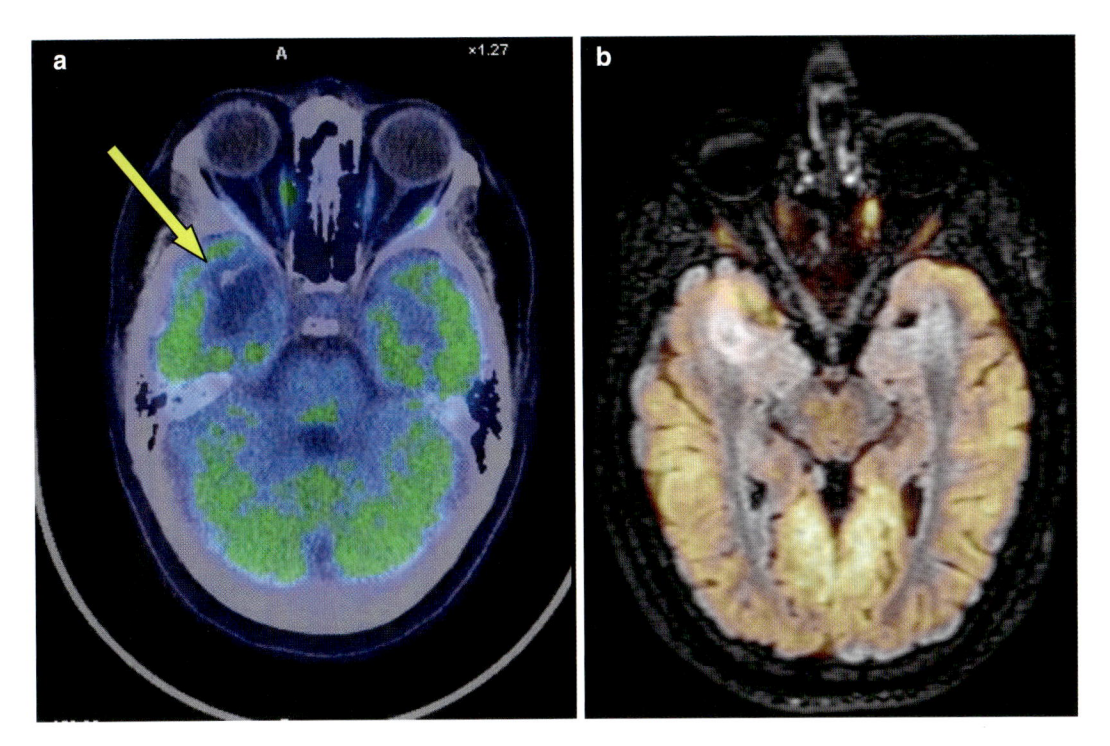

Fig. 20.2 Same patient. Axial ¹⁸F-FDG–PET/CT (**a**) and PET/MRI (**b**) fusion images show no significant radiocompound fixation in the temporal lesion (low metabolic lesion). On brain window CT, the lesion is well demarcated and hypodense (*yellow arrow* in **a**)

Case 2

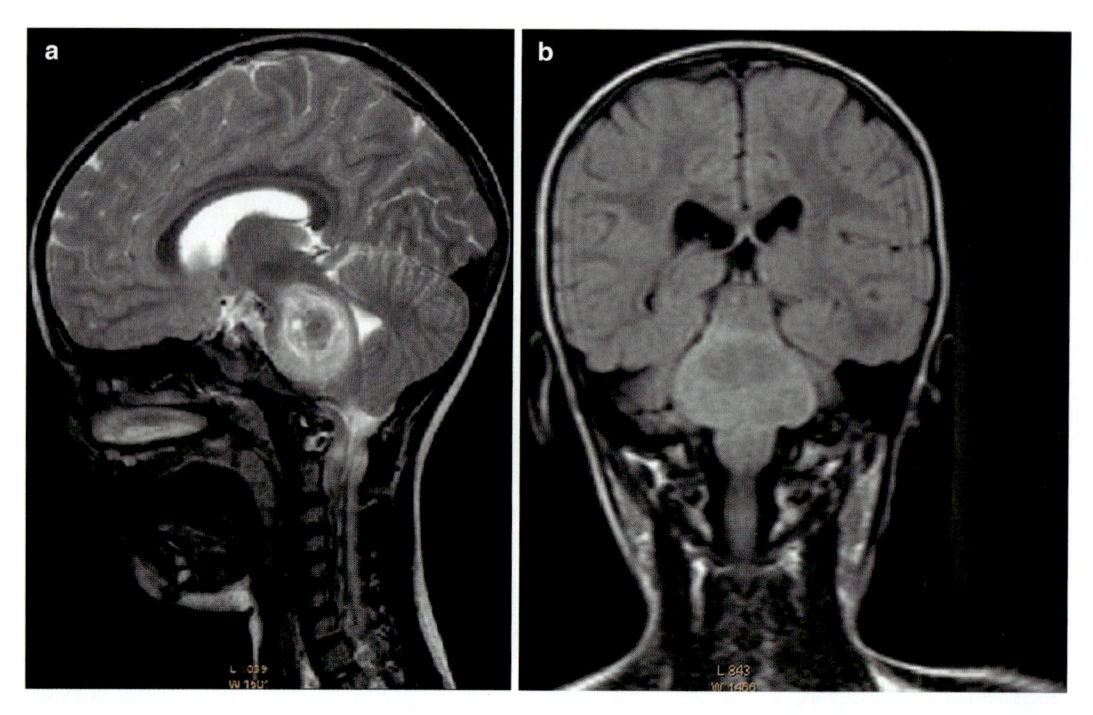

Fig. 20.3 A 5-year-old boy with headache, otalgia, diplopia, and strabismus, ataxic. (**a, b**) Sagittal and coronal MRI shows a large lesion of the pons that has caused its dimensional increase. The lesion appears inhomogeneous, with a parenchymal part and hemosiderin deposits. A glial tumor was suspected, but a vascular origin could not be excluded

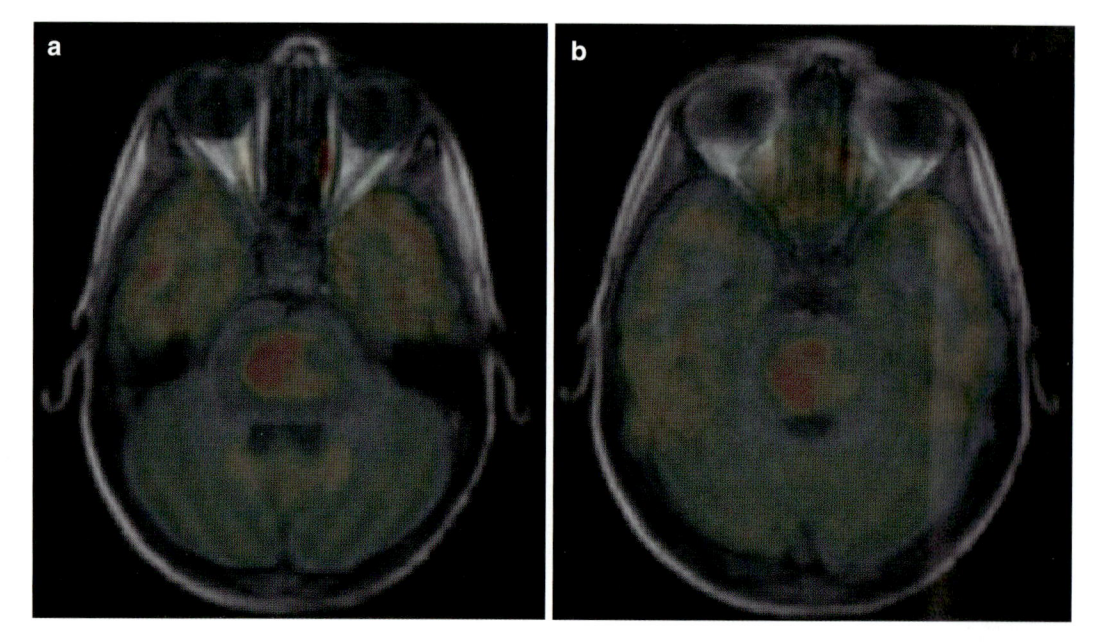

Fig. 20.4 Same patient as in Fig. 20.3. Axial PET/MRI fusion images (**a, b**) show the ^{18}F-FDG-avid lesion in the pons (highly metabolic lesion); neurological view

Case 2 (continued)

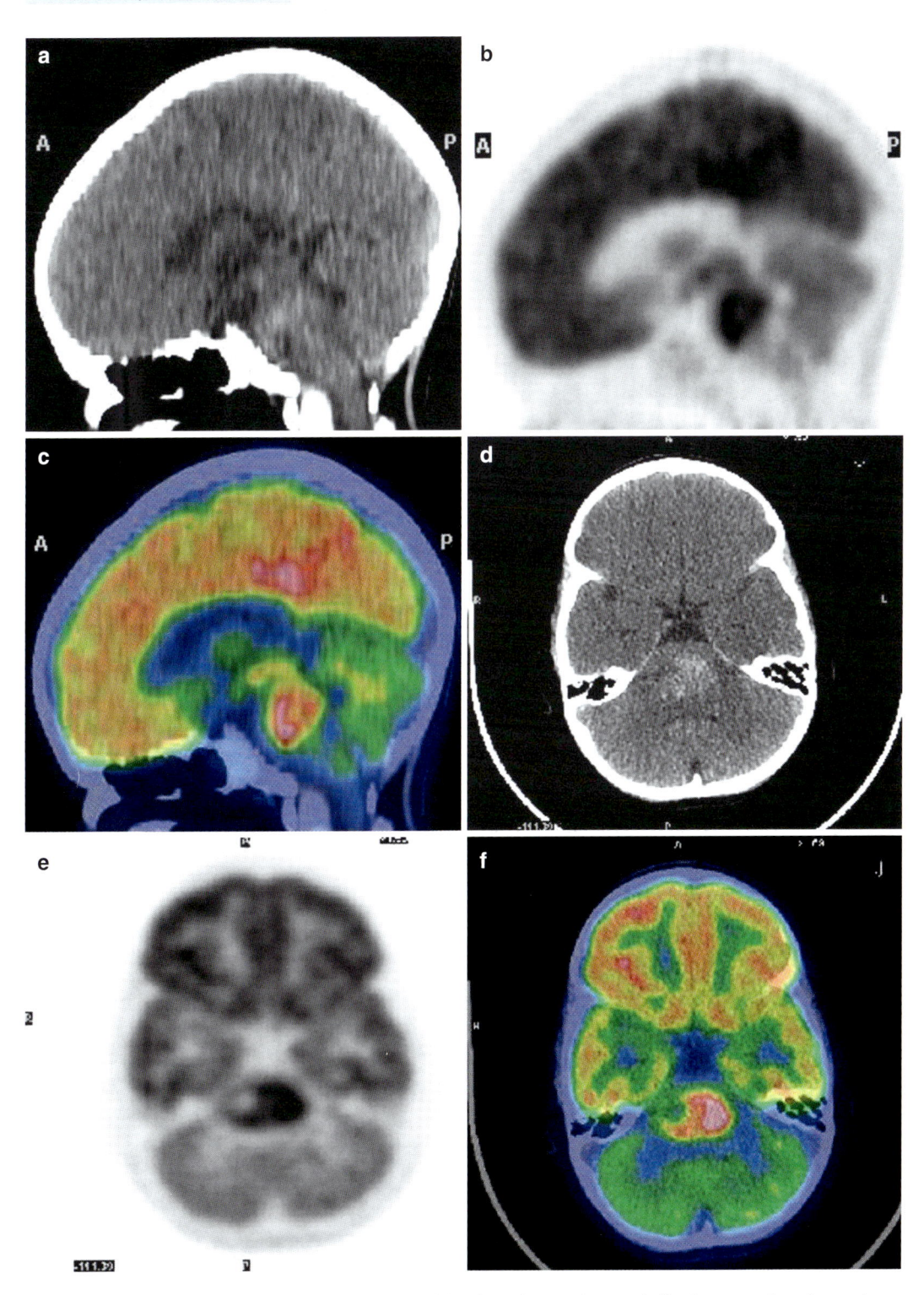

Fig. 20.5 Same patient as above. Sagittal (**a–c**) and axial (**d–f**) CT (**a**, **d**), PET (**b**, **e**) and PET/CT fusion (**c**, **f**) images show an intense FDG accumulation in the pons (SUV$_{max}$ 6.19), above the cortex. To the right of the lesion is a photopenic area, indicating necrosis or hemorrhage. The high FDG accumulation suggests an aggressive lesion; neuroradiologic view. The patient died 2 months later

Teaching Point

^{18}F-FDG–PET can be used in the differential diagnosis between high serial glial tumor and low grade and benign, e.g. vascular, lesions

Case 3

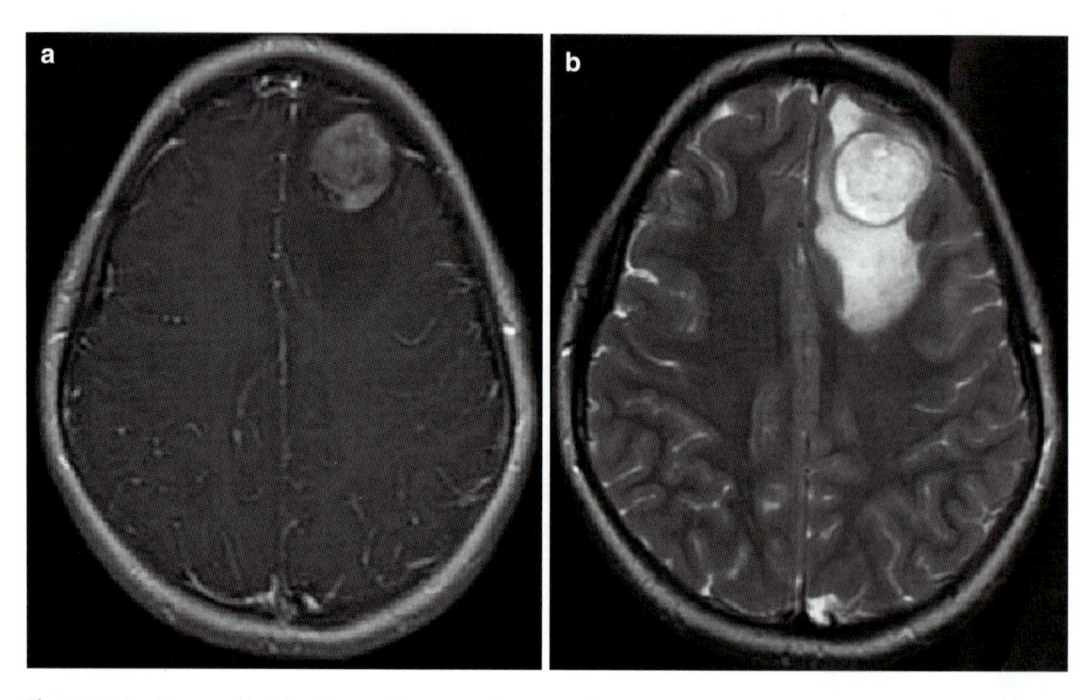

Fig. 20.6 An 11-year-old girl underwent liver transplantation 6 years earlier due to biliary atresia. Following a loss of consciousness, she was evaluated by MRI. Axial T1 (**a**) and T2 fast spin-echo (**b**) sequences show a superior frontal gyrus lesion, with a large edema component, surfacing the cortex. Spectroscopy and perfusion analysis showed an increase in the Cho/Cr ratio, a decrease in the NAA/Cr ratio, and an increase in relative cerebral blood volume (rCBV)

Case 3 (continued)

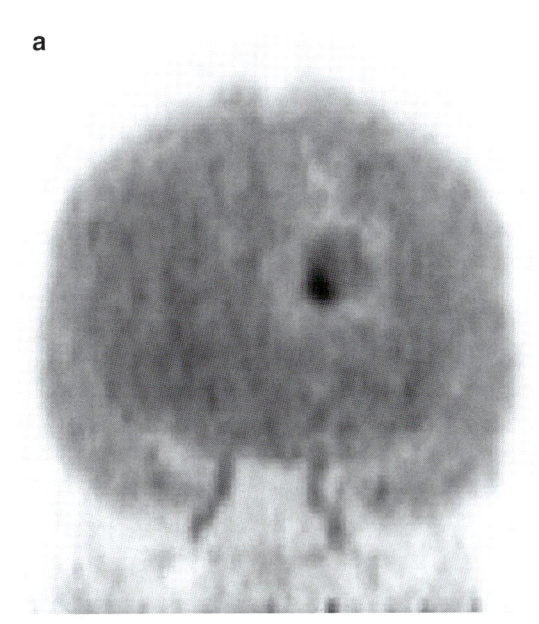

a

b

Fig.20.7 (**a**) Maximum imaging projection (MIP) and (**b**) axial PET/CT fusion images show the FDG-avid lesion in the left frontal lobe. On the MIP, note the photopenic area surrounding the highly metabolic component of the lesion due to edema. The patient underwent surgery. The finding was ganglioglioma

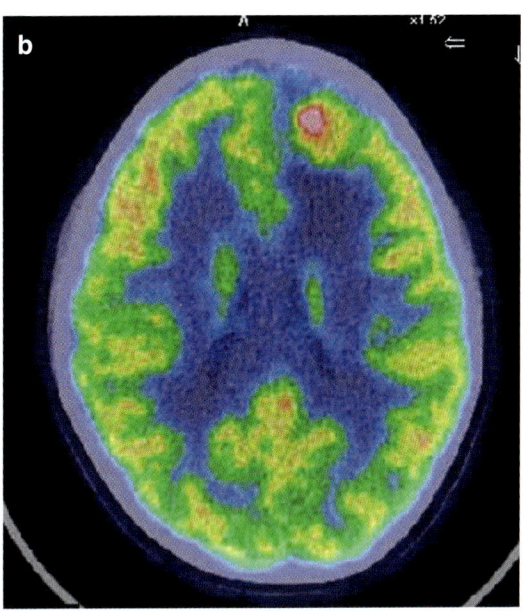

Teaching Point

Ganglioglioma is the second most common cause of spinal cord tumors in children [4]. It arises from ganglion cells in the central nervous system and most often occurs in the temporal lobe, but it can develop anywhere in the brain or in the spinal cord. Gangliogliomas are generally benign tumors, composed of transformed neuronal and glial elements, with rare malignant progression of the glial component.

Differential Diagnosis: Recurrent High-Grade Brain Tumor and Radionecrosis

Case 1

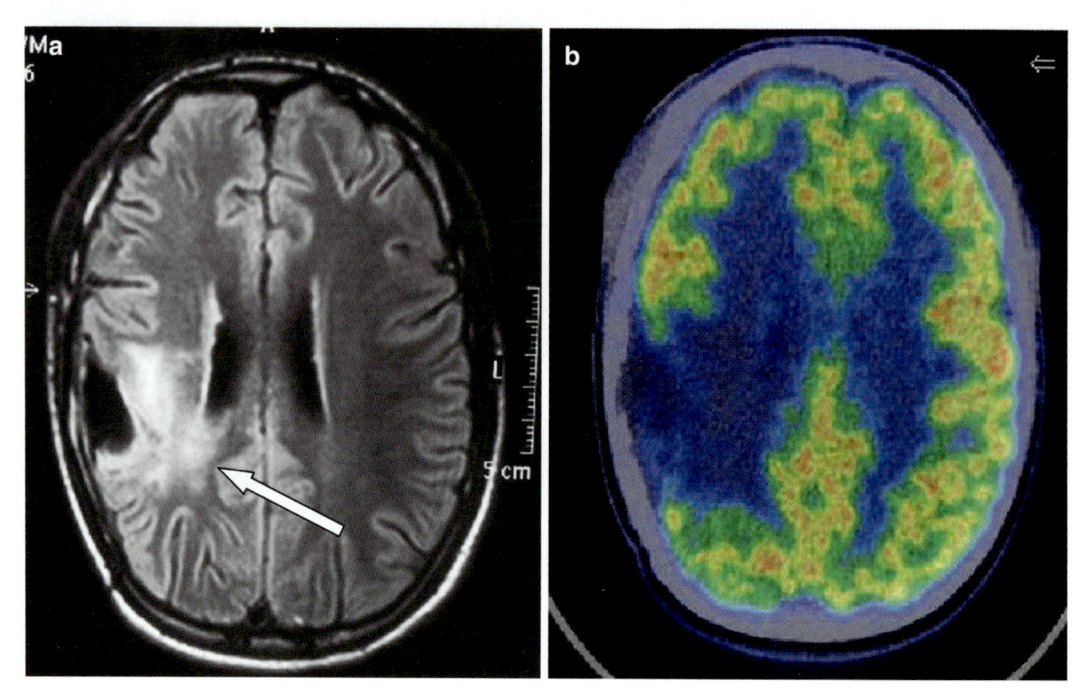

Fig. 20.8 A 16-year-old underwent surgery and radiotherapy 8 months earlier for right parietal anaplastic oligoastrocytoma. The MRI (**a**) during temozolomide therapy shows dubious disease relapse (*white arrow* in **a**). ^{18}F-FDG–PET/CT (**b**) does not demonstrate pathological uptake. The final diagnosis was radionecrosis

Case 2

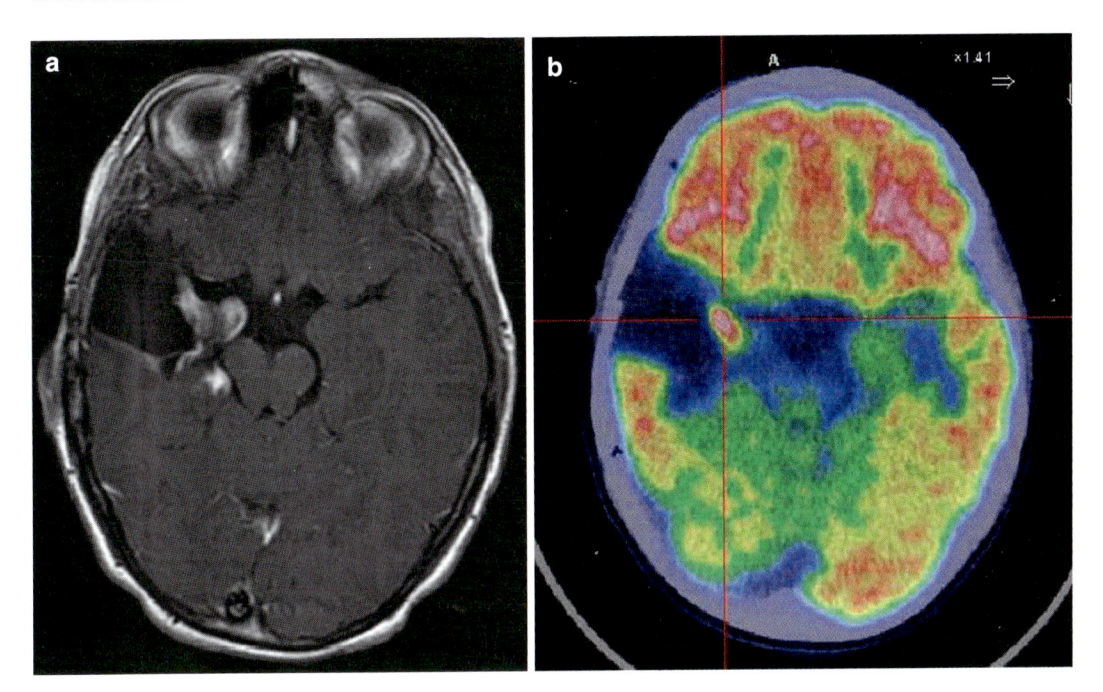

Fig. 20.9 A 9-year-old boy underwent surgery 2 years earlier for right temporal anaplastic astrocytoma and was treated with temozolomide. (**a**) Axial T1 sequence MRI shows signal alteration extending to the amygdala and the posterior portion of the para-hippocampus. (**b**) Axial ^{18}F-FDG–PET/CT fusion image confirms the suspected disease relapse, showing intense focal uptake within the medial part of the surgical cavity

Case 3

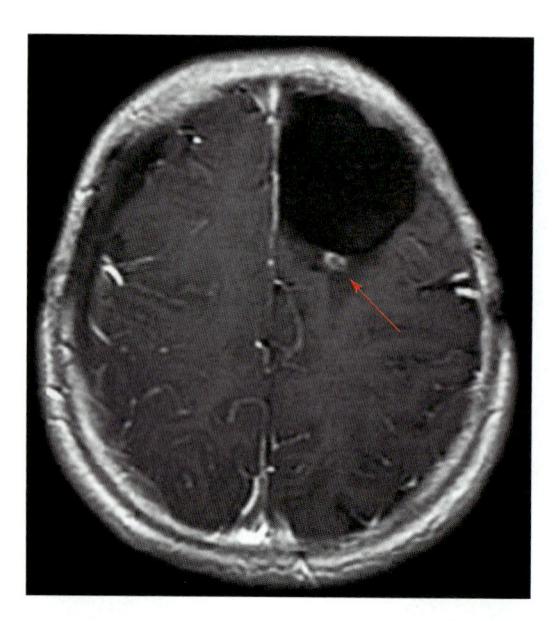

Fig. 20.10 A 9-year-old girl underwent surgery and radiotherapy 4 years earlier for a left frontal ependymoma grade II. Axial T1 sequence MRI after gadolinium injection shows a small nodule along the posterior profile of the surgical cavity (*red arrow*). Disease recurrence or radionecrosis was suspected

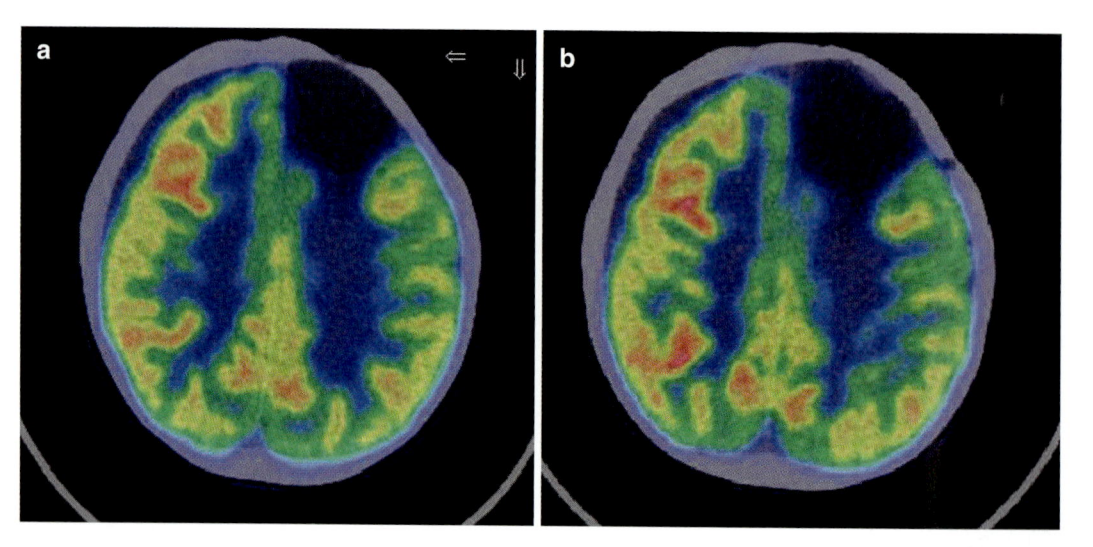

Fig. 20.11 Same patient as in Fig. 20.10. Axial brain window PET/CT fusion images at one (**a**) and four (**b**) hours after tracer injection do not show any pathological FDG accumulation corresponding to the signal alteration seen on the MRI. The patient is off therapy and has been free of disease for 2 years

Case 4

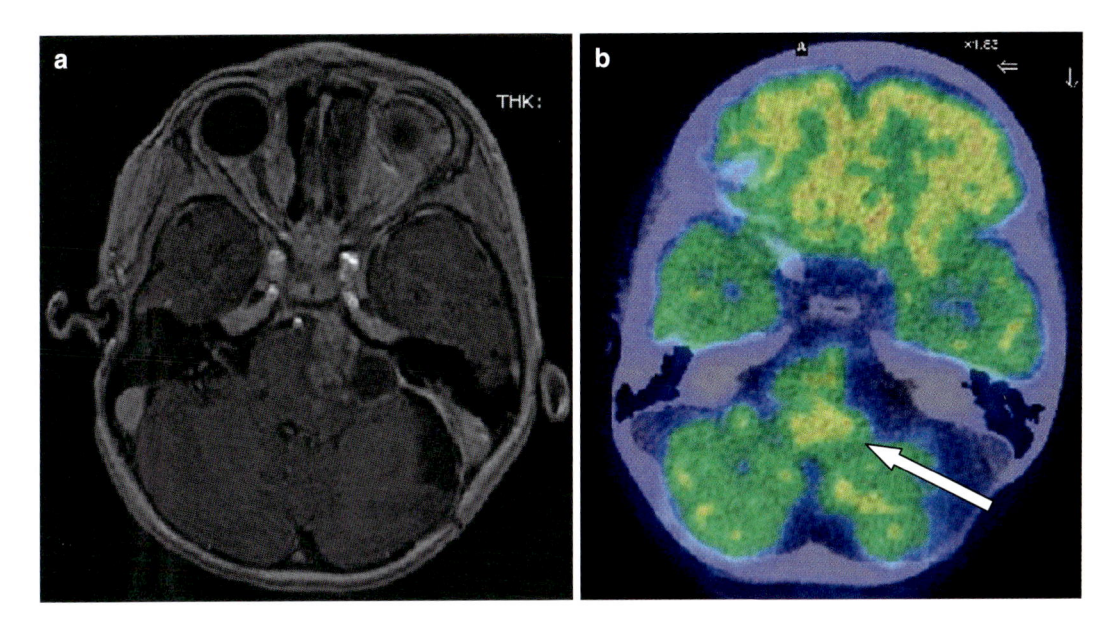

Fig. 20.12 A 5-year-old girl who 2 years earlier underwent surgery, chemotherapy, and radiotherapy for anaplastic astrocytoma of the pons and cerebellum. Following the development of diplopia, she was evaluated by MRI, based on a suspicion of disease recurrence. Spoiled gradient recalled (SPGR) sequence MRI after gadolinium (**a**) injection shows irregular impregnation of the residual tissue at the brainstem on the left side, with cystic and/or necrotic areas. The axial ^{18}F-FDG–PET/CT fusion image 1 h after tracer injection (**b**) shows a mild nonhomogeneous increase of radiocompound uptake in the brainstem (*white arrow*), with a photopenic left lateral area indicative of the cystic or necrotic component

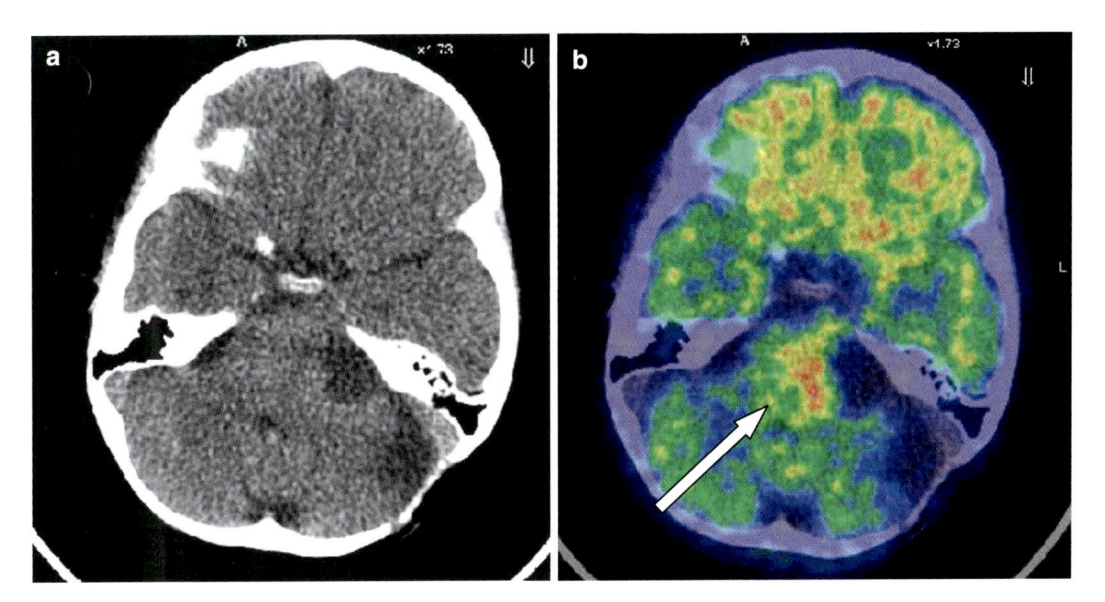

Fig. 20.13 Same patient as in Fig. 20.12. Axial brain window CT (**a**) and PET/CT (**b**) at 4 h after FDG injection. Note the improvement in the visual analysis on delayed image. The lesion is better rendered (*white arrow*)

Teaching Point

It is advisable to repeat a delayed acquisition at a later time point when the image at 1 h after FDG injection is negative or doubtful.

Case 5

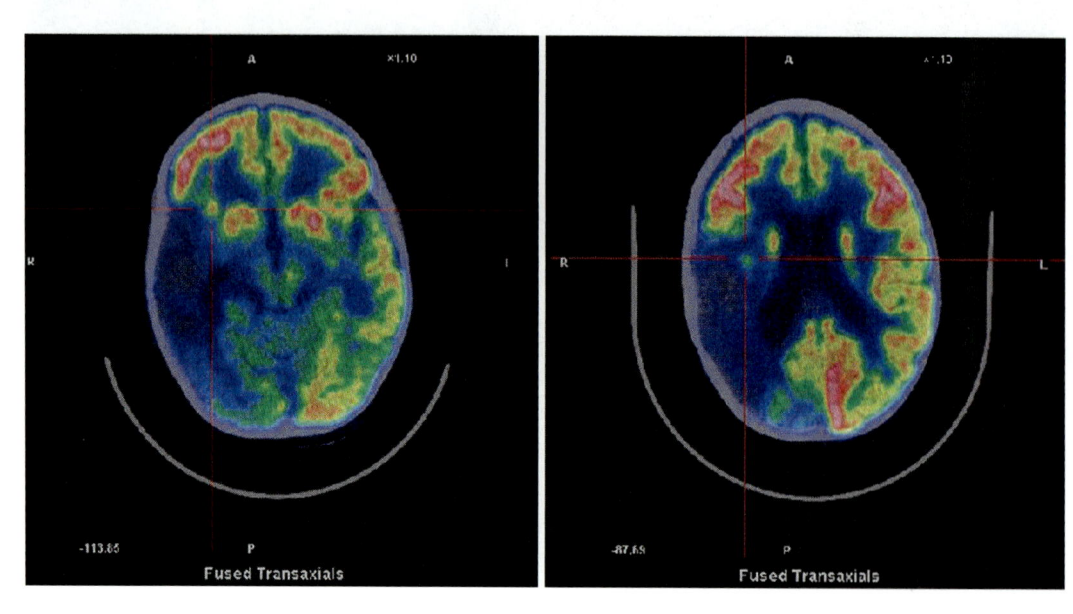

Fig. 20.14 A 3-year-old treated for a right parietotemporal pineal germinoma underwent restaging for suspected disease recurrence. Two different levels of axial brain window PET/CT images show two small areas of FDG uptake, indicative of relapse. Note the large photopenic area due to the previous round of therapy and recent intralesional bleeding

Case 6

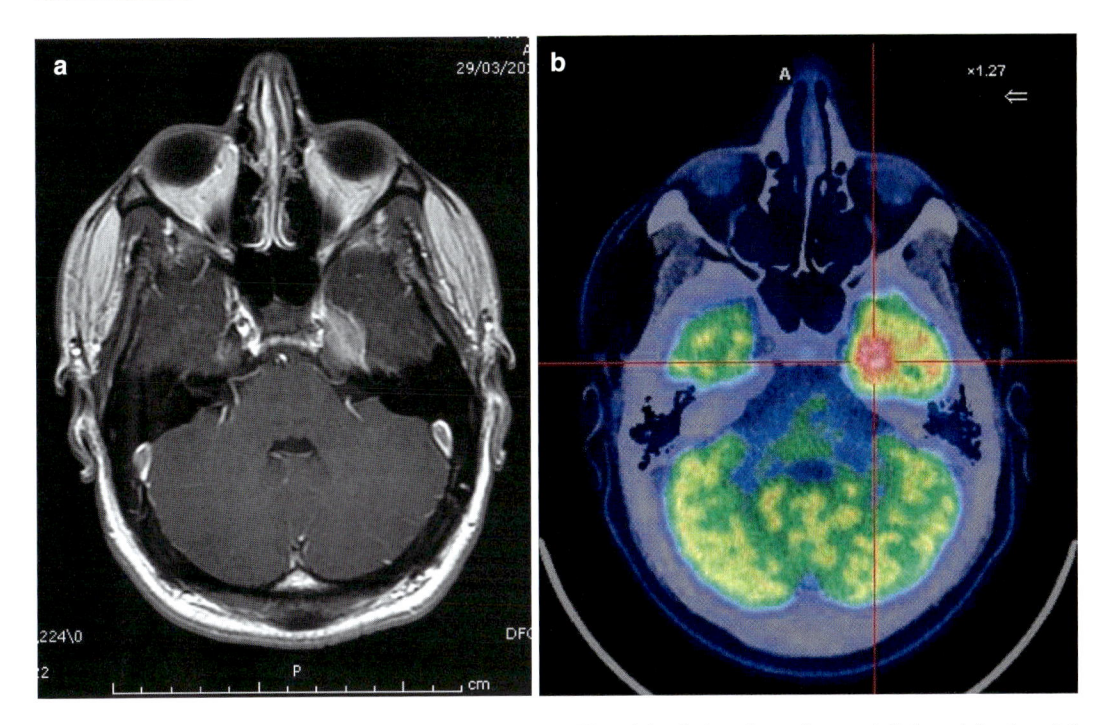

Fig. 20.15 A 16-year-old with suspected systemic disease recurrence following treatment for T-cell lymphoblastic lymphoma. Following episodes of vomiting and headache extending from the left parietotemporal area to the upper part of the lower jaw, she underwent MRI. Axial T1-weighted imaging after gadolinium injection (**a**) shows signal attenuation involving the left cavernous sinus and cranial nerve V ipsilaterally. The PET/CT fusion image (**b**) confirms disease recurrence in the brain

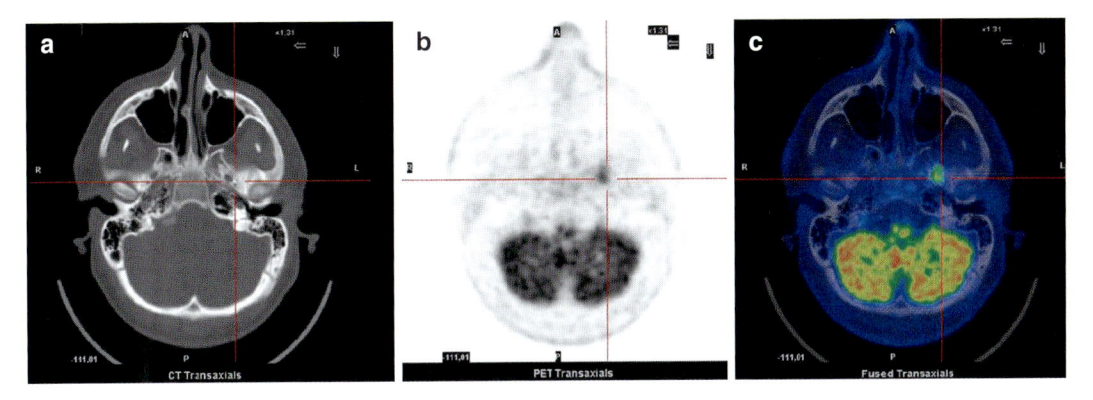

Fig. 20.16 Same patient as in Fig. 20.15. Axial bone window CT (**a**), PET (**b**), and PET/CT (**c**). Note the small area of FDG uptake in the left oval foramina, through which the III branch of cranial nerve V passes. This finding correlated with the clinical signs of pain in the upper branch of the lower jaw

Case 7

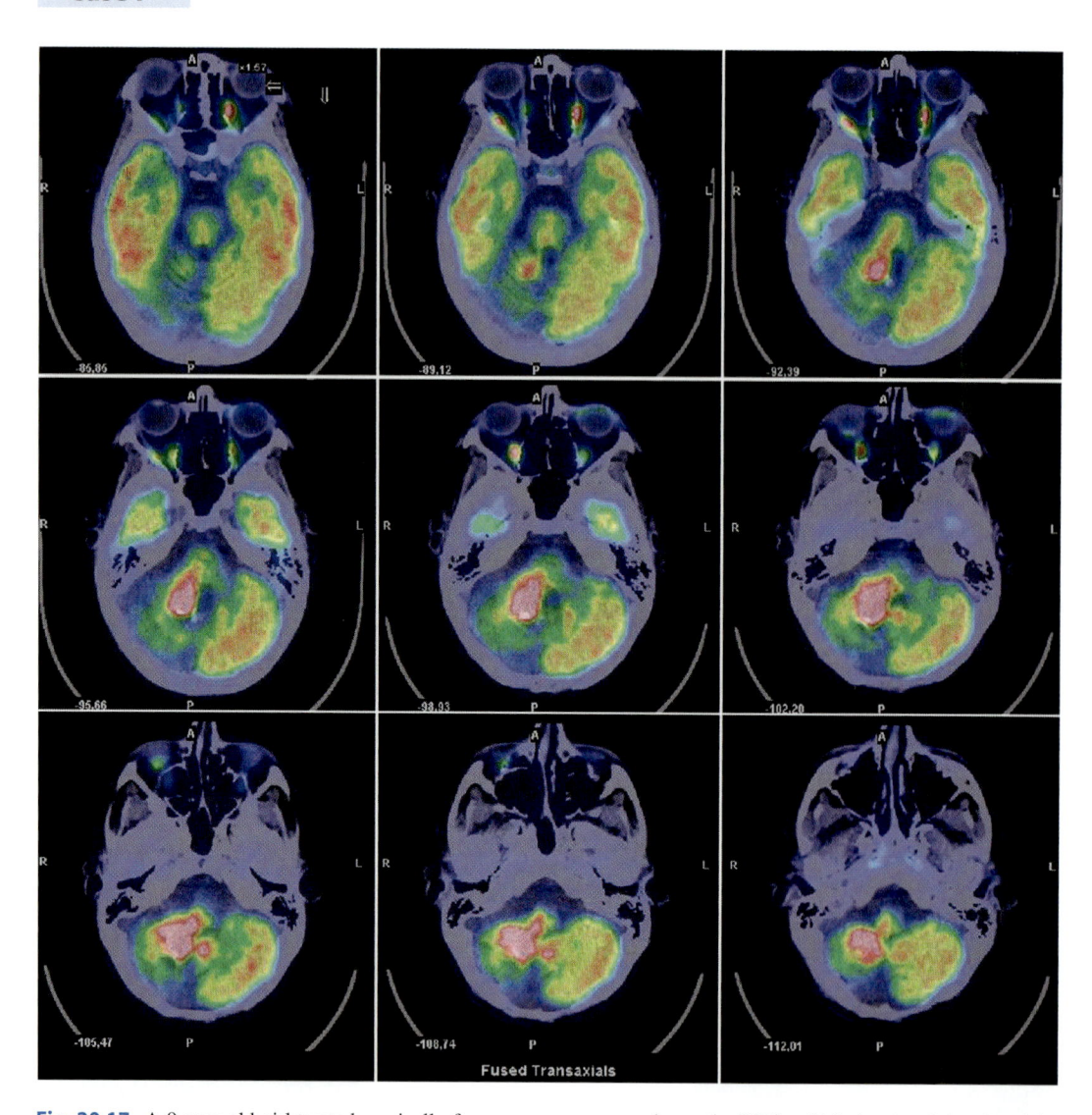

Fig. 20.17 A 9-year-old girl treated surgically for cerebellar medulloblastoma underwent ^{18}F-FDG evaluation for suspected disease relapse. Axial PET/CT fusion image sequence shows the FDG-avid lesion involving the right cerebellar peduncle, pons, and olfactory bulb

Case 7 (continued)

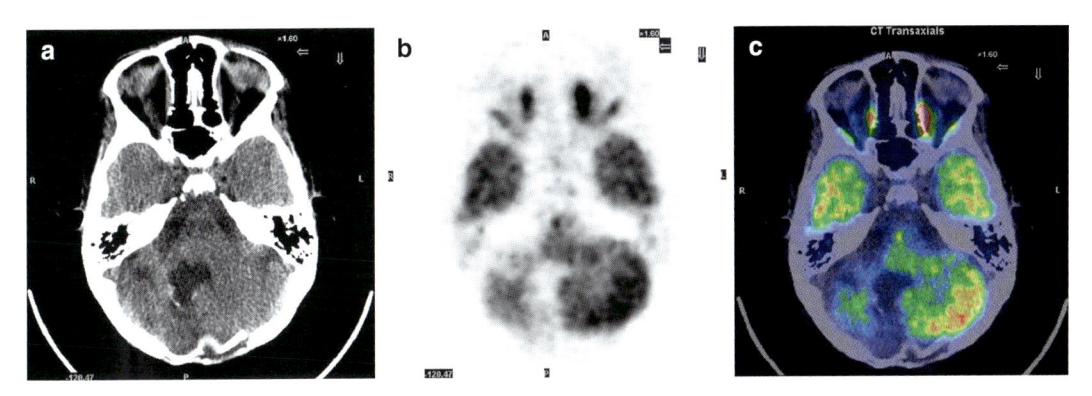

Fig. 20.18 Same patient after repeat surgery. (**a**) CT, (**b**) PET, and (**c**) PET/CT fusion images

References

1. Dumas-Duport C (1993) Dysembryoplastic neuroepithelial tumours. Brain Pathol 3:283–295
2. Kleihues P, Burger PC, Scheithauer BW (1993) The new WHO classification of brain tumours. Brain Pathol 3:255–268
3. Louis DN, Ohgaki H, Wiestler OD et al (2007) The 2007 WHO classification of tumours of the central nervous system. Acta Neuropathol 114:97–109
4. Pandita A, Balasubramaniam A, Perrin R, Shannon P, Guha A (2007) Malignant and benign ganglioglioma: a pathological and molecular study. Neuro Oncol 9(2):124–134

PET/CT in the Clinical Evaluation of Pediatric Epilepsy

21

Valentina Garibotto, Maria Isabel Vargas, Margitta Seeck, and Fabienne Picard

21.1 Introduction

FDG–PET is a well-established functional imaging modality in the evaluation of pediatric patients with epilepsy [1, 12]. While ictal scans can be useful, the long duration required to reach steady-state glucose uptake (on the order of many minutes compared with partial seizures, which usually last <2 min) often leads to scans that contain a difficult-to-interpret mixture of interictal, ictal, and postictal states. In addition, the practical realization of an ictal FDG–PET study requires the coordination of radiotracer availability with the ictal event, which is difficult to assure. Consequently, ictal PET studies are rarely performed, and ictal SPECT perfusion studies are preferred instead. However, if ictal injection is feasible, ictal PET images may clearly depict the cortical area responsible for the epileptic event (Fig. 21.1).

V. Garibotto (✉)
Nuclear Medicine Division,
Department of Medical Imaging,
Geneva University and Geneva University Hospitals,
Rue Gabrielle-Perret-Gentil 4,
Geneva 1211, Switzerland
e-mail: valentina.garibotto@hcuge.ch

M.I. Vargas
Neuroradiology Division,
Department of Medical Imaging,
Geneva University and Geneva University Hospitals,
Rue Gabrielle-Perret-Gentil 4,
Geneva 1211, Switzerland
e-mail: maria.vargas@hcuge.ch

M. Seeck • F. Picard
EEG and Epilepsy Unit, Neurology Division,
Department of Clinical Neurosciences,
Geneva University and Geneva University Hospitals,
Rue Gabrielle-Perret-Gentil 4,
Geneva 1211, Switzerland
e-mail: margitta.seeck@hcuge.ch;
fabienne.picard@hcuge.ch

Presurgical FDG–PET scans in epilepsy patients are typically obtained when the patient is in the interictal state, with the goal of detecting focal areas of decreased metabolism, i.e., relative hypometabolism, as these presumably reflect focal functional disturbances of cerebral activity associated with epileptogenic tissue. Nonetheless, the specific cause of hypometabolism in and near epileptogenic regions of the brain remains unclear [3].

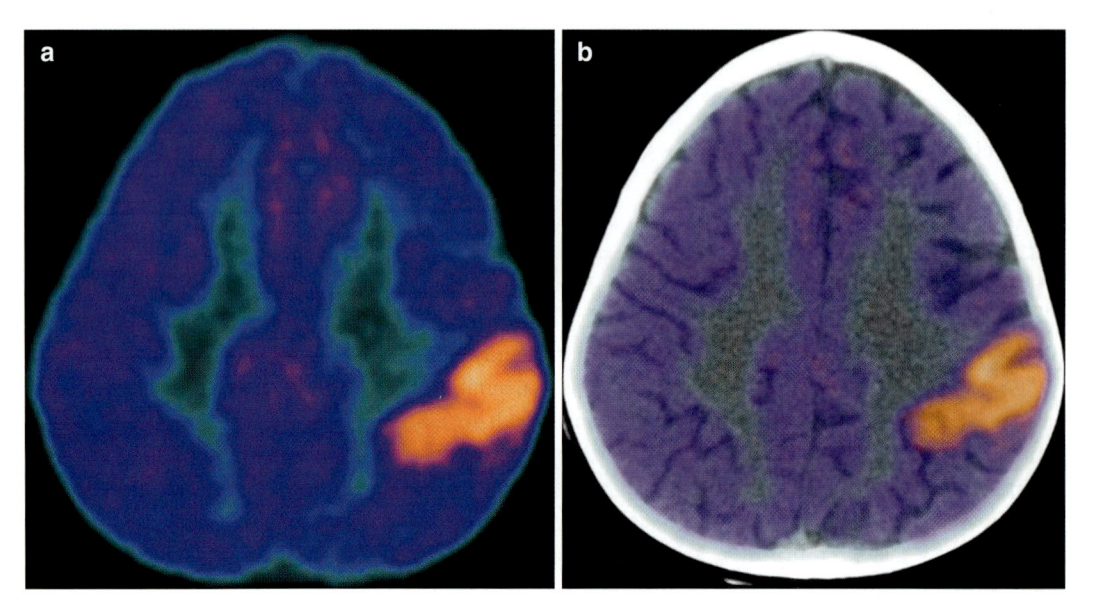

Fig. 21.1 A 5-year-old girl with Rasmussen's encephalitis and partial seizures since the age of 3 years. (**a**) Axial PET image, (**b**) PET/MRI fusion. FDG was fortuitously administered during a seizure and shows, with very high spatial resolution and excellent image contrast, the involved cortex in the left hemisphere

21.2 FDG–PET in Temporal Lobe Epilepsy

The value of FDG–PET has been best proven in the evaluation of medically refractory epilepsy patients who are candidates for surgery, specifically those with clinically suspected temporal lobe epilepsy. In this setting, the sensitivity of FDG–PET is between 80 and 90 % [1–4]. Only a few studies have addressed the sensitivity and specificity of FDG–PET in medial temporal lobe epilepsy patients with and without evidence of hippocampal sclerosis on MRI. However, FDG–PET is still considered to be reliable in lateralizing the epileptogenic temporal lobe even in MRI-negative patients, as shown in Fig. 21.2 [5]. Of course, MRI techniques are constantly evolving, and new sequences and new analytical approaches may one day allow the identification of focal alterations in cases previously considered to be "MRI negative."

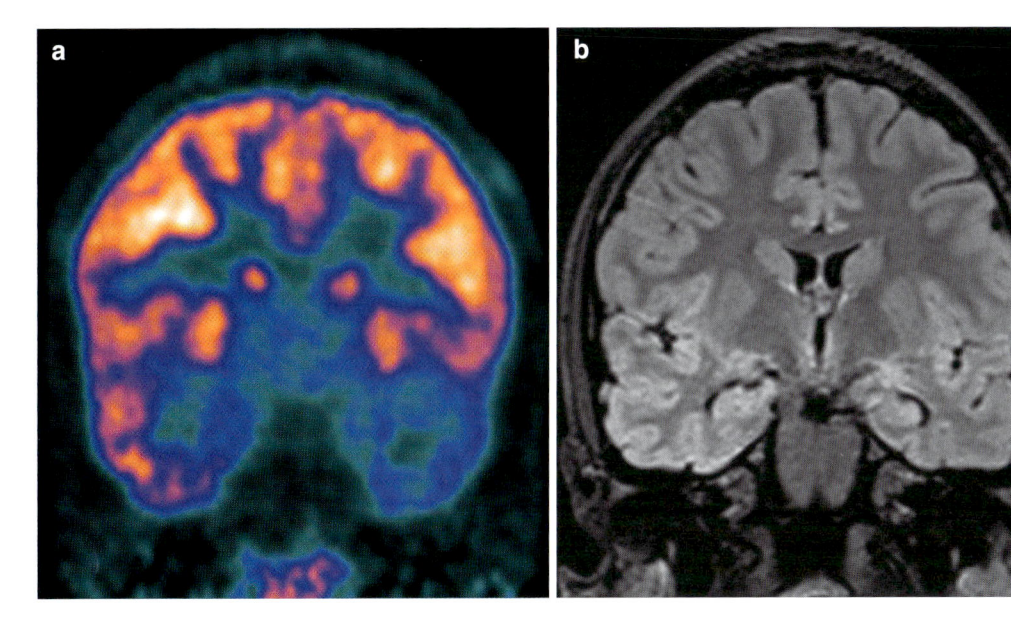

Fig. 21.2 A 13-year-old boy with partial complex epileptic seizures. (**a**) Coronal PET image, (**b**) MRI image. MRI does not show any clear abnormality, while on the PET image, there is marked hypometabolism in the left temporal pole. A repeated MRI investigation identified an area of probable cortical dysplasia. A left anterior temporal lobectomy was planned

21.3 FDG–PET in Extratemporal Epilepsy

The clinical value of FDG–PET in neocortical epilepsy is less clear. The larger reported series consist of observational retrospective studies, and only a few were performed in the era of advanced MRI techniques [1, 6]. Most importantly, the FDG–PET findings in nonlesional neocortical epilepsy are often obtained from heterogeneous patients and patient groups. An example of the FDG pattern in a specific syndrome such as tuberous sclerosis is provided in Fig. 21.3 [7].

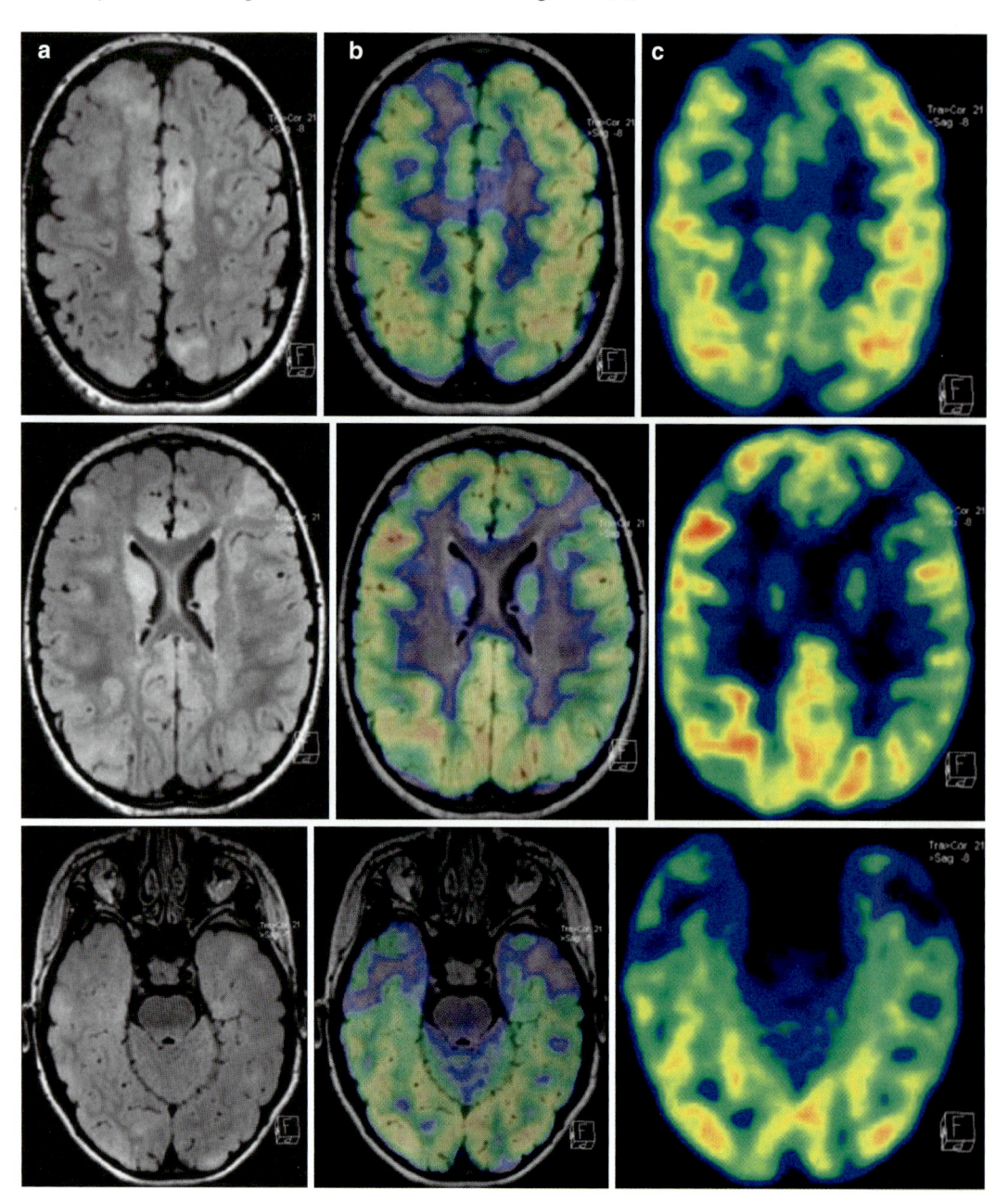

Fig. 21.3 A 5-year-old girl who at the age of 5 months was diagnosed with tuberous sclerosis and generalized epileptic seizures. (**a**) Axial MRI, (**b**) PET/MRI fusion, and (**c**) PET images. The PET/MRI fusion images show multiple cortical lesions in the two hemispheres, typically hypometabolic on FDG–PET imaging. However, these imaging modalities do not allow localization of the lesion generating the epileptic seizures. Instead, promising results were obtained using α-[^{11}C]methyl-L-tryptophan (AMT), a tracer specific for the serotonergic system

In tuberous sclerosis typically FDG-PET shows hypometabolism in and around tubers, believed to be due to decreased neuronal number and simplified dendritic pattern. A tuber with a disproportionately large area of hypometabolism compared with its size on MR images is most likely epileptogenic [8]. However, both epileptic and nonepileptic tubers show reduced uptake on FDG-PET, while promising results have been obtained using a tracer specific for the serotonergic system, the α-[11C]methyl-l-tryptophan (AMT). AMT-PET shows increased AMT uptake interictally in epileptic but not quiescent tubers in almost two-thirds of children with tuberous sclerosis and intractable epilepsy: all tubers with at least 10% AMT increase were found to be epileptogenic [11].

Co-registered multimodality imaging may provide other supportive localizing information confirming that a questionable PET metabolic abnormality is indeed a true disturbance reflective of the epileptogenic zone, thus emphasizing the added value of imaging fusion or hybrid imaging, when available [9, 13, 14].

21.4 Other PET Tracers

Many tracers have shown promising results in the molecular imaging of epilepsy, especially those targeting the GABAergic system (^{11}C-flumazenil), the serotonergic system (^{11}C-WAY and α-^{11}C-methyl-L-tryptophan), the dopaminergic system, the glutamatergic system, nicotinic receptors, adenosine receptors, and opioid-based ligands. However, these tracers, mostly based on carbon-11 chemistry and on the availability of an on-site cyclotron, are still limited to dedicated research centers, and their description is beyond the scope of this chapter. The results obtained with these tracers were recently summarized in two reviews [10, 11, 12].

References

1. Kurian M, Spinelli L, Delavelle J et al (2007) Multimodality imaging for focus localization in pediatric pharmacoresistant epilepsy. Epileptic Disord 9:20–31
2. Ryvlin P, Bouvard S, Le Bars D et al (1998) Clinical utility of flumazenil-PET versus [18F] fluorodeoxyglucose-PET and MRI in refractory partial epilepsy. A prospective study in 100 patients. Brain 121:2067–2081
3. Knowlton RC (2006) The role of FDG-PET, ictal SPECT, and MEG in the epilepsy surgery evaluation. Epilepsy Behav 8:91–101
4. Henry TR, Engel J Jr, Mazziotta JC (1993) Clinical evaluation of interictal fluorine-18-fluorodeoxyglucose PET in partial epilepsy. J Nucl Med 34:1892–1898
5. Carne RP, O'Brien TJ, Kilpatrick CJ et al (2004) MRI-negative PET-positive temporal lobe epilepsy: a distinct surgically remediable syndrome. Brain 127:2276–2285
6. Juhasz C, Chugani DC, Muzik O et al (2001) Relationship of flumazenil and glucose PET abnormalities to neocortical epilepsy surgery outcome. Neurology 56:1650–1658
7. Luat AF, Makki M, Chugani HT (2007) Neuroimaging in tuberous sclerosis complex. Curr Opin Neurol 20:142–150
8. Chandra PS, Salamon N, Huang J, et al (2006) FDG-PET/MRI coregistration and diffusion-tensor imaging distinguish epileptogenic tubers and cortex in patients with tuberous sclerosis complex: a preliminary report. Epilepsia 47:1543–1549
9. Garibotto V, Heinzer S, Vulliemoz S et al (2013) Clinical applications of hybrid PET/MRI in neuroimaging. Clin Nucl Med 38:e13–e18
10. Garibotto V, Picard F (2013) Nuclear medicine imaging in epilepsy. Epileptologie 30:109–121
11. Chugani DC (2011) Alpha-methyl-L-tryptophan: mechanisms for tracer localization of epileptogenic brain regions. Biomark Med 5:567–575
12. Kumar A, Semah F, Chugani HT, et al (2012) Epilepsy diagnosis: positron emission tomography. Handb Clin Neurol 107:409–424
13. Salamon N, Kung J, Shaw SJ, et al (2008) FDG-PET/MRI coregistration improves detection of cortical dysplasia in patients with epilepsy. Neurology 71: 1594–1601
14. Rubi S, Setoain X, Donaire A, et al (2011) Validation of FDG-PET/MRI coregistration in nonlesional refractory childhood epilepsy. Epilepsia 52:2216–2224

Epilepsia Partialis Continua

Silvia Morbelli

22.1 Introduction

Epilepsia partialis continua (EPC) is a rare form of focal status epilepticus. The clonic jerks can affect any single muscle or muscle group or extend to widespread muscular involvement [1]. Electrophysiological studies have demonstrated electroencephalography (EEG) abnormalities, including giant somatosensory-evoked potentials that prove the cortical origin of the muscle jerks [2]. In childhood, the most frequent cause of EPC is Rasmussen's encephalitis [3], but vascular, immune-mediated, neoplastic, or metabolic–toxic causes have also been described [4]. In case of hyperglycemia-induced EPC, the status epilepticus may cease following the normalization of blood glucose levels, although there are reports of its evolution into drug-resistant epilepsy [5].

22.2 Clinical Case

Type 1 diabetes mellitus was diagnosed in a 3-year-old boy following an episode of diabetic ketoacidosis (polyuria, polydipsia, and weight loss). After 5 months of unsatisfactory metabolic glycemic control despite intensive insulin replacement, he developed continuous myoclonic jerks of the left hand and arm, with partial attenuation during sleep. Despite intensive anticonvulsive drug therapy (carbamazepine, valproic acid, ethosuccimide, clobazam), focal seizures persisted in the following years. Given the drug resistance of the disease, surgical treatment was proposed when the child reached 11 years of age. EEG and MRI were performed to localize the epileptic focus, thus guiding surgical treatment.

EEG showed abnormal theta-delta rhythms together with spike-wave abnormalities over the right frontotemporal cortex. The MRI showed hypotrophy and mild hyperintensities of both hippocampi, suggesting mesial temporal sclerosis, without clear lateralization.

Since the results of the MRI scan were inconclusive, the brain ^{18}F-FDG–PET with simultaneous EEG recording was proposed in order to localize the epileptic focus.

The EEG recorded during the 30 min of FDG uptake during the PET scan showed repeated episodes of the above-described abnormalities (Fig. 22.1). Accordingly, the brain FDG–PET scan was considered as "ictal." The PET-derived information shown in Fig. 22.1 supported the EEG evidence and helped to guide surgery.

S. Morbelli, MD
Nuclear Medicine Unit,
IRCCS AOU San Martino – IST, Genoa,
Largo R. Benzi 10, Genoa 16132, Italy
e-mail: silviadaniela.morbelli@hsanmartino.it

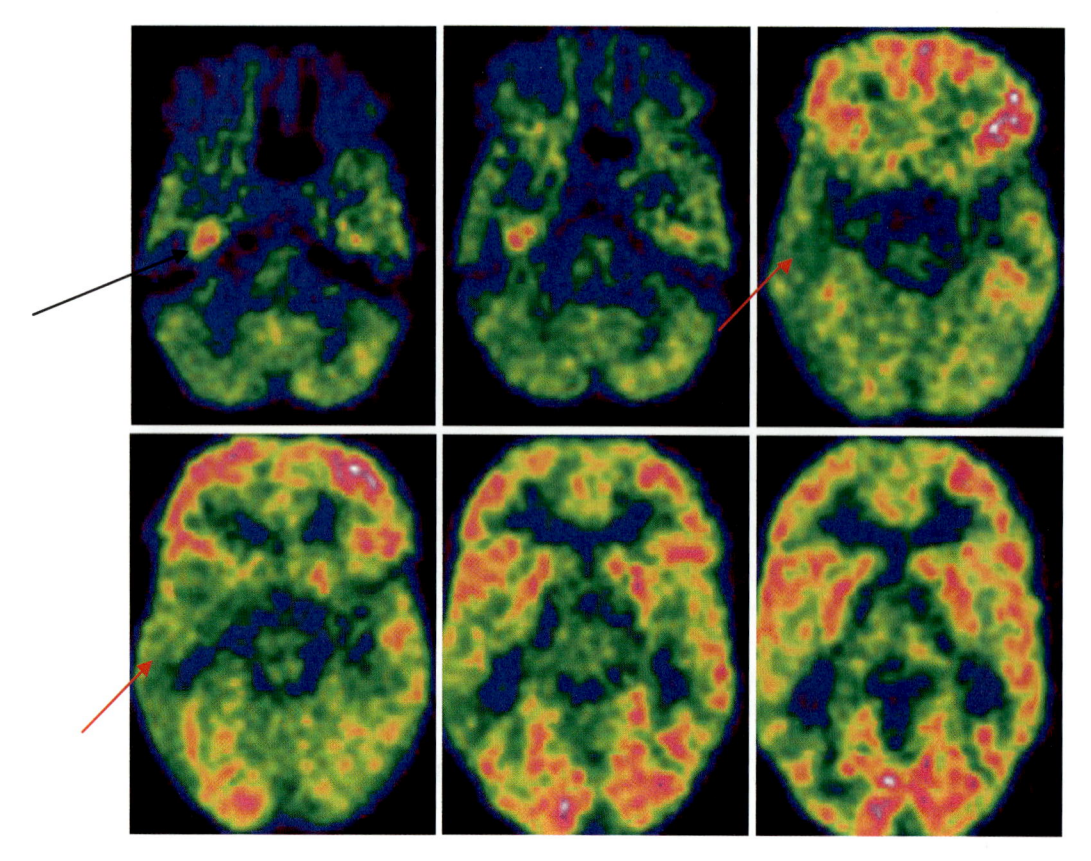

Fig. 22.1 Transaxial FDG–PET scan slices show a hypermetabolic focus in the right temporal mesial cortex (*black arrow*) and hypometabolism in the ipsilateral lateral and posterior temporal cortex (intra-hemispheric diaschisis, *red arrows*)

Teaching Point

In patients who are candidates for the surgical treatment of epilepsy and whose MRI study is inconclusive, the brain ^{18}F-FDG–PET may provide relevant information about the site and side of the epileptic focus. Simultaneous EEG recording during the FDG distribution time is mandatory. The epileptic focus will appear as a hypermetabolic site in the unusual case of ictal PET (as in the case described above) and as a hypometabolic area during an interictal (i.e., in the absence of a sustained epileptic discharge as seen on EEG) acquisition.

References

1. Obeso JA, Rothwell JC, Marsden CD (1985) The spectrum of cortical myoclonus. From focal reflex jerks to spontaneous motor epilepsy. Brain 108:193–224
2. Cockerell OC, Rothwell J, Thompson PD et al (1996) Clinical and physiological features of epilepsia partialis continua. Cases ascertained in the UK. Brain 119:393–407
3. Schomer DL (1993) Focal status epilepticus and epilepsia partialis continua in adults and children. Epilepsia 34(Suppl 1):S29–S36
4. Bien CG, Elger CE (2008) Epilepsia partialis continua: semiology and differential diagnoses. Epileptic Disord 10(1):3–7
5. Baglietto MG, Mancardi MM, Giannattasio A, Minuto N, Rossi A, Capovilla G, Veneselli E, Lorini R, d'Annunzio G (2009) Epilepsia partialis continua in type 1 diabetes: evolution into epileptic encephalopathy with continuous spike-waves during slow sleep. Neurol Sci 30(6):509–512

Brain ¹⁸F-FDG–PET/CT Imaging in Hemolytic Uremic Syndrome During and After the Acute Phase

23

Riccardo Benti and Angelina Cistaro

Hemolytic uremic syndrome (HUS) is a multisystemic disease clinically characterized by uremia, thrombocytopenia, and hemolytic anemia. It is the most common cause of acute renal failure in children between 1 and 4 years of age [1]. Besides the kidneys, the central nervous system (CNS) is clinically involved in 20–50 % of HUS patients. Common signs of severe CNS injury are seizures, alteration of consciousness, hemiparesis, visual disturbances, and brainstem symptoms. Acute mortality rates are 4–10 %.

The pathogenesis of typical HUS (90 % of pediatric cases) is related to gastrointestinal infections caused by Shiga-toxin-producing *Escherichia coli* (e.g., *E. coli* 0157:H7). Two main mechanisms have been postulated to explain the brain damage reflecting the neuronal and endothelial cytotoxicity of Shiga toxin seen in HUS-associated microangiopathy: gray matter injury and/or diffuse endothelial damage, with complement activation, resulting in perivascular edema and thrombotic vasculitis. These events can also occur when endothelial damage evolves to induce the gross activation of platelets in larger terminal arteries, leading to acute ischemic occlusion with important ischemic damage and a poor prognosis [2, 3].

Morphological brain imaging, i.e., CT [4] and MRI [5], and MRI parametric imaging [6] show structural changes in the basal ganglia, cerebellum, thalami, and brainstem in 20–60 % of HUS patients with clinically severe CNS involvement. The clinical resolution of HUS-related neurological symptoms and signs often precedes the complete normalization of these imaging patterns, such that their long-term prognostic value is debated.

Functional imaging of brain perfusion/metabolism has only rarely been applied in HUS. However, we have found that in patients in the acute phase of HUS who do not exhibit the main neurological symptoms, ¹⁸F-FDG–PET/CT shows mild to discrete reductions in cortical metabolism in the posterior cortex of the cerebral hemispheres. Specifically, there is a significant and diffuse/symmetric impairment of perfusion/metabolism in the posterior cortex and cerebellum, with minor impairment of the basal ganglia and recovery after clinical healing. In addition, a mild increase in FDG uptake is seen in subcortical gray matter in some cases. A focal/asymmetric pattern of cortical hypoperfusion/hypometabolism in HUS seems to be associated with the presence of relevant neurological symptoms/signs in the acute phase. PET studies carried out after clinical resolution (1–12 months later) show

R. Benti, MD
Department of Nuclear Medicine, Fondazione IRCCS,
Maggiore-Policlinico Mangiagalli Hospital,
Regina Elena, Via Francesco Sforza 35,
Milan 20122, Italy
e-mail: rbenti@policlinico.mi.it

A. Cistaro, MD (✉)
Department of Nuclear Medicine, Positron Emission Tomography Center IRMET S.p.A., Euromedic Inc.,
Via Onorato Vigliani 89, Turin 10100, Italy

Institute of Cognitive Sciences and Technologies,
National Research Council, Rome, Italy
e-mail: a.cistaro@irmet.com

perfusion/metabolism recovery in the previously affected areas, albeit with the persistence of a significant degree of functional cerebellar hypometabolism (Figs. 23.1, 23.2, 23.3, 23.4, and 23.5).

Our PET results are consistent with both models of brain injury suggested in HUS: (a) mild/symmetric and long-time reversible involvement of the gray matter in most patients (metabolic injury) and (b) further focal/asymmetric cortical involvement in patients with relevant neurological symptoms in the acute phase and different recovery patterns of perfusion/metabolism in gray matter (thrombotic focal vascular damage).

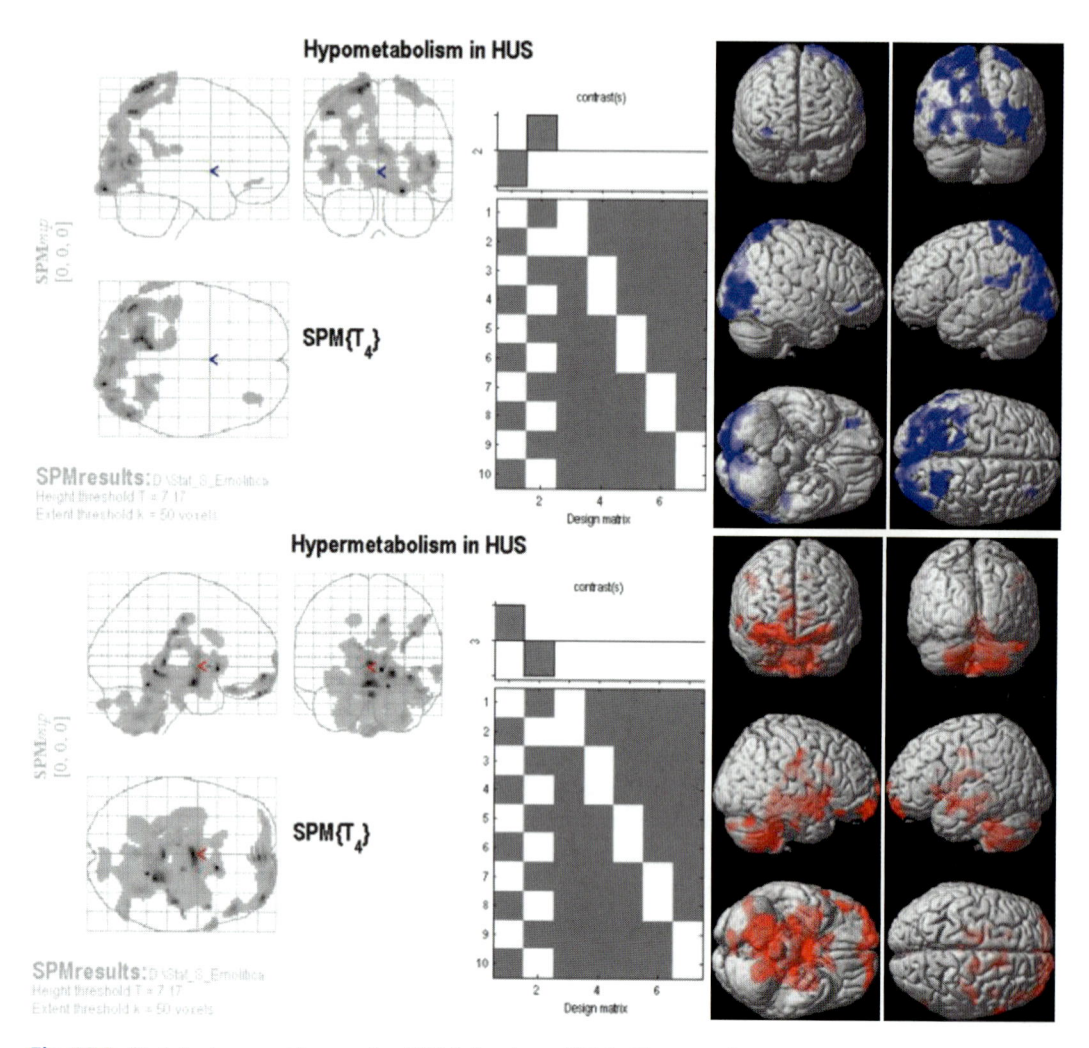

Fig. 23.1 Statistical parametric mapping (*SPM*) data in five HUS patients without neurological symptoms (paired data *t* test): acute vs. late PET studies. Volume-of-interest (VOI)-based analyses of PET data were performed by comparing serial PET studies; processing included the normalization of PET brain volumes to 3D templates (SPM). The normalized brain volumes were analyzed for regional specific FDG uptake, with SPM2 processing applied using the analysis of acute vs. recovery PET/CT studies. Hypometabolic regions are shown in *blue* and hypermetabolic regions in *red*

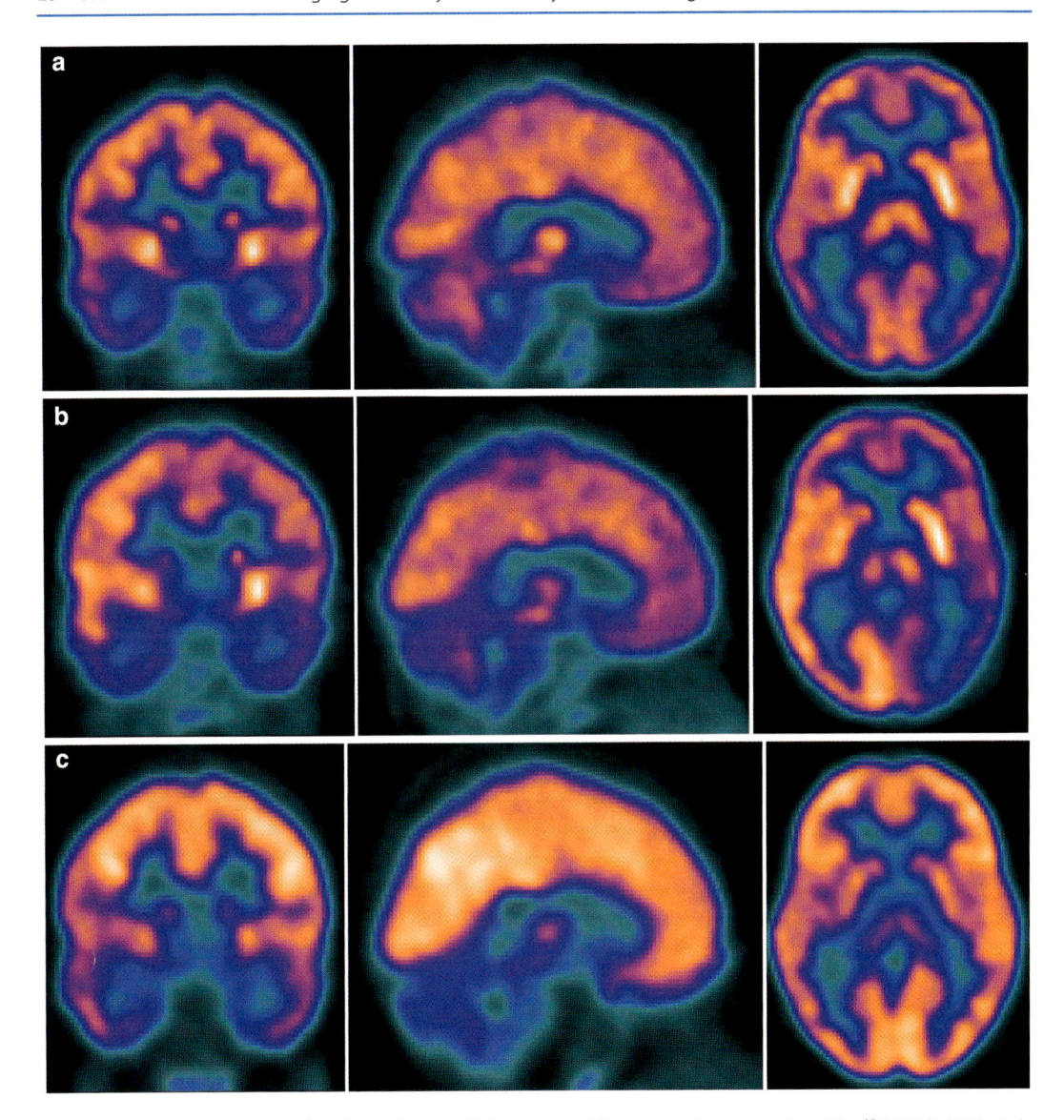

Fig. 23.2 PET/CT brain imaging in an 8-year-old boy. The ^{18}F-FDG–PET study (Biograph TruePoint PET/CT, Siemens, Erlangen, Germany) was conducted 40–60 min after intravenous ^{18}F-FDG administration (100–120 MBq). Low-dose CT sections of the head were used for attenuation correction. The ^{18}F-FDG–PET study was performed on day 3, during acute HUS without neurological symptoms (**a**); on day 12, during acute HUS with neurological symptoms (**b**); and 3 months later, after clinical resolution (**c**)

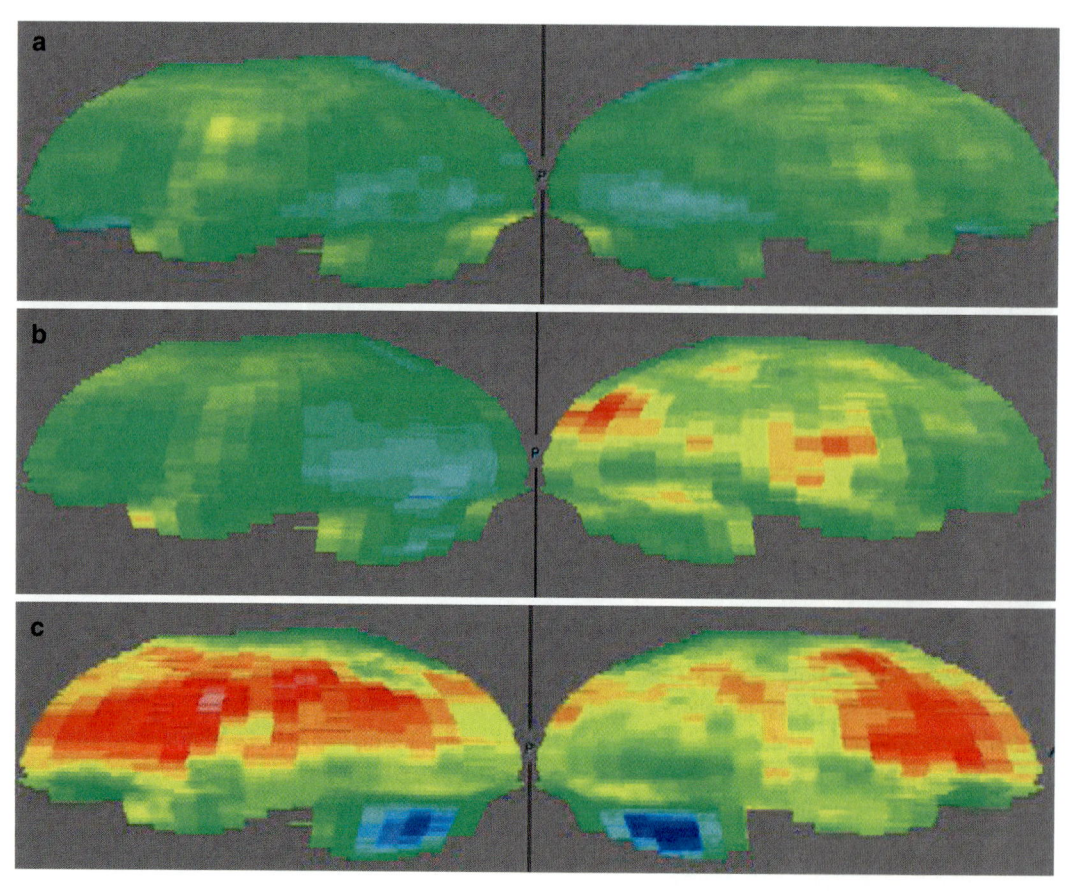

Fig. 23.3 ^{18}F-FDG–PET studies on day 3, during acute HUS without neurological symptoms (**a**); on day 12, during acute HUS with neurological symptoms (**b**); and 3 months later, after clinical resolution (**c**). The studies are compared with those in a healthy adult and were normalized to the Scenium brain volumetric template

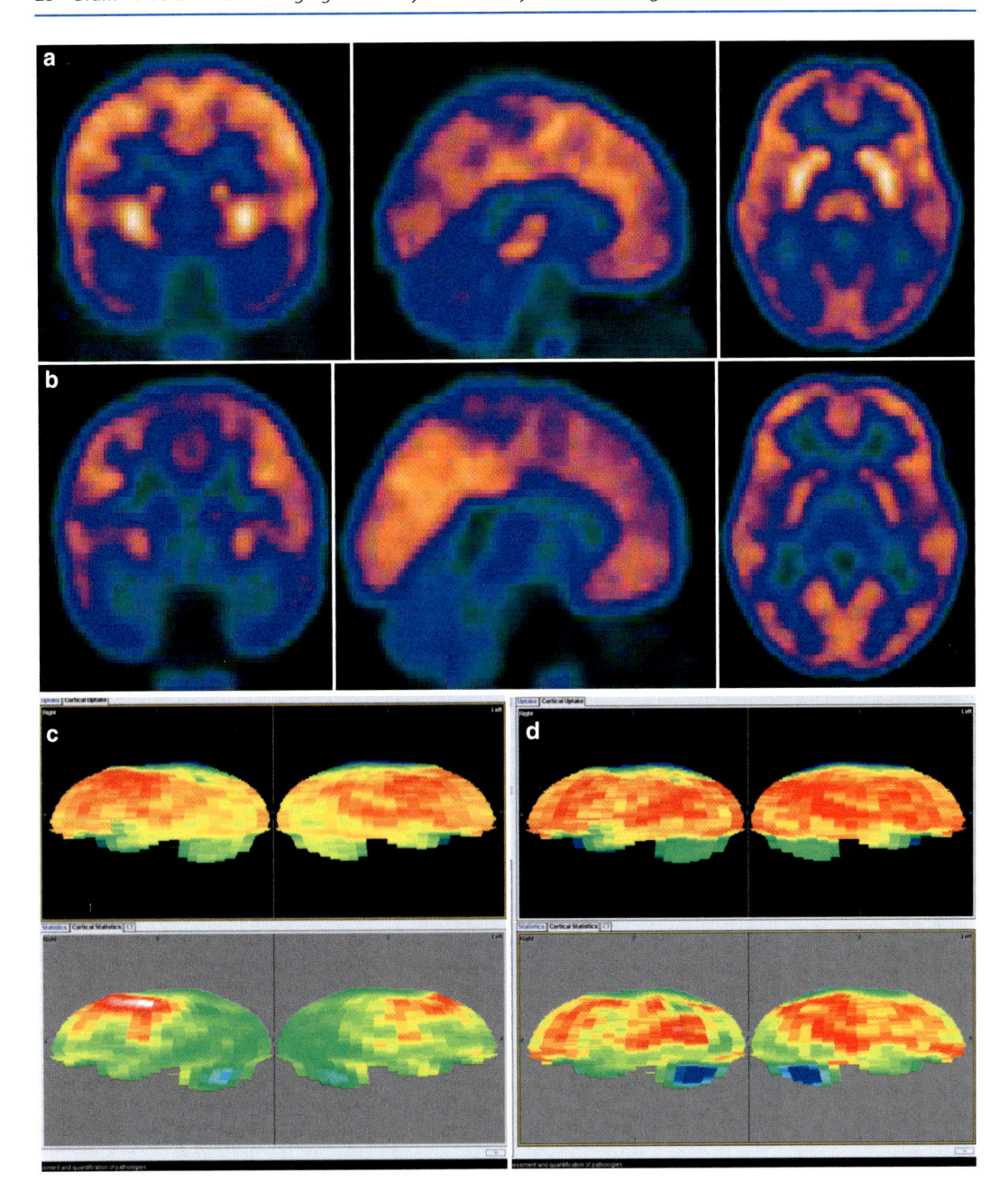

Fig. 23.4 ¹⁸F-FDG–PET studies (Biograph TruePoint PET/CT tomograph, Siemens, Erlangen, Germany) in a 4-year-old girl during acute HUS (**a**) and 3 months later (**b**). (**c, d**) ¹⁸F-FDG–PET study in the same patient during acute HUS (**c**) and 3 months later, after clinical resolution (**d**), compared to the findings in a healthy adult and normalized to the Scenium™ brain volumetric template

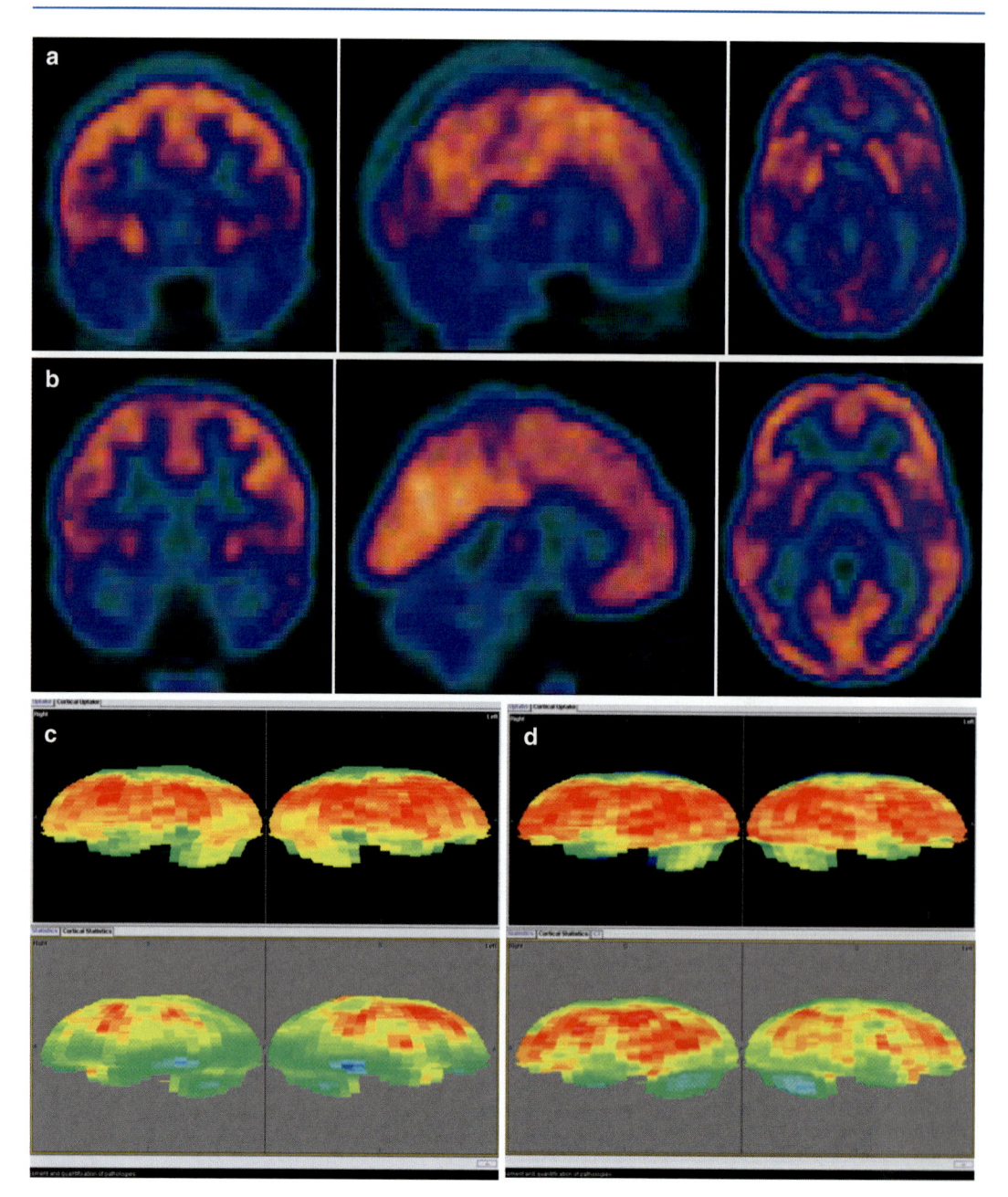

Fig. 23.5 ^{18}F-FDG–PET study (Biograph TruePoint PET/CT tomograph, Siemens, Erlangen, Germany) in a 7-year-old boy during acute HUS (**a**) and 3 months later, after clinical resolution (**b**). ^{18}F-FDG–PET study in the same patient during acute HUS (**c**) and 3 months later, after clinical resolution (**d**) compared to the findings in a healthy adult and normalized to the Scenium brain volumetric template

References

1. Herrera P, Valenzuela C, Skarmeta M, Méndez M, Bustos-González A (2012) Enterocolitis, antimicrobials and hemolytic-uremic syndrome in children: Review of a concept. Rev Chilena Infectol 29(3):313–316
2. Rota S, Cravedi P, Remuzzi G, Ruggenenti P (2005) Hemolytic uremic syndrome. G Ital Nefrol 22(Suppl 33):S57–S64
3. Landoni VI, Schierloh P, de Campos Nebel M, Fernández GC, Calatayud C, Lapponi MJ, Isturiz MA (2012) Shiga toxin 1 induces on lipopolysaccharide-treated astrocytes the release of tumor necrosis factor-alpha that alter brain-like endothelium integrity. PLoS Pathog 8(3):e1002632. Epub 2012 Mar 29
4. Steinborn M, Leiz S, Rüdisser K, Griebel M, Harder T, Hahn H (2004) CT and MRI in haemolytic uraemic syndrome with central nervous system involvement: distribution of lesions and prognostic value of imaging findings. Pediatr Radiol 34(10):805–810
5. Gómez-Lado C, Martinón-Torres F, Alvarez-Moreno A et al (2007) Reversible posterior leukoencephalopathy syndrome: an infrequent complication in the course of haemolytic-uremic syndrome. Rev Neurol 44(8):475–478
6. Toldo I, Manara R, Cogo P, Sartori S, Murer L, Battistella PA, Laverda AM (2009) Diffusion-weighted imagng findings in hemolytic uremic syndrome with central nervous system involvement. J Child Neurol 24(2):247–250

Part V

Infection and Inflammation

Inflammatory Bowel Diseases

24

Giorgio Treglia and Pierpaolo Alongi

24.1 Introduction

Inflammatory bowel diseases (IBDs) are multifactorial chronic diseases resulting from the complex interaction of genetic, immunological, and microbial factors [1]. They involve the gastrointestinal tract and comprise two related entities: Crohn's disease (CD) and ulcerative colitis (UC). The incidence of IBDs in children (<18 years of age) reported in the past decade varies between 1 and 9 per 100,000 for CD and between 0 and 5 per 100,000 for UC. The two forms of IBD can be differentiated by their inflammatory patterns. UC is characterized by chronic inflammation of the colonic mucosa; the rectum is primarily involved, but the disease may also extend into proximal colonic segments in a continuous fashion. CD may involve any segment of the gastrointestinal tract, but it most commonly affects the distal small bowel and terminal ileum. The inflammation associated with CD can be limited to the intestinal mucosa or involve the entire thickness of the bowel wall. CD is further characterized by "skip" lesions, consisting of inflammatory lesions with normal mucosa between affected segments [2, 3].

The symptoms of IBD correlate with the relapse and remission of disease activity and with the involved segment of the intestinal tract. In addition, patients with CD or UC may have extraintestinal manifestations. Current management of the two diseases is similar and is aimed at controlling the inflammation and in maintaining symptom remission using medical therapy. Surgery is useful for the treatment of complications, which include fulminant colitis, abscesses, fistulas, strictures, and cancer [2, 3].

IBDs are usually diagnosed based on a detailed patient history, physical examination, laboratory tests, and radiological studies including CT, MRI, ultrasonography, and endoscopic evaluation. A challenge for clinicians in the management of IBD is to determine whether the patient's symptoms are related to inflammation in the intestinal tract or to complications such as fibrotic strictures. A noninvasive test able to detect active inflammation in the intestinal tract would therefore be useful in the evaluation and management of IBDs [3, 4]. In this respect, the use of nuclear imaging technologies in the diagnosis and management of IBDs is ever increasing.

G. Treglia, MD (✉)
Department of Nuclear Medicine,
Oncology Institute of Southern Switzerland,
Via Ospedale, 12, Bellinzona Ticino CH-6500,
Switzerland
e-mail: giorgiomednuc@libero.it

P. Alongi, MD
Nuclear Medicine Unit,
IRCCS Scientific Institute San Raffaele,
Milan, Italy

^{18}F-FDG–PET and PET/CT have been proposed as noninvasive imaging methods to assess the extent, location, and activity of IBDs in adult and pediatric patients [5–9].

Clinical Case

A 12-year-old boy with a clinical history of IBD, previously treated, suffered symptom relapse after a period of clinical remission, suggesting disease reactivation. Since bowel strictures hampered a complete endoscopic evaluation, disease activity and extent were evaluated by a ^{18}F-FDG-PET/CT study. The resulting scan showed diffuse and intense radiopharmaceutical uptake in the large bowel, indicative of active IBD (Fig. 24.1).

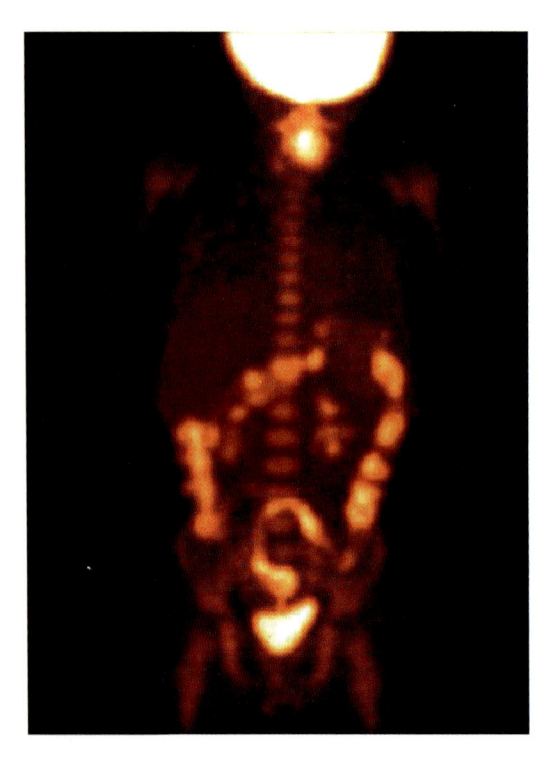

Fig. 24.1 The maximum intensity projection ^{18}F-FDG–PET image shows diffuse and intense radiopharmaceutical uptake in the large bowel

Teaching Point
^{18}F-FDG–PET/CT may be a useful noninvasive tool for identifying and localizing active intestinal inflammation, not only in adult but also in pediatric patients with IBD. Even if ^{18}F-FDG–PET/CT currently does not replace conventional studies, this functional approach may be useful when conventional studies either cannot be performed or fail to be completed.

References

1. Löffler M, Weckesser M, Franzius C et al (2006) High diagnostic value of 18F-FDG-PET in pediatric patients with chronic inflammatory bowel disease. Ann N Y Acad Sci 1072:379–385
2. Baumgart DC, Sandborn WJ (2007) Inflammatory bowel disease: clinical aspects and established and evolving therapies. Lancet 369:1641–1657
3. Chandler MB, Zeddun SM, Borum ML (2011) The role of positron emission tomography in the evaluation of inflammatory bowel disease. Ann N Y Acad Sci 1228:59–63
4. Al-Hawary M, Zimmermann EM (2012) A new look at Crohn's disease: novel imaging techniques. Curr Opin Gastroenterol 28:334–340
5. Treglia G, Quartuccio N, Sadeghi R et al (2013) Diagnostic performance of Fluorine-18-Fluorodeoxyglucose positron emission tomography in patients with chronic inflammatory bowel disease: a systematic review and a meta-analysis. J Crohn Colitis 7:345–354
6. Skehan SJ, Issenman R, Mernagh J et al (1999) 18F-fluorodeoxyglucose positron tomography in diagnosis of paediatric inflammatory bowel disease. Lancet 354:836–837
7. Lemberg DA, Issenman RM, Cawdron R et al (2005) Positron emission tomography in the investigation of pediatric inflammatory bowel disease. Inflamm Bowel Dis 11:733–738
8. Däbritz J, Jasper N, Loeffler M et al (2011) Noninvasive assessment of pediatric inflammatory bowel disease with 18F-fluorodeoxyglucose-positron emission tomography and computed tomography. Eur J Gastroenterol Hepatol 23:81–89
9. Cistaro A, Quartuccio N, Mansi L et al (2012) The role of positron emission tomography in inflammatory bowel disease. Eur J Inflam 10(3):251–256

Appendicitis

Mariapaola Cucinotta and Angelina Cistaro

In children, appendicitis is the most frequent pathology causing an acute abdomen and requiring surgical treatment [1, 2]. Its incidence is higher among preadolescents/adolescents and young adults, whereas it is uncommon in preschool-aged children ($\leq$5 years old) [1].

The etiology and pathogenesis of appendicitis are unclear although various conditions have been suggested as causative, such as obstruction of the appendiceal lumen by a fecalith, hyperplasia of the lymphoid follicles in the appendiceal wall, primary bacterial and viral infections, or even blunt abdominal trauma and ischemia of the appendix [1, 3]. A diet low in fiber and high in refined carbohydrates, a genetic predisposition, and type I hypersensitivity reactions also have been implicated in the pathogenesis [1]. Yet, while appendicitis is a very common and well-known disease, its diagnosis is frequently difficult, as demonstrated by the high rate of negative laparotomies reported in several studies [2, 4, 5].

To aid in the diagnosis of appendicitis and thereby guide therapeutic decision-making, numerous scores have been developed over the years, based on clinical and laboratory parameters such as neutrophilic leukocytosis [2, 4, 5]. In 2008, the Appendicitis Inflammatory Response (AIR) score was introduced. It considers, besides the usual parameters, another diagnostically important laboratory measurement: C-reactive protein [5]. Both white blood cell count and CRP, despite their low specificity, have a high sensitivity and positive predictive value in the diagnosis of acute appendicitis. Together they result in a significant specificity (~70 %) [6].

A timely and correct diagnosis is important when appendicitis is suspected, not only to avoid unnecessary surgery (and consequent associated morbidity and hospital costs) in patients negative for the disease but also in positive cases to prevent the potentially life-threatening complications (perforation, evolution to a gangrenous form) that can result from a diagnostic delay [7, 8].

Consequently, there is increasing use of noninvasive imaging exams such as ultrasonography, MRI, and CT, which are of high accuracy in the diagnosis of appendicitis and alternative causes of abdominal pain [7, 8]. As for PET, there have been few studies on its role in the detection of appendicitis. Some of them reported high ^{18}F-FDG uptake in the right iliac fossa, subsequently related to the presence of appendicitis,

---

M. Cucinotta, MD
Nuclear Medicine Unit,
Department of Radiological Sciences,
Policlinico Gaetano Martino Hospital,
University of Messina, Via Consolare Valeria, 1,
Messina 98125, Italy
e-mail: mariapaola.cucinotta@gmail.com

A. Cistaro, MD (✉)
Department of Nuclear Medicine, Positron Emission Tomography Center IRMET S.p.A., Euromedic Inc.,
Via Onorato Vigliani 89, Turin 10100, Italy

Institute of Cognitive Sciences and Technologies,
National Research Council, Rome, Italy
e-mail: a.cistaro@irmet.com

as an incidental finding during exams to determine or evaluate malignancies [9, 10].

This avid uptake of ^{18}F-FDG by inflammatory lesions is problematic and misleading in the differential diagnosis of tumors (Fig. 25.1) [11, 12]. Accordingly, familiarity with the normal pattern and physiological variations of ^{18}F-FDG distribution and with clinical data relevant to the patient can aid in correctly diagnosing appendicitis [11]. To reduce the likelihood of false-positives, studies have been conducted in which the behaviors of ^{18}F-FDG and other radiolabeled PET tracers (e.g., amino acids) was compared; their higher specificity for tumor diagnosis was reported [11, 12]. Another option is to use a dual-phase ^{18}F-FDG scan, as the SUV significantly increases in tumors over time but decreases in inflammatory lesions [11, 12].

Nonetheless, the high resolution of PET (especially when combined with CT or MRI) together with the high concentration of ^{18}F-FDG taken up by inflammatory tissues makes PET a potentially useful tool in the earlier detection of appendicitis and other abdominal inflammatory diseases [11].

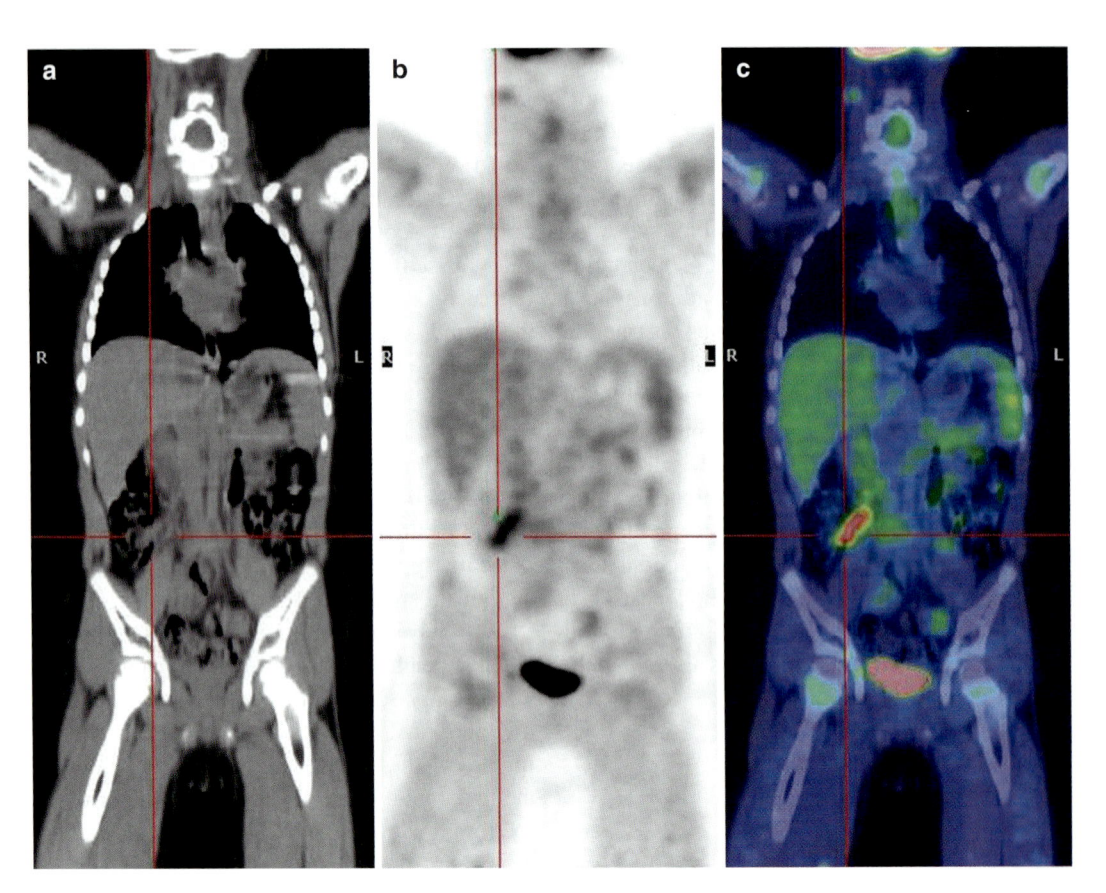

Fig. 25.1 A 12-year-old boy treated for acute lymphoblastic leukemia, t(12;21) positive. CT (**a**), PET (**b**), and PET/CT fusion (**c**) images show FDG accumulation in the right abdomen, corresponding to appendiceal inflammation

References

1. Gardikis S, Giatromanolaki A, Kambouri K, Tripsianis G, Sivridis E, Vaos G (2011) Acute appendicitis in preschoolers: a study of two different populations of children. Ital J Pediatr 37:35
2. Shreef KS, Waly AH, Abd-Elrahman S, Abd Elhafez MA (2010) Alvarado score as an admission criterion in children with pain in right iliac fossa. Afr J Paediatr Surg 7(3):163–165
3. Toumi Z, Chan A, Hadfield MB, Hulton NR (2010) Systematic review of blunt abdominal trauma as a cause of acute appendicitis. Ann R Coll Surg Engl 92(6):477–482
4. Gonçalves JP, Cerqueira A, Martins S (2011) The Alvarado score validation in diagnosing acute appendicitis in children at Braga Hospital. Acta Med Port 24(2):583–588
5. De Castro SSM, Ünlü Ç, Steller EP, Van Wagensveld BA, Vrouenraets BC (2012) Evaluation of the appendicitis inflammatory response score for patients with acute appendicitis. World J Surg 36(7):1540–1545
6. Mekhail P, Naguib N, Yanni F, Izzidien A (2011) Appendicitis in paediatric age group: correlation between preoperative inflammatory markers and postoperative histological diagnosis. Afr J Paediatr Surg 8(3):309–312
7. Toorenvliet BR, Wiersma F, Bakker RF, Merkus JW, Breslau PJ, Hamming JF (2010) Routine ultrasound and limited computed tomography for the diagnosis of acute appendicitis. World J Surg 34(10):2278–2285
8. Purysko AS, Remer EM, Leão Filho HM, Bittencourt LK, Lima RV, Racy DJ (2011) Beyond appendicitis: common and uncommon gastrointestinal causes of right lower quadrant abdominal pain at multidetector CT. Radiographics 31:927–947
9. Torigian DA (2009) Utility of ^{18}F-FDG-PET/CT imaging in the diagnosis of appendicitis. Hell J Nucl Med 12(3):281–282
10. Koff SG, Sterbis JR, Davison JM, Montilla-Soler JL (2006) A unique presentation of appendicitis: F-18 FDG PET/CT. Clin Nucl Med 31(11):704–706
11. Günal O, Doğn S, Gürleyik E (2009) Appendicular mass imitating a malignant cecal tumor on f18-FDG PET/CT study: a case report. Cases J 2:8420
12. Ogawa S, Itabashi M, Kameoka S (2009) Significance of FDG-PET in identification of diseases of the appendix – based on experience of two cases falsely positive for FDG accumulation. Case Rep Gastroenterol 3:125–130

Spondylodiscitis

Mariapaola Cucinotta and Angelina Cistaro

Spondylodiscitis is an inflammatory process involving the vertebral bodies and the cartilaginous disks between them. It is generally caused by microorganisms, most commonly *Staphylococcus aureus*, followed by *Kingella kingae* and other, rarer bacteria [1–4]. Involvement of the spine generally occurs by hematogenous spread from the site of primary infection [1]. Spondylodiscitis is rare in childhood and mostly affects toddlers (0–3 years old), probably because of a more copious blood supply to the cartilaginous disks [5, 6]. Unfortunately, in these very young patients, the diagnosis is difficult as the children are unable to describe their symptoms and may be uncooperative [3, 6]. Moreover, the clinical course can be insidious, with uncertain laboratory results and negative radiographs [4, 6]. The most commonly affected site in toddlers is the lumbar region, such that the children may present with back stiffness, refusal to sit or walk, limping, increased irritability or crying, gait disturbances, or back or abdominal pain [3, 4]. An MRI study is generally fundamental to reach a correct and early diagnosis, which is crucial in order to avoid the severe complications that require surgical treatment, such as epidural abscess and spinal cord compression along with vertebral bone destruction and spinal instability [1, 4, 5]. In addition, PET/CT with ^{18}F-FDG is a very useful tool in the early diagnosis of spondylodiscitis and in evaluating the response to treatment, based on, for example, comparisons of the SUV_{max} determined in exams performed before and after antibiotic therapy [7, 8].

M. Cucinotta, MD
Nuclear Medicine Unit,
Department of Radiological Sciences,
Policlinico Gaetano Martino Hospital,
University of Messina, Via Consolare Valeria, 1,
Messina 98125, Italy
e-mail: mariapaola.cucinotta@gmail.com

A. Cistaro, MD (✉)
Department of Nuclear Medicine, Positron Emission Tomography Center IRMET S.p.A., Euromedic Inc.,
Via Onorato Vigliani 89, Turin 10100, Italy

Institute of Cognitive Sciences and Technologies,
National Research Council, Rome, Italy
e-mail: a.cistaro@irmet.com

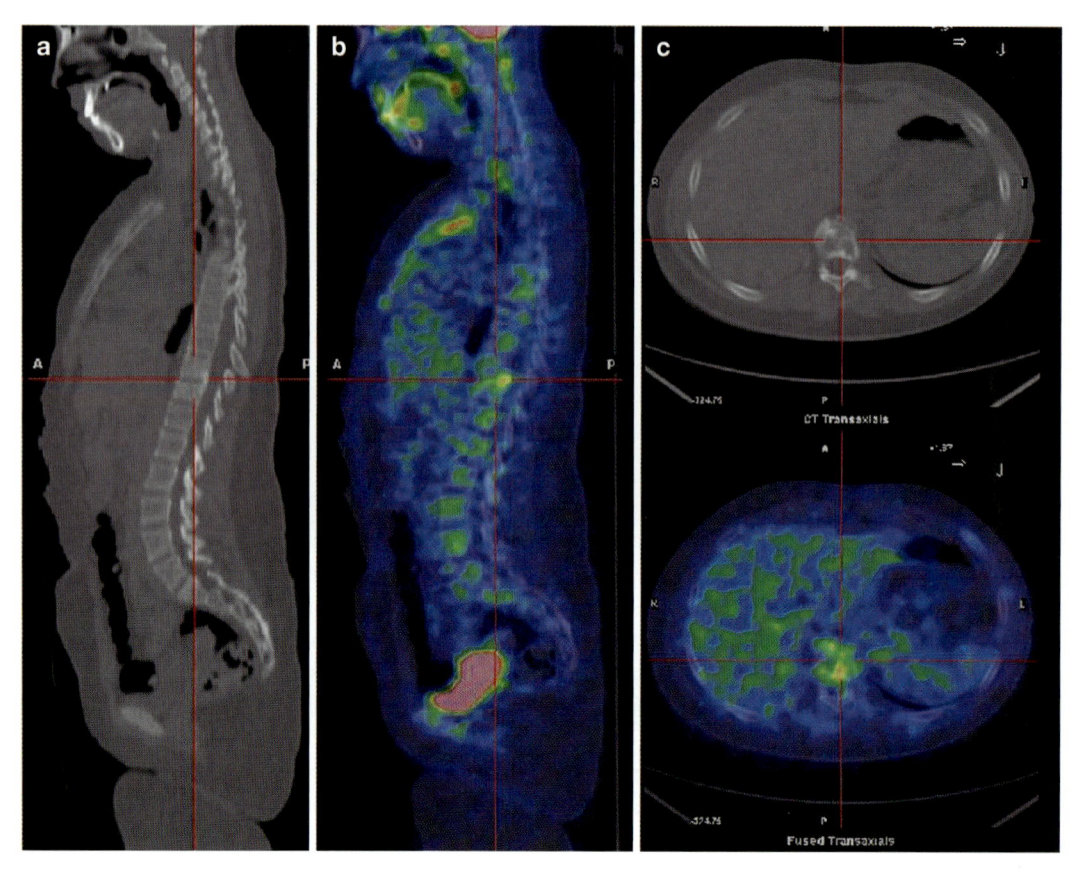

Fig. 26.1 A 12-year-old girl with spondylodiscitis was evaluated in a PET study, performed while she was on antibiotic therapy. Sagittal (**a**, **b**) and axial (**c**) CT and PET/CT fusion images with bone window show inhomogeneous FDG uptake corresponding to the intervertebral disk between the tenth and eleventh vertebrae. Antibiotic treatment was continued

Teaching Point

PET and MRI are of similar accuracy in the diagnosis of spondylodiscitis, supporting the use of PET when MRI findings are doubtful or the exam is not possible [9]. PET is more accurate and more specific than MRI in assessing the therapeutic response of spondylodiscitis and in some cases is preferable to MRI in the determination of when medical treatment can be safely discontinued.

References

1. Ziegelbein J, El-Khoury GY (2011) Early spondylodiscitis presenting with single vertebral body involvement: a report of two cases. Iowa Orthop J 31: 219–224
2. Budnik I, Porte L, Arce JD, Vial S, Zamorano J (2011) Espondilodiskitis caused by Kingella kingae in children: a case report. Rev Chilena Infectol 28(4):369–373
3. Ceroni D, Cherkaoui A, Kaelin A, Schrenzel J (2010) Kingella kingae spondylodiscitis in young children: toward a new approach for bacteriological investigations? A preliminary report. J Child Orthop 4(2): 173–175
4. Bining HJS, Saigal G, Chankowsky J, Rubin EE, Camlioglu EB (2006) Kingella kingae spondylodiscitis in a child. Br J Radiol 79:181–183
5. Tapia Moreno R, Espinosa Fernández MG, Martínez León MI, González Gómez JM, Moreno Pascual P (2009) Spondylodiscitis: diagnosis and medium-long term follow up of 18 cases. An Pediatr 71(5): 391–399
6. Brown R, Hussain M, McHugh K, Novelli V, Jones D (2001) Discitis in young children. J Bone Joint Surg Br 83(1):106–111
7. Gemmel F, Rijk PC, Collins JMP, Parlevliet T, Stumpe KD, Palestro CJ (2009) Expanding role of ^{18}F-fluoro-d-deoxyglucose PET and PET/CT in spinal infections. Eur Spine J 19(4):540–551
8. Nanni C, Boriani L, Salvadori C, Zamparini E, Rorato G, Ambrosini V, Gasbarrini A, Tumietto F, Cristini F, Scudeller L, Boriani S, Viale P, Fanti S (2012) FDG PET/CT is useful for the interim evaluation of response to therapy in patients affected by haematogenous spondylodiscitis. Eur J Nucl Med Mol Imaging 39(10):1538–1544
9. Skanjeti A, Penna D, Douroukas A, Cistaro A et al (2012) PET in the clinical work-up of patients with spondylodiscitis: a new tool for the clinician? Q J Nucl Med Mol Imaging 56(1):1–8

Other Bone Lesions

27

Angelina Cistaro

An acute traumatic fracture can be present with a level of ^{18}F-FDG uptake generally considered indicative of neoplasm. It is important to recognize that increased FDG-PET activity in bone should not be accepted as definitive evidence of neoplastic or metastatic disease.

Nevertheless, FDG-PET/CT is useful in differentiating some rare benign form of bone disease, such as eosinophilic granuloma, from more aggressive manifestation.

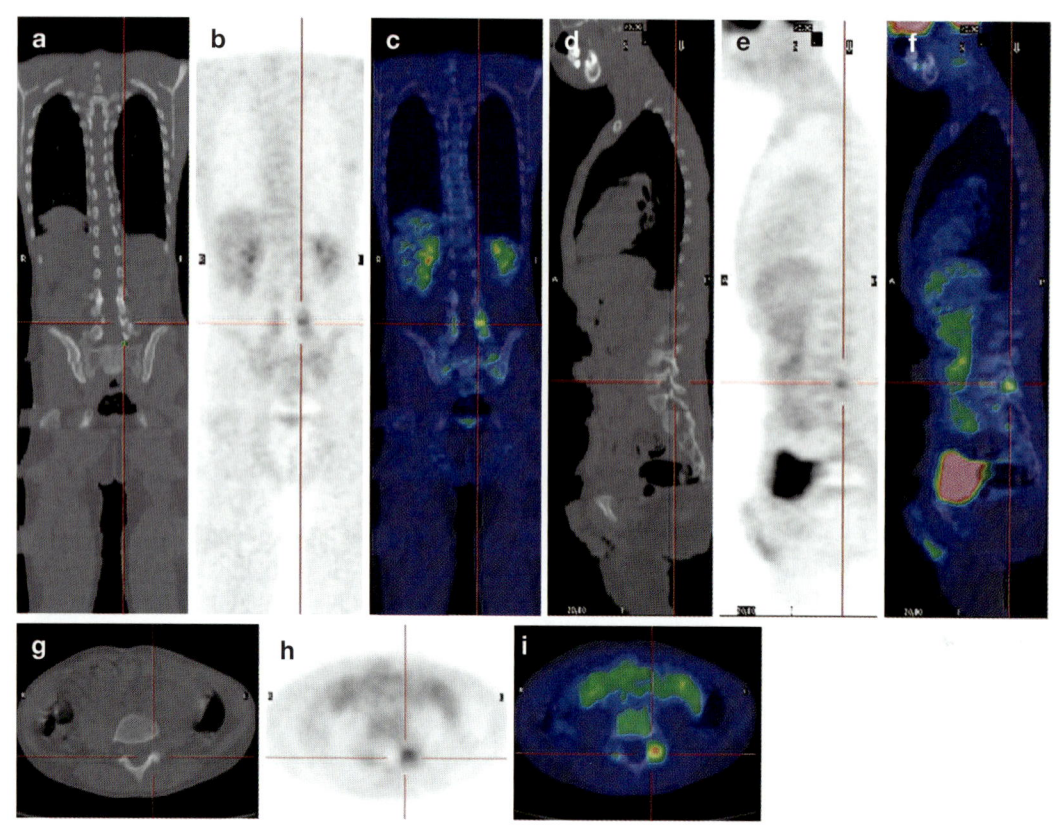

Fig. 27.1 A 13-year-old boy suffered a traumatic fracture of the left superior articular process of the fifth vertebra while playing football. Coronal (**a–c**), sagittal (**d–f**), and axial (**g–i**) CT with bone window (**a, d, g**), PET (**b, e, h**), and PET/CT fusion (**c, f, i**) images show focal FDG uptake corresponding to the fracture site

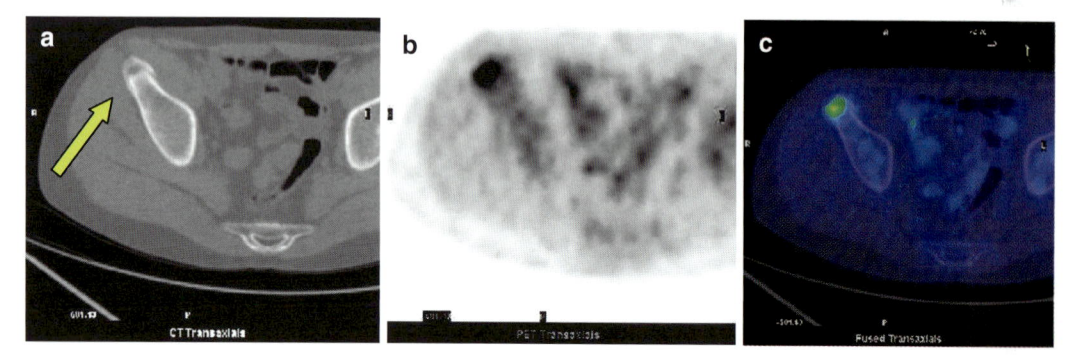

Fig. 27.2 A 15-year-old boy underwent a PET evaluation during chemotherapy for Hodgkin's lymphoma, stage III. Axial bone window CT (**a**), PET (**b**), and PET/CT fusion (**c**) images show ^{18}F-FDG uptake in the left anterior iliac spine (*yellow arrow* in **a**). The diagnosis was a traumatic fracture subsequent to bone marrow biopsy

27 Other Bone Lesions 211

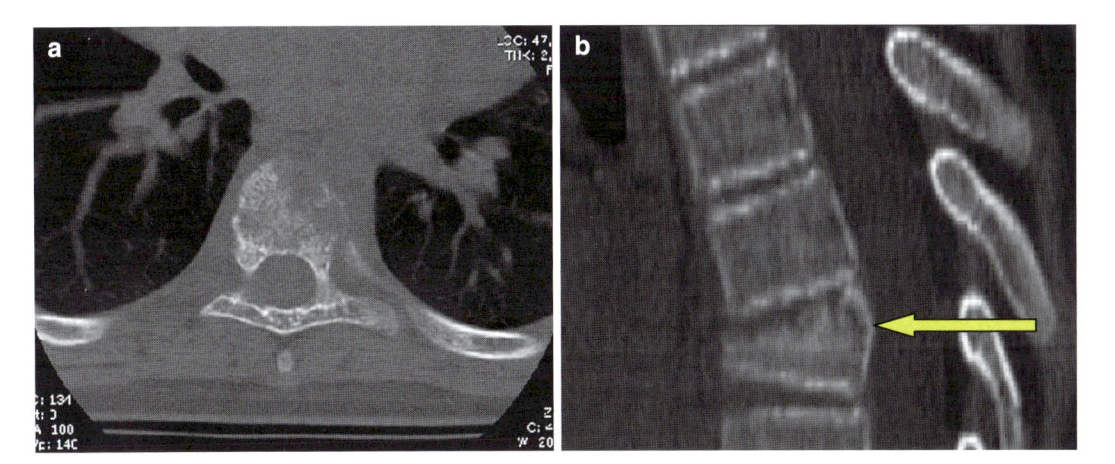

Fig. 27.3 An 11-year-old girl was admitted for dorsal pain, without trauma. Bone scintigraphy showed an accumulation in the fifth and sixth vertebrae. Axial (**a**) and sagittal (**b**) bone window CT shows a lytic lesion in the sixth dorsal vertebra (*yellow arrow* in **b**), with pathological findings in the left paravertebral soft tissues

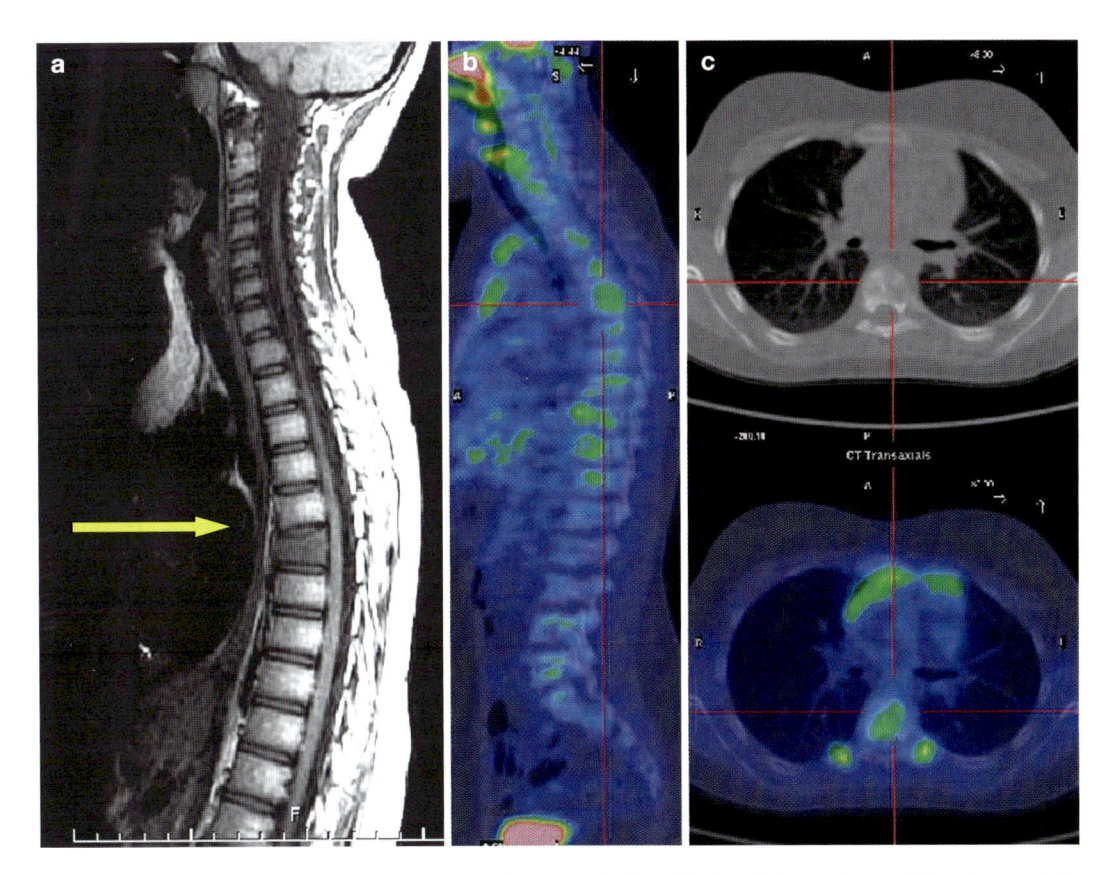

Fig. 27.4 T1 MRI (**a**) conducted for suspected bone fracture, probably secondary to bone marrow disease such as lymphoproliferative conditions (*yellow arrow* in **a**). Alternatively, an eosinophilic granuloma was considered. The patient was referred to our center for metabolic characterization of the bone lesion and to search for other metabolically active areas, more accessible to biopsy and with lower risk of late-onset damage. The PET/CT (**b**, **c**) study shows an inhomogeneous lesion with low metabolic activity in the sixth dorsal vertebra, confirming the second hypothesis

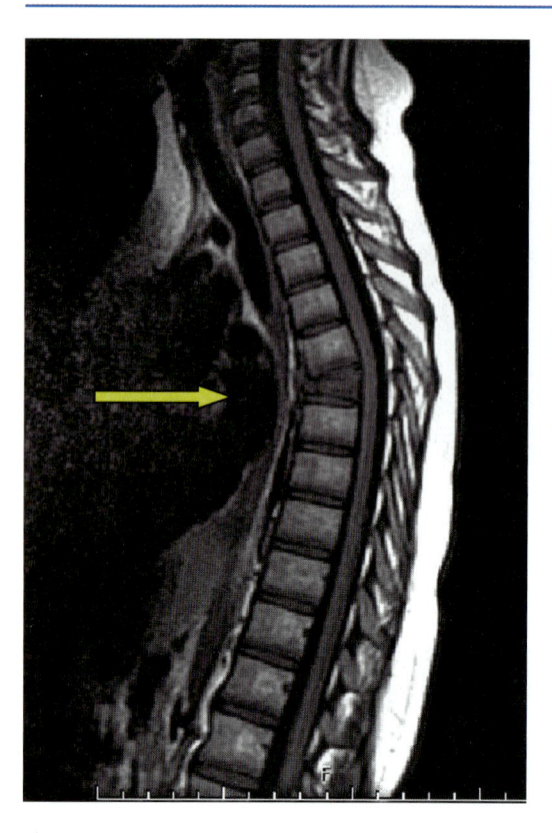

Fig. 27.5 Same patient as in Fig. 27.4. Sagittal T1 MRI follow-up at 3 months showed stabilization of the lesion and an area of tissue thickening, indicative of a reparative process (*yellow arrow*)

Teaching Point

It is important to consider that although eosinophilic granuloma is usually a benign form of bone disease, in rare cases, it may be the presenting manifestation of the more serious, multifocal, Langerhans cell histiocytosis. In these patients, the prognosis is more guarded.

Suggested Reading

1. Cho WI, Chang UK (2011) Comparison of MR imaging and FDG-PET/CT in the differential diagnosis of benign and malignant vertebral compression fractures. J Neurosurg Spine 14(2):177–183, Epub 2011
2. Shammas A (2009) Nuclear medicine imaging of the pediatric musculoskeletal system. Semin Musculoskelet Radiol 13(3):159–180
3. Thakur NA, Daniels AH, Schiller J, Valdes MA, Czerwein JK, Schiller A, Esmende S, Terek RMJ (2012) Benign tumors of the spine. J Am Acad Orthop Surg 20(11):715–724

Pulmonary Aspergillosis

28

Mariapaola Cucinotta and Angelina Cistaro

Pulmonary aspergillosis is the most frequent clinical manifestation of the infection caused by *Aspergillus* spp. in immunosuppressed patients. Several conditions have been identified as risk factors for the development of the disease, all of which either substantially promote exposure to fungal spores or compromise the patient's immune system. Among the various risk factors, severe and persistent neutropenia and impaired cell-mediated immunity are the most important. Consequently, individuals at highest risk of developing aspergillosis are those with acute myeloid leukemia and other malignant diseases as well as recipients of hematopoietic stem cell or solid-organ transplants [1, 2].

Aspergillus spp. are the second most common cause of invasive fungal infections (IFIs) in children, after *Candida* spp. infections. Within the past 20 years, the incidence of IFIs has considerably increased, paralleling the improved quality of treatment and survival rate of immunocompromised patients [3]. IFIs are associated with high morbidity and mortality, which can mainly be attributed to the difficulties and delays in diagnosing their occurrence [3, 4]. A favorable prognosis in affected patients therefore largely depends on early diagnosis as well as timely and correct pharmacological treatment [4, 5].

Today, IFIs are detected based on clinical signs, laboratory tests, and radiological exams. The definitive diagnosis relies on the microbiological findings from cultures and/or biopsies, but these methods are characterized by their low sensitivity, especially in the earlier phases of infection [4]. A useful laboratory test is the detection of galactomannan antigen in biological fluids [5]. Among imaging exams, chest X-rays and CT can provide important diagnostic information. CT findings include the "halo sign," i.e., a ground-glass opacity surrounding a nodule or mass. However, this radiological finding has a low specificity because it is seen not only in IFIs but also in other infections and in several noninfectious diseases [6]. Moreover, the "halo sign" does not allow discrimination between infections caused by *Aspergillus fumigatus* and those due to other invasive molds [7].

Nuclear medicine contributes significantly to the detection of invasive aspergillosis. Among the many radiopharmaceuticals proposed for this purpose is ^{67}Ga-citrate, although its use is limited by its unfavorable pharmacokinetics and failure to distinguish between infections and malignant

M. Cucinotta, MD
Nuclear Medicine Unit,
Department of Radiological Sciences,
Policlinico Gaetano Martino Hospital,
University of Messina,
Via Consolare Valeria, 1, Messina 98125, Italy
e-mail: mariapaola.cucinotta@gmail.com

A. Cistaro, MD (✉)
Department of Nuclear Medicine,
Positron Emission Tomography Center
IRMET S.p.A., Euromedic Inc.,
Via Onorato Vigliani 89, Turin 10100, Italy

Institute of Cognitive Sciences and Technologies,
National Research Council, Rome, Italy
e-mail: a.cistaro@irmet.com

diseases. Other radiotracers have been studied, such as ^{99m}Tc-labeled polyethyleneglycol liposomes, ^{99m}Tc-interleukin-8, ^{99m}Tc-fluconazole, and ^{99m}Tc-antimicrobial peptides such as ubiquicidin, but none has demonstrated significant specificity for aspergillosis [4].

The need for sensitive and specific radiocompounds has led to the development of an ^{111}In-labeled cyclic peptide targeting *Aspergillus fumigatus*. ^{111}In-DTPA-c(CGGRLGPFC)-NH(2) was shown to be taken up in significantly higher amounts in the lungs of mice infected with the fungus than in those of healthy mice, but clinical trials are still needed [8].

PET with ^{18}F-FDG, despite its low specificity because it follows glucose metabolism, remains

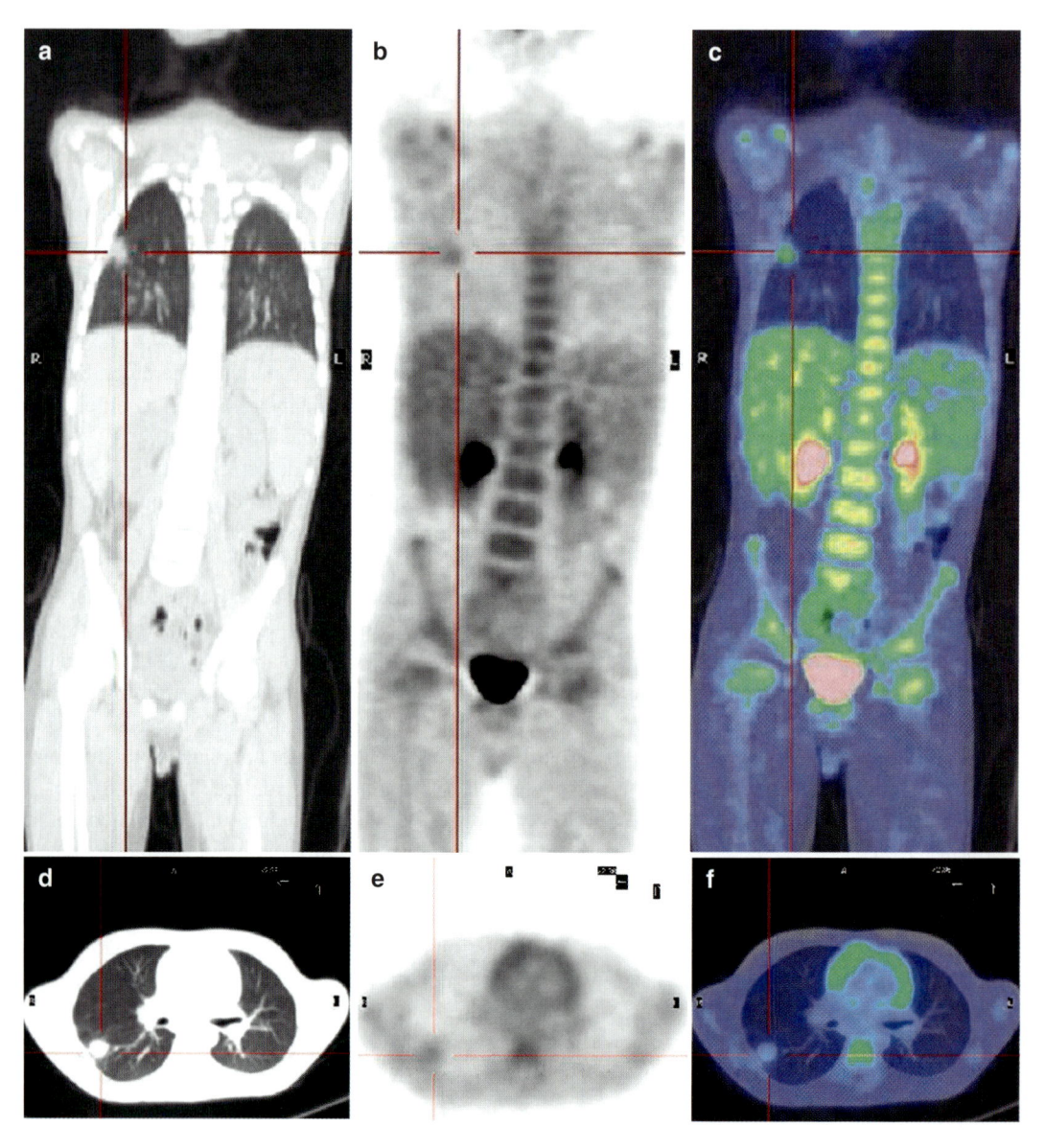

Fig. 28.1 An 8-year-old boy treated for Epstein–Barr-virus-associated hemophagocytic lympho-histiocytosis complicated by aspergillosis. Coronal (**a–c**) and axial (**d–f**) CT with lung window (**a, d**), PET (**b, e**), and PET/CT fusion (**c, f**) images show mild FDG accumulation corresponding to the aspergillosis lesion in the lower lobe of the right lung. On the coronal PET/CT fusion image (**c**), note the splenic and bone marrow activation

Fig. 28.2 A 5-year-old girl who underwent hematopoietic stem cell transplantation for T-cell immunodeficiency syndrome. Seven days after transplantation, she developed a fever. Axial CT (**a**), PET (**b**), and PET/CT fusion (**c**) images show mild inhomogeneous FDG uptake in the anterior segment of the upper lobe of the left lung. Aspergillus antigenemia was positive and therapy with amphotericin B was initiated

a promising tool in the initial diagnosis and staging of active invasive fungal infection. According to a recent prospective study of 30 patients with IFIs (ten with acute invasive aspergillosis) [9], ^{18}F-FDG uptake in all fungal lesions previously identified by CT and/or MRI was higher than in noninfected tissues [9]. In addition, preclinical evaluations in mouse models demonstrated the high sensitivity of the new PET radiotracers specific for aspergillosis. These compounds are low molecular mass iron chelators, termed siderophores, and they are used by *Aspergillus fumigatus* in iron acquisition, which is fundamental for the growth and virulence of the fungus. Triacetylfusarinine (TAFC) and ferrioxamine E (FOXE), both labeled with ^{68}Ga, showed high focal uptake that corresponded to the pathological findings in infected lung tissue seen on CT [4].

References

1. Pagano L, Akova M, Dimopoulos G, Herbrecht R, Drgona L, Blijlevens N (2011) Risk assessment and prognostic factors for mould-related diseases in immunocompromised patients. J Antimicrob Chemother 66(1):5–14
2. Ramos ER, Jiang Y, Hachem R, Kassis C, Kontoyiannis DP, Raad I (2011) Outcome analysis of invasive aspergillosis in hematologic malignancy and hematopoietic stem cell transplant patients: the role of novel antimold azoles. Oncologist 16(7):1049–1060
3. Brissaud O, Guichoux J, Harambat J, Tandonnet O, Zaoutis T (2012) Invasive fungal disease in PICU: epidemiology and risk factors. Ann Intensive Care 2(1):6
4. Petrik M, Franssen GM, Haas H, Laverman P, Hörtnagl C, Schrettl M, Helbok A, Lass- Flörl C, Decristoforo C (2012) Preclinical evaluation of two ^{68}Ga-siderophores as potential radiopharmaceuticals for Aspergillus fumigatus infection imaging. Eur J Nucl Med Mol Imaging 39(7):1175–1183
5. Zou M, Tang L, Zhao S, Zhao Z, Chen L, Chen P, Huang Z, Li J, Chen L, Fan X (2012) Systematic review and meta-analysis of detecting galactomannan in bronchoalveolar lavage fluid for diagnosing invasive aspergillosis. PLoS One 7(8):43347
6. Georgiadou SP, Sipsas NV, Marom EM, Kontoyiannis DP (2011) The diagnostic value of halo and reversed halo signs for invasive mold infections in compromised hosts. Clin Infect Dis 52(9):1144–1155
7. Li XS, Zhu HX, Fan HX, Zhu L, Wang HX, Song YL (2011) Pulmonary fungal infections after bone marrow transplantation: the value of high-resolution computed tomography in predicting their etiology. Chin Med J 124(20):3249–3254
8. Yang Z, Kontoyiannis DP, Wen X, Xiong C, Zhang R, Albert ND et al (2009) Gamma scintigraphy imaging of murine invasive pulmonary aspergillosis with a ^{111}In-labeled cyclic peptide. Nucl Med Biol 36(3):259–266
9. Hot A, Maunoury C, Poiree S, Lanternier F, Viard JP, Loulergue P, Coignard H, Bougnoux ME, Suarez F, Rubio MT, Mahlaoui N, Dupont B, Lecuit M, Faraggi M, Lortholary O (2011) Diagnostic contribution of positron emission tomography with [^{18}F]fluorodeoxyglucose for invasive fungal infections. Clin Microbiol Infect 17(3):409–417

Mycobacteriosis

29

Giorgio Treglia and Angelina Cistaro

29.1 Introduction

Tuberculosis is a common, and in many cases lethal, infectious disease caused by *Mycobacterium tuberculosis*. The bacterium is transmitted by aerosol (e.g., coughing) and infected individuals usually present with respiratory symptoms. While pulmonary TBC is the most common presentation, the infection can spread to virtually any tissue or organ of the body, either by hematogenous or lymphatic dissemination or contiguity. TBC remains a major worldwide cause of morbidity and mortality. In addition, the incidence of non-tuberculous mycobacterial infections, especially *Mycobacterium avium intracellulare* complex (MAC), is increasing [1].

Despite various improvements in imaging technology, surgical resection is still required to differentiate malignant from benign lesions, such as mycobacteriosis, in a significant number of patients. Sputum culture and radiological examinations are not useful as tools in diagnosing latent and active disease or for monitoring the response to therapy in patients with bacillus-unproven mycobacteriosis (including smear-negative pulmonary and most cases of extrapulmonary mycobacteriosis) [2].

While ^{18}F-FDG–PET and PET/CT are sensitive techniques in oncological imaging, it is well known that inflammatory and infectious lesions, including mycobacteriosis, can cause false-positive results at ^{18}F-FDG–PET [3–5]. Macrophages, lymphocytes, neutrophil granulocytes, and other inflammatory cells as well as fibroblasts avidly take up ^{18}F-FDG, especially under active conditions [4]. Both lymphocytes and especially macrophages are intensely present at sites of active TBC.

G. Treglia, MD
Department of Nuclear Medicine,
Oncology Institute of Southern Switzerland,
Via Ospedale, 12, Bellinzona CH-6500, Switzerland
e-mail: giorgiomednuc@libero.it

A. Cistaro, MD (✉)
Department of Nuclear Medicine,
Positron Emission Tomography Center
IRMET S.p.A., Euromedic Inc.,
Via Onorato Vigliani 89, Turin 10100, Italy

Institute of Cognitive Sciences and Technologies,
National Research Council, Rome, Italy
e-mail: a.cistaro@irmet.com

Clinical Case

A 13-year-old girl with history of Hodgkin's lymphoma, previously treated, underwent ^{18}F-FDG–PET/CT for disease restaging. The ^{18}F-FDG–PET/CT scan showed multiple areas of increased radiopharmaceutical uptake in the thoracic and upper abdominal regions, corresponding to several lymphadenopathies, multiple bilateral pulmonary nodules, and multiple hypodense areas in the liver (Fig. 29.1).

These PET findings were strongly suggestive of neoplastic disease. The patient underwent liver, pulmonary, and thoracic lymph nodal biopsy. Histology of the biopsy specimens showed the presence of granulomatous disease without neoplastic cells. Laboratory data revealed the presence of TBC infection. Consequently, the final diagnosis, made on the basis of radiological and laboratory data, was active TBC. The patient was treated with an antimycobacterial agent.

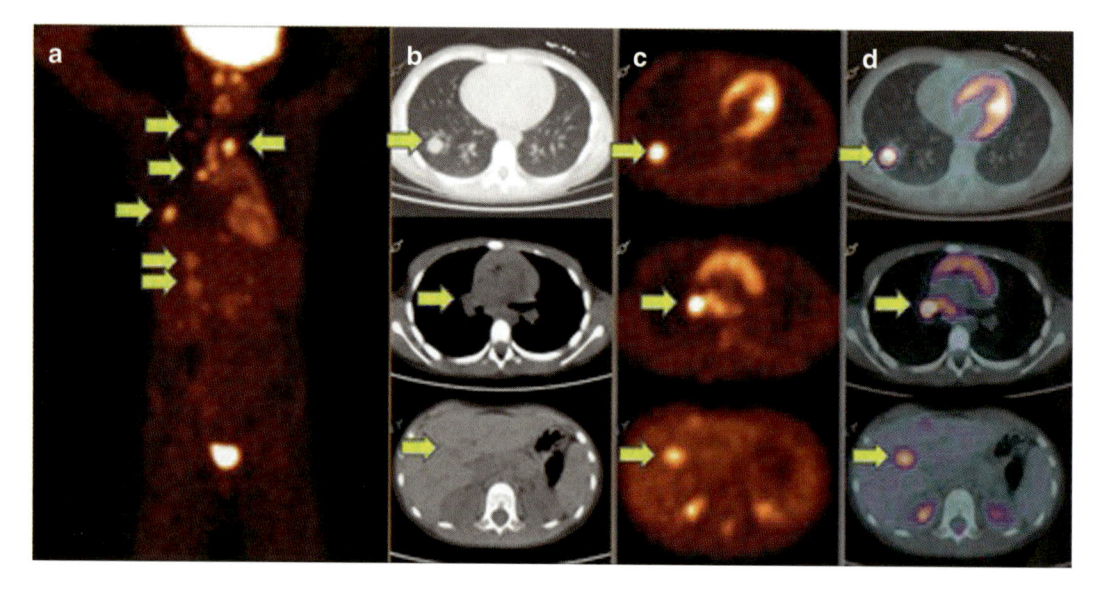

Fig. 29.1 Maximum intensity projection ^{18}F-FDG–PET image (**a**) shows multiple areas of increased radiopharmaceutical uptake in the thoracic region and in the upper abdomen (*arrows*). The axial CT (**b**), PET (**c**), and PET/CT (**d**) images show increased radiopharmaceutical uptake corresponding to pulmonary (**b–d**, *first row*), lymph node (**b–d**, *second row*), and liver (**b–d**, *third row*) lesions (*arrows*). These findings were suspicious for malignancy but histology demonstrated the presence of granulomatous disease and laboratory data suggested a TBC infection

Teaching Point

Mycobacteriosis (including TBC) frequently causes an increased ^{18}F-FDG uptake in affected organs. Thus, in geographic regions with a high prevalence of granulomatous diseases, positive ^{18}F-FDG–PET results should be interpreted with caution in differentiating benign from malignant abnormalities.

^{18}F-FDG–PET and PET/CT may be useful in the detection of foci of mycobacteriosis, allowing the accurate localization of biopsy sites for subsequent histological examination, and in the evaluation of disease activity in patients with mycobacteriosis, including pediatric patients.

References

1. Grandjean L, Moore D (2008) Tuberculosis in the developing world: recent advances in diagnosis with special consideration of the extensively drug-resistant tuberculosis. Curr Opin Infect Dis 21:454–461
2. Winer-Muram HT (2006) The solitary pulmonary nodule. Radiology 239:34–49
3. Bakheet S, Powe J (2000) Benign causes of 18-FDG uptake on whole-body imaging. Semin Nucl Med 28:352–358
4. Kubota R, Yamada S, Kubota K et al (1992) Intratumoral distribution of fluorine-18-deoxyglucose in vivo: high accumulation in macrophages and granulation tissues studied by microautoradiography. J Nucl Med 33:1972–1980
5. Treglia G, Taralli S, Calcagni ML et al (2011) Is there a role for fluorine 18 fluorodeoxyglucose-positron emission tomography and positron emission tomography/computed tomography in evaluating patients with mycobacteriosis? A systematic review. J Comput Assist Tomogr 35:387–393

Part VI

Other Applications

Sarcoidosis

30

Giorgio Treglia and Angelina Cistaro

30.1 Introduction

Sarcoidosis is a systemic inflammatory disease of unknown etiology that affects the lungs (in >90 % of sarcoidosis patients), salivary glands, eyes, lymph nodes, liver, heart, and in some cases the subcutaneous tissues, joints, and the skeletal muscle system [1, 2]. In affected organs, there is an accumulation of T lymphocytes and mononuclear phagocytes. Noncaseating epithelioid granulomas are the characteristic histopathological lesions [1–3]. Considering the protean clinical manifestations of sarcoidosis as well as its multiple localizations, its natural history and course are variable and unpredictable. The majority of granulomas eventually resolve, but in some patients, fibrosis ensues, giving rise to tissue dysfunction [1, 2, 4].

Imaging methods, particularly chest radiography and CT, play an important role in the diagnosis and treatment of sarcoidosis, in primary staging of the disease, and in patient follow-up. Bilateral pulmonary hilar lymphadenopathy and mediastinal lymph nodes are the most common radiological findings, often associated with pulmonary infiltrates [1, 2, 5]. Disease activity in sarcoidosis can be monitored by detecting and quantifying the degree of inflammatory and granulomatous reactions that occur in the lungs and elsewhere in the body. The ability to visualize ^{18}F-FDG accumulation by activated inflammatory cells makes whole-body ^{18}F-FDG–PET/CT a promising modality in the assessment of disease activity in sarcoidosis patients [6].

G. Treglia, MD
Department of Nuclear Medicine,
Oncology Institute of Southern Switzerland,
Via Ospedale, 12, Bellinzona CH-6500, Switzerland
e-mail: giorgiomednuc@libero.it

A. Cistaro, MD (✉)
Department of Nuclear Medicine,
Positron Emission Tomography Center
IRMET S.p.A., Euromedic Inc.,
Via Onorato Vigliani 89, Turin 10100, Italy

Institute of Cognitive Sciences and Technologies,
National Research Council, Rome, Italy
e-mail: a.cistaro@irmet.com

Case 1

A 14-year-old boy underwent ^{18}F-FDG–PET/CT for a fever of unknown origin. The scan showed multiple areas of increased radiopharmaceutical uptake in the thoracic region, corresponding to several bilateral lymph nodes in the mediastinum and pulmonary hilar region. He therefore underwent mediastinal lymph node biopsy. Histology showed the presence of granulomatous disease, compatible with sarcoidosis. Based on the radiological and histology findings, the diagnosis was active sarcoidosis (Fig. 30.1).

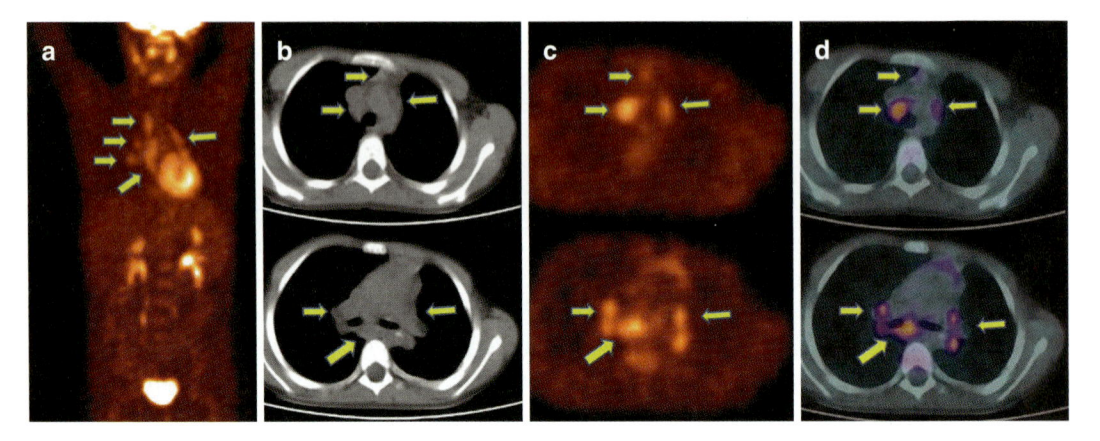

Fig. 30.1 Maximum intensity projection ^{18}F-FDG–PET image (**a**) shows multiple areas of increased radiopharmaceutical uptake in the thoracic region (*arrows*). Axial CT (**b**), PET (**c**), and PET/CT (**d**) images show the presence of increased radiopharmaceutical uptake corresponding to several lymph nodes located bilaterally in the mediastinum and in the pulmonary hilar region

Teaching Point

Sarcoidosis typically causes increased ^{18}F-FDG uptake. Thus, in differentiating benign from malignant abnormalities, positive ^{18}F-FDG–PET findings should be interpreted with caution. ^{18}F-FDG–PET/CT is a very useful molecular imaging method in assessing disease activity and in identifying the occult sites of disease in patients with sarcoidosis, including pediatric patients.

Case 2

One year before presenting to our clinic, a 17-year-old boy without a remarkable disease history had an EBV infection, with the appearance of lymph nodes in the left lateral cervical region and, on his right side, in the trochlear area. Concurrently, he reported occasional skeletal pain and swelling in the right knee and both feet, progressive rhinitis with anosmia, and polydipsia–polyuria. Due to the persistence of a fever of unknown origin, the patient underwent a ^{18}F-FDG–PET/CT which showed multiple areas of increased tracer uptake in the body (Figs. 30.2, 30.3, 30.4, and 30.5). Histology on some of the ^{18}F-FDG-avid lesions demonstrated granulomatous disease compatible with sarcoidosis. The patient underwent immunosuppressive therapy. A repeated ^{18}F-FDG–PET/CT demonstrated an excellent response to the treatment (Fig. 30.6).

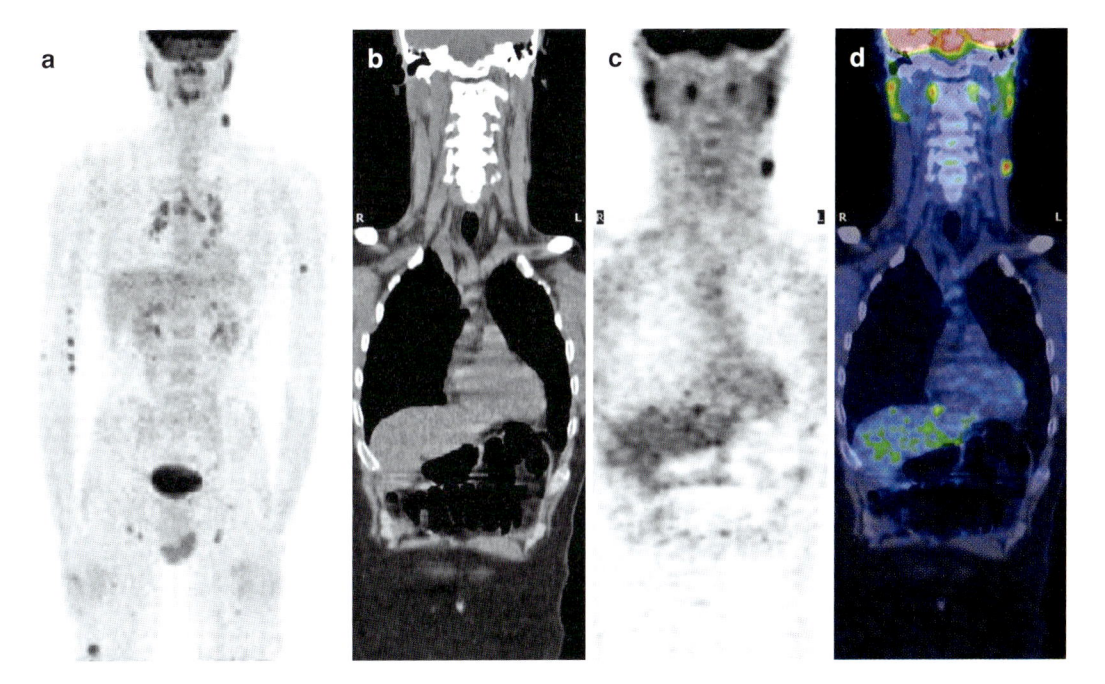

Fig. 30.2 Maximum intensity projection PET image (**a**) showing ^{18}F-FDG uptake in the lymph nodes of the left laterocervical region, arms, mediastinum, pulmonary hilar and inguinal regions, and in the right leg. Coronal CT with mediastinal window (**b**), PET (**c**), and PET/CT fusion (**d**) images show a ^{18}F-FDG-avid left laterocervical lymph node

Case 2 (continued)

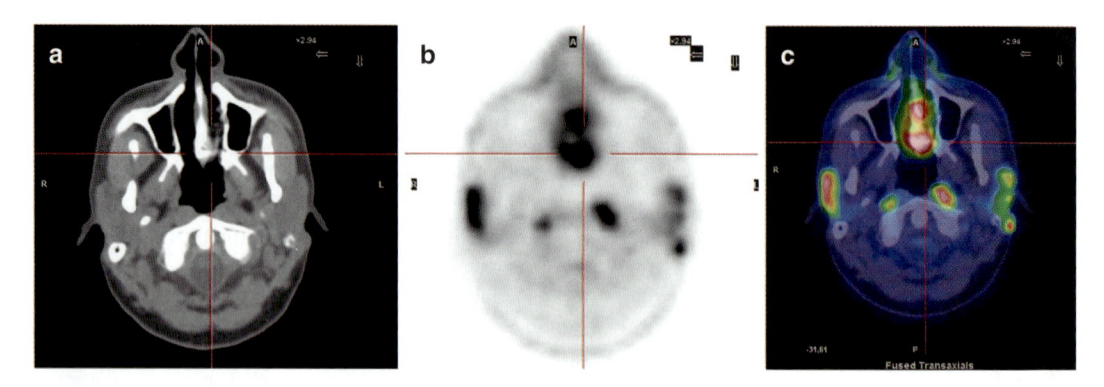

Fig. 30.3 Axial CT (**a**), PET (**b**), and PET/CT fusion (**c**) images show intense and inhomogeneous ^{18}F-FDG uptake by the nasal cavity and parotid glands, consistent with the ultrasound findings of numerous hypoechoic solid areas, partially confluent

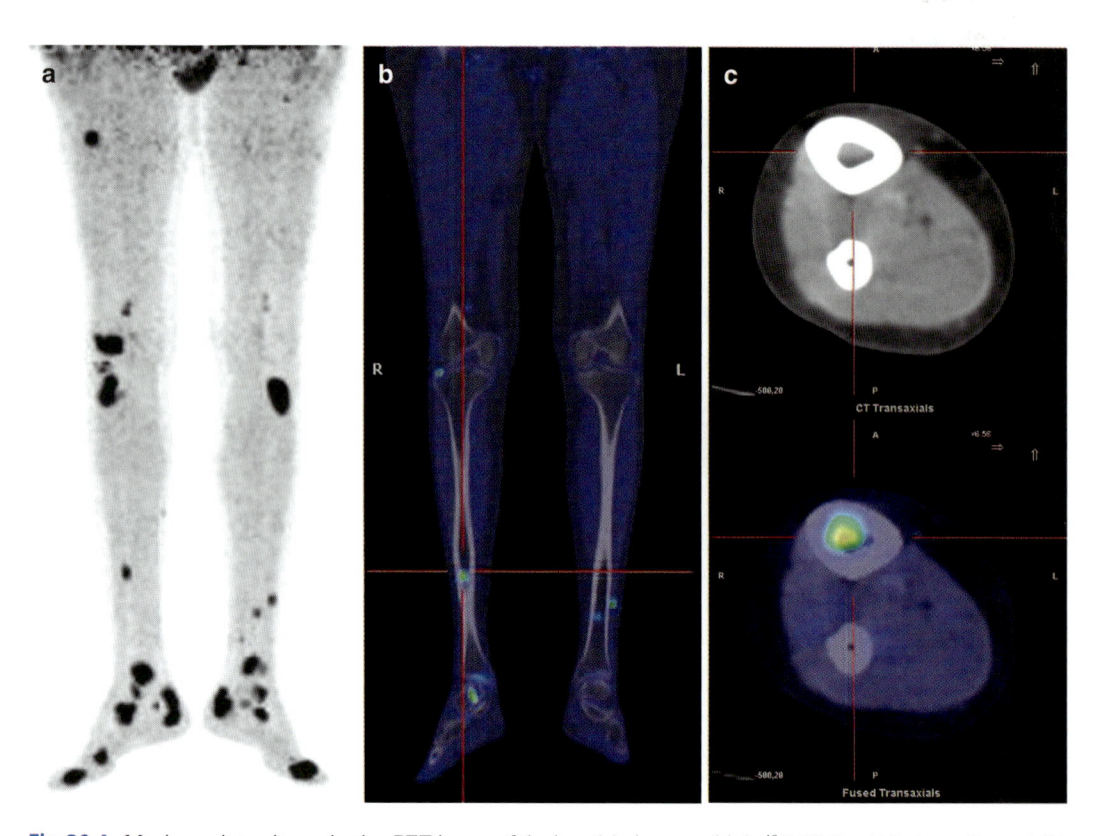

Fig. 30.4 Maximum intensity projection PET image of the legs (**a**) shows multiple ^{18}F-FDG-avid lesions. Coronal (**b**) and axial (**c**) fusion PET images corresponding to an intramedullary lesion of the right tibia

30 Sarcoidosis

Case 2 (continued)

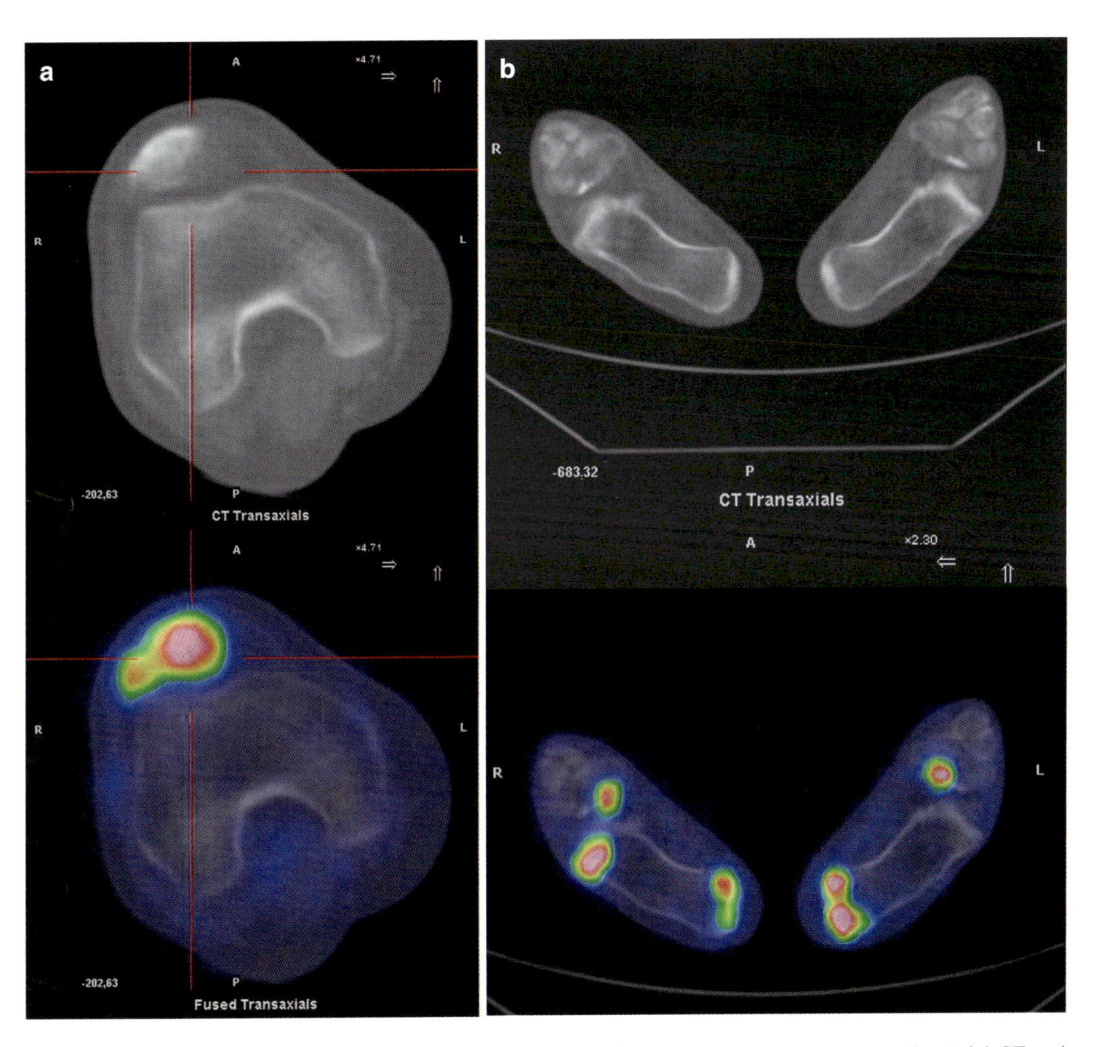

Fig. 30.5 Axial CT and PET/CT of the right knee (**a**) show a ^{18}F-FDG-avid lesion on the patella. Axial CT and PET/CT of the feet (**b**) show other bone lesions

Case 2 (continued)

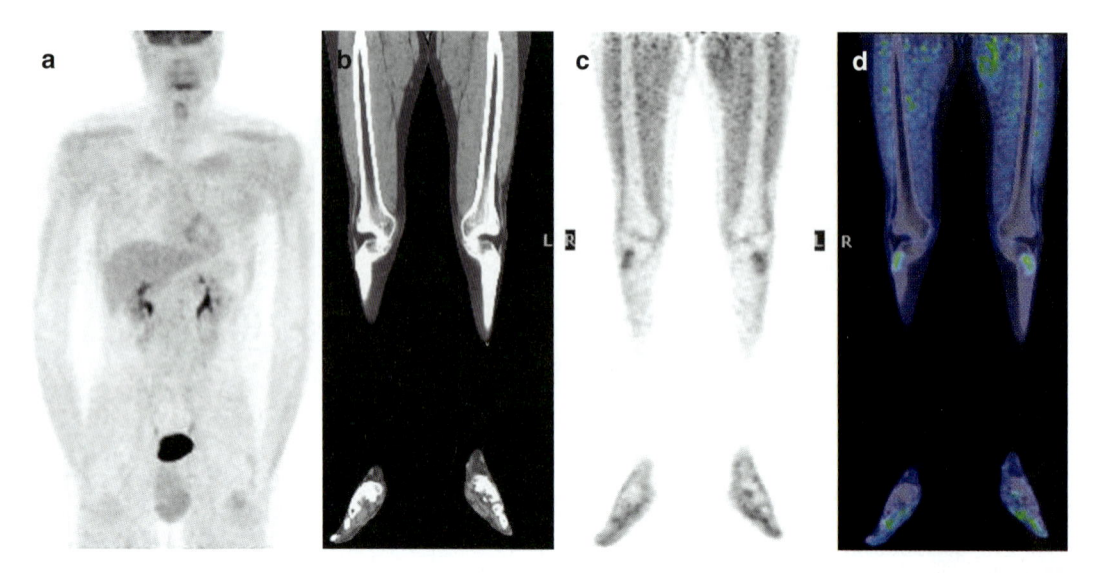

Fig. 30.6 Maximum intensity projection PET image of the body (**a**) and coronal CT (**b**), PET (**c**), and PET/CT fusion (**d**) images of the legs show a complete response to immunosuppressive drugs, except for persisting mild patellar uptake bilaterally

Teaching Point

The degree of inflammatory and granulomatous reactions in sarcoidosis can be detected and estimated by means of ^{18}F-FDG–PET throughout the body. The same method can be used to evaluate the response to therapy.

References

1. Morgenthau AS, Iannuzzi MC (2011) Recent advances in sarcoidosis. Chest 139:174–182
2. Iannuzzi MC, Rybicki BA, Teirstein AS (2007) Sarcoidosis. N Engl J Med 357:2153–2165
3. Müller-Quernheim J (1998) Sarcoidosis: immunopathogenetic concepts and their clinical application. Eur Respir J 12:716–738
4. Nunes H, Soler P, Valeyre D (2005) Pulmonary sarcoidosis. Allergy 60:565–582
5. Koyama T, Ueda H, Togashi K et al (2004) Radiologic manifestations of sarcoidosis in various organs. Radiographics 24:87–104
6. Treglia G, Taralli S, Giordano A (2011) Emerging role of whole-body 18F-fluorodeoxyglucose positron emission tomography as a marker of disease activity in patients with sarcoidosis: a systematic review. Sarcoidosis Vasc Diffuse Lung Dis 28:87–94

Neurofibromatosis

31

Giorgio Treglia and Angelina Cistaro

Neurofibromatosis type 1 (NF1) is an autosomal dominant disease in which the most common tumor is neurofibroma. This benign tumor of the peripheral nerve sheath may present as a focal nodular cutaneous or subcutaneous lesion, an intraforaminal spinal nerve root tumor, or as plexiform neurofibroma (PNF). In addition, patients with NF1 are at high risk of developing malignant peripheral nerve sheath tumors (MPNST) [1–6]. Accordingly, differentiating between benign and malignant tumors in NF1 patients has important prognostic and therapeutic implications, but it can be difficult, especially in individuals with multiple benign tumors. MRI and CT can be used to determine the site and extent of the PNF, but these methods are not reliable in discriminating with high accuracy between benign PNF and tumors that have degenerated into MPNST [1–6].

Histology remains the gold standard for identifying malignant transformation within a PNF. However, it requires complete excision, which in many patients is not technically feasible. If a core biopsy is performed, the focus of malignant change, particularly within a large heterogeneous tumor, may be missed. Moreover, histopathology and tumor grading of MPNST do not strictly correlate with the prognosis [1–6].

Several studies have shown the potential role of whole-body FDG-PET and PET/CT in patients with NF1 for detecting malignant change in PNF, for predicting tumor progression in these patients, for predicting survival in patients with MPNST, and for surveillance in pediatric patients with NF1 (Figs. 31.1, 31.2, and 31.3). An overview of the literature on the role of FDG-PET and PET/CT in patients with NF1 has been recently provided [7]. Its conclusions can be summarized as follows: (a) FDG-PET and PET/CT are useful and highly sensitive noninvasive methods to identify malignant change in neurogenic tumors in patients with NF1; (b) FDG-PET and PET/CT allow the discrimination of MPNST from benign neurogenic lesions in NF1; nevertheless, an overlap between these two disease manifestations regarding their SUVs should be considered. Early and delayed imaging (at 4 h) and the use of a SUV_{max} cutoff of 3.5 in the

G. Treglia, MD
Department of Nuclear Medicine,
Oncology Institute of Southern Switzerland,
Via Ospedale, 12, Bellinzona CH-6500, Switzerland
e-mail: giorgiomednuc@libero.it

A. Cistaro, MD (✉)
Department of Nuclear Medicine, Positron Emission Tomography Center IRMET S.p.A., Euromedic Inc.,
Via Onorato Vigliani 89, Turin 10100, Italy

Institute of Cognitive Sciences and Technologies,
National Research Council, Rome, Italy
e-mail: a.cistaro@irmet.com

latter allow accurate lesion characterization with maximal sensitivity; (c) FDG-PET and PET/CT may improve preoperative tumor staging, guide biopsy, and influence treatment, thereby reducing the number of surgical procedures for benign neurogenic lesions or allowing early intervention in NF1 patients whose tumors have a high probability of progression.

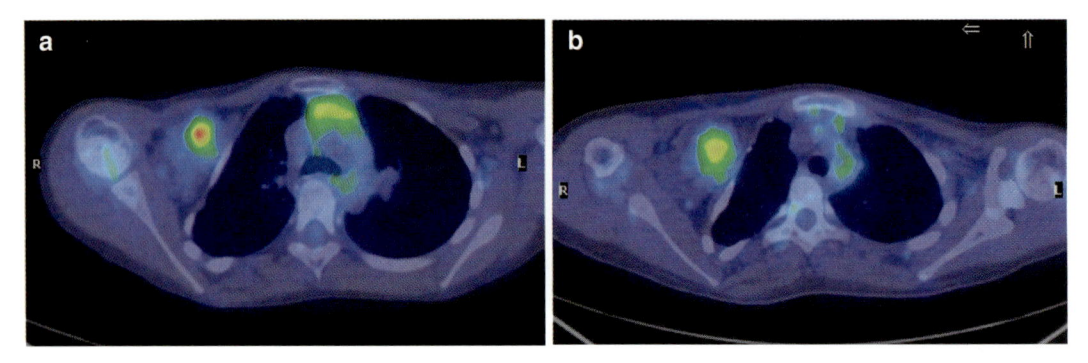

Fig. 31.1 A 10-year-old girl with neurofibromatosis type 1. The plexiform neurofibroma involved the right cervical and axillary region. (**a**) Axial PET/CT study and (**b**) axial PET/CT control after 2 years (March 2010) show a mild nonhomogeneous ^{18}F-FDG uptake (SUV$_{max}$ 1.7) with a focal much intense radiotracer accumulation (SUV$_{max}$ 3.9)

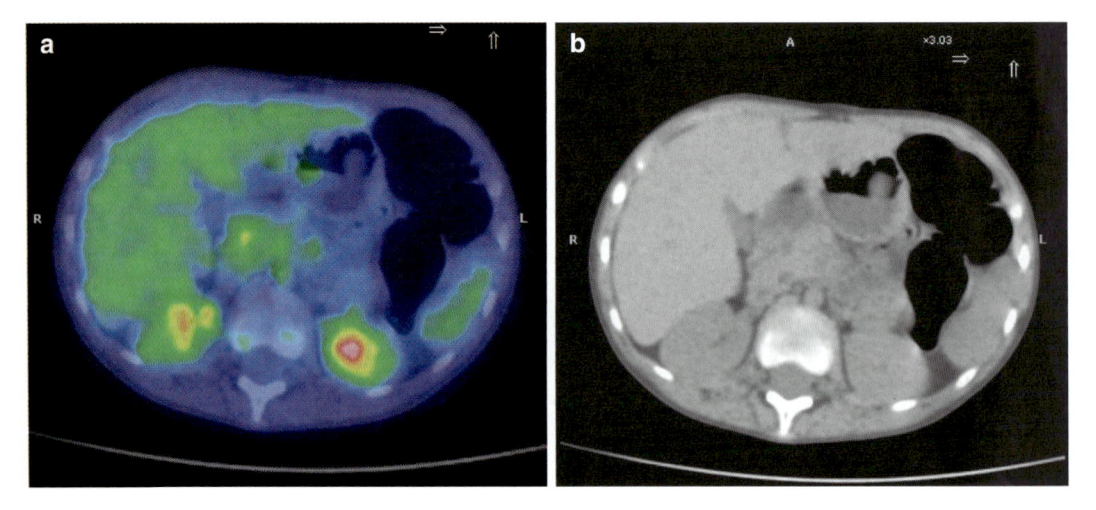

Fig. 31.2 A 9-year-old girl with neurofibromatosis type I and multiple neurofibromas extending from the mediastinum to the cardias. In abdomen the neurofibromas enclose the celiac trunk reaching the porta hepatis. (**a**) Axial PET/CT and (**b**) CT images show a mass surrounding the celiac trunk (SUV$_{max}$ 1.8)

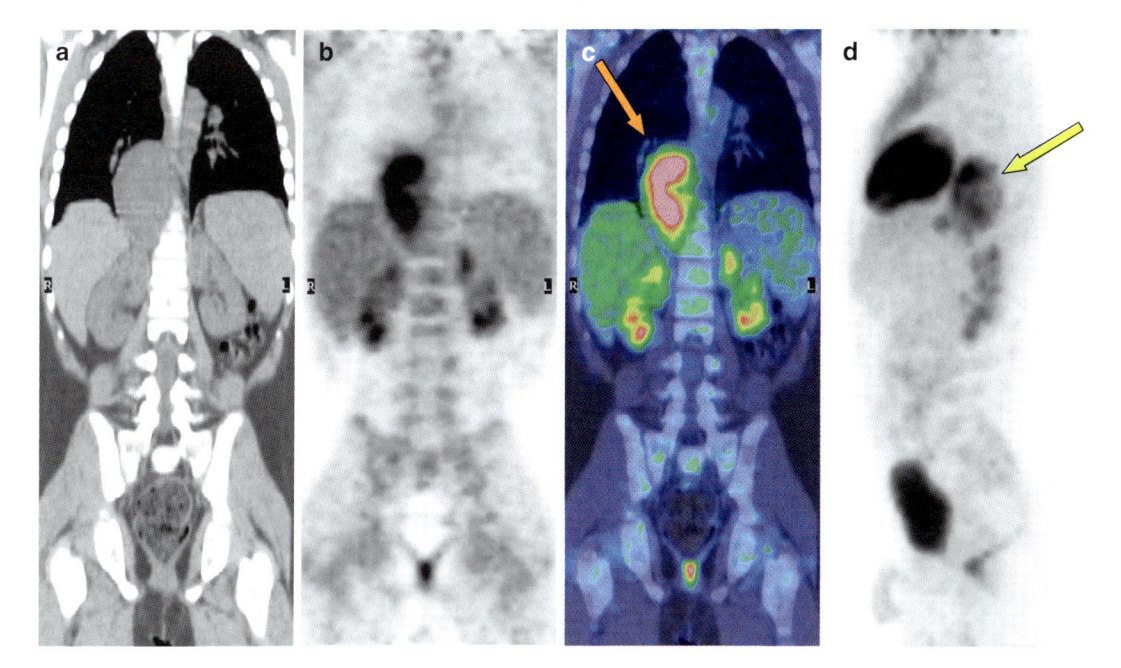

Fig. 31.3 A 7-year-old boy with neurofibromatosis type I. (**a**) Coronal CT, (**b**) PET, (**c**) PET/CT fusion, and (**d**) sagittal maximum intensity projection PET images show increased FDG uptake corresponding to a paravertebral mass in the left posterior mediastinum (*orange arrow* in **c** and *yellow arrow* in **d**) between seventh and tenth dorsal vertebrae (SUV$_{max}$ 9.5). Histology demonstrated the presence of a malignant nerve sheath tumor

Teaching Point

FDG-PET and PET/CT are useful methods to identify malignant change in neurogenic tumors in NF1 and to discriminate malignant from benign neurogenic lesions. Both FDG-PET and PET/CT may improve preoperative tumor staging, guide biopsy, and influence treatment planning [7].

References

1. Ferner RE (2007) Neurofibromatosis 1 and neurofibromatosis 2: a twenty first century perspective. Lancet Neurol 6:340–351
2. Tonsgard JH (2006) Clinical manifestations and management of neurofibromatosis type 1. Semin Pediatr Neurol 13:2–7
3. Ferner RE, Gutmann DH (2002) International consensus statement on malignant peripheral nerve sheath tumours in neurofibromatosis 1. Cancer Res 62:1573–1577
4. Evans DG, Baser ME, McGaughran J et al (2002) Malignant peripheral nerve sheath tumours in neurofibromatosis 1. J Med Genet 39:311–314
5. Ferner RE (2007) Neurofibromatosis 1. Eur J Hum Genet 15:131–138
6. Carli M, Ferrari A, Mattke A et al (2005) Pediatric malignant peripheral nerve sheath tumor: the Italian and German soft tissue sarcoma cooperative group. J Clin Oncol 23:8422–8430
7. Treglia G, Taralli S, Bertagna F et al (2012) Usefulness of whole-body fluorine-18-fluorodeoxyglucose positron emission tomography in patients with neurofibromatosis type 1: an overview. Radiol Res Pract 2012:431029

Autoimmune Lymphoproliferative Syndrome

Angelina Cistaro

32.1 Introduction

Autoimmune lymphoproliferative syndrome (ALPS) is a rare disorder arising from a genetic mutation in the *Fas* gene. This gene encodes a cell-death receptor that belongs to the tumor necrosis factor receptor (TNFR) superfamily and induces cell death trigged by FasL [1]. *Fas* (also called Apo-1 and CD95) is also a member of the superfamily of nerve growth factor receptors expressed by activated effector lymphocytes. It is involved in switching off the immune response, limiting the clonal expansion of lymphocytes, favoring peripheral tolerance, and inducing apoptosis in lymphocytes when triggered by its ligand (FasL), which is expressed by cytotoxic T cells and NK cells [2].

The Fas–FasL system maintains lymphocyte homeostasis and plays a role in preventing cancer [2, 3]. Patients with ALPS have a defect in this apoptotic pathway, leading to chronic lymph proliferation, autoimmune manifestations, and a propensity to develop malignancies [4, 5]. The risk of developing malignancies is unknown but is estimated to be 10–20 %. Most commonly, patients develop B-cell lymphomas (non-Hodgkin's or Hodgkin's), but leukemia and a number of solid tumors (thyroid, breast, and liver carcinoma) have been described as well [4, 5].

Clinical Case

A young patient with low back pain underwent CT and MRI studies, which showed enhancing vertebral lesions, pulmonary nodules, and diffuse laterocervical lymphadenopathy. The ^{18}F-FDG–PET/CT exam showed many areas of intense tracer uptake in multiple vertebrae, several ribs, the sacrum, liver, and both lungs, and multiple lymph nodes at cervical, thoracic, and abdominal sites. A bone marrow biopsy determined a "lymphomatoid granulomatosis," a rare variant of B-cell non-Hodgkin's lymphoma (LNH), while a genetic analysis identified a *Fas* gene mutation. After treatment, the ^{18}F-FDG–PET/CT scan showed complete regression of the disease (Figs. 32.1, 32.2, 32.3, 32.4, 32.5, 32.6, and 32.7).

Clinical Case (continued)

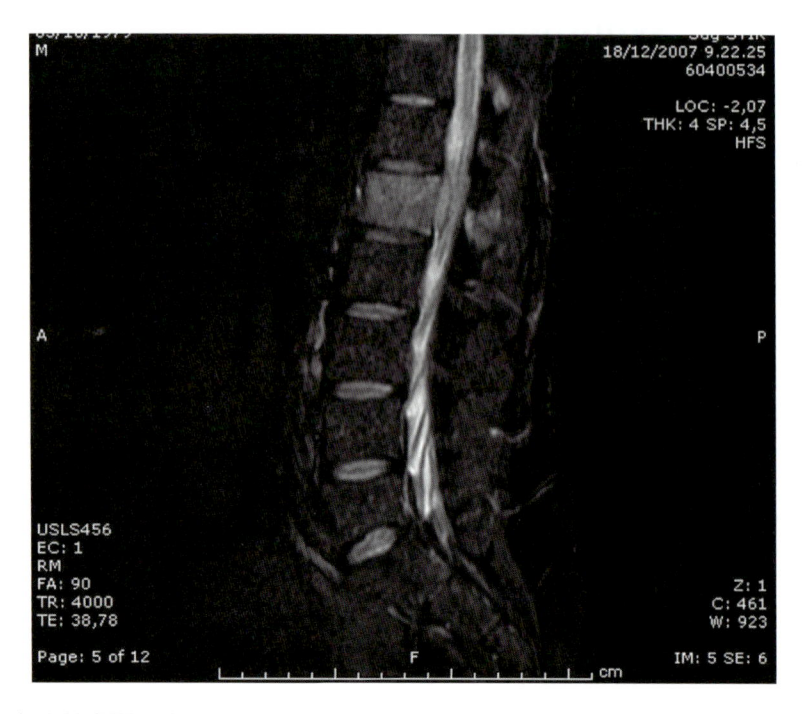

Fig. 32.1 Sagittal T2 STIR MRI shows significant signal alteration involving the first lumbar vertebral body, with epidural pathologic tissue and slight dural sac compression

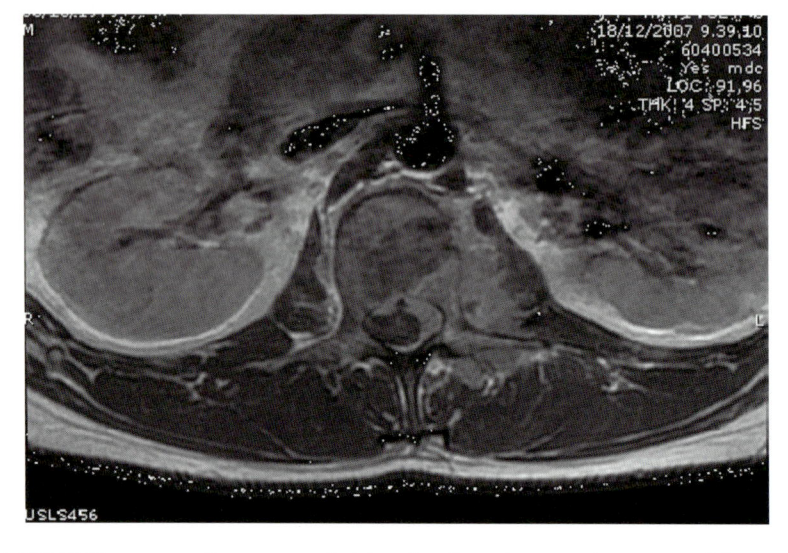

Fig. 32.2 Axial T1 MRI sequence after contrast administration shows intense enhancement of the vertebral body and epidural tissue

32 Autoimmune Lymphoproliferative Syndrome

Clinical Case (continued)

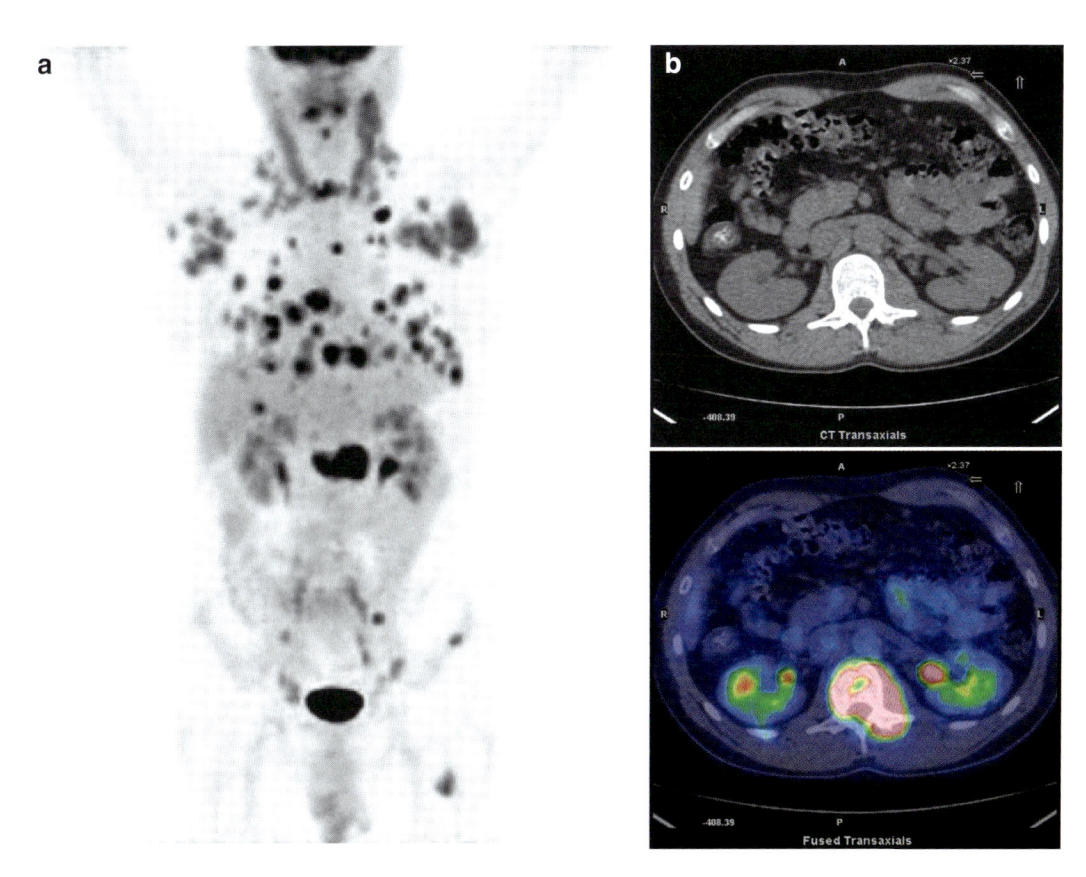

Fig. 32.3 Maximum intensity projection (**a**) shows intense FDG uptake in the vertebrae, ribs, sacrum, left femur, liver, and both lungs. Further uptake was detected in multiple lymph nodes distributed at cervical, thoracic, and abdominal stations. Axial CT and PET/CT fusion images (**b**) show intense FDG uptake in the first lumbar vertebral body

Clinical Case (continued)

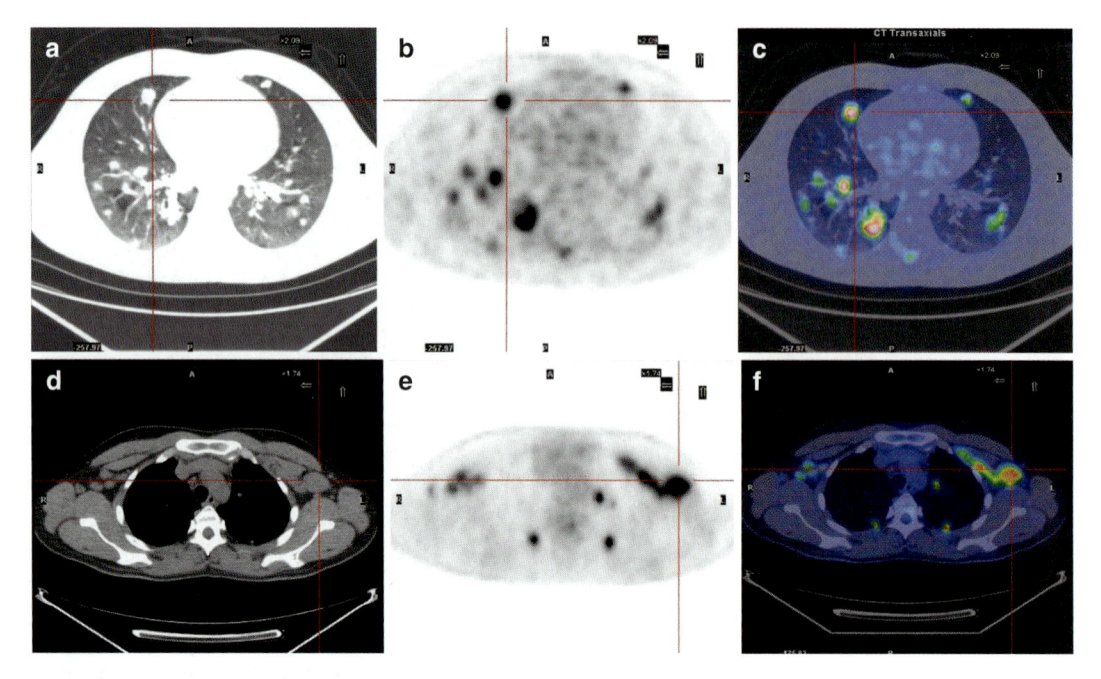

Fig. 32.4 (**a–c**) Axial CT with lung window (**a**), PET (**b**), and PET/CT fusion (**c**) images show multiple uptake in both lungs. (**d–f**) Axial CT with mediastinal window (**d**), PET (**e**), and PET/CT fusion (**f**) images show tracer accumulation in the axillary lymph nodes

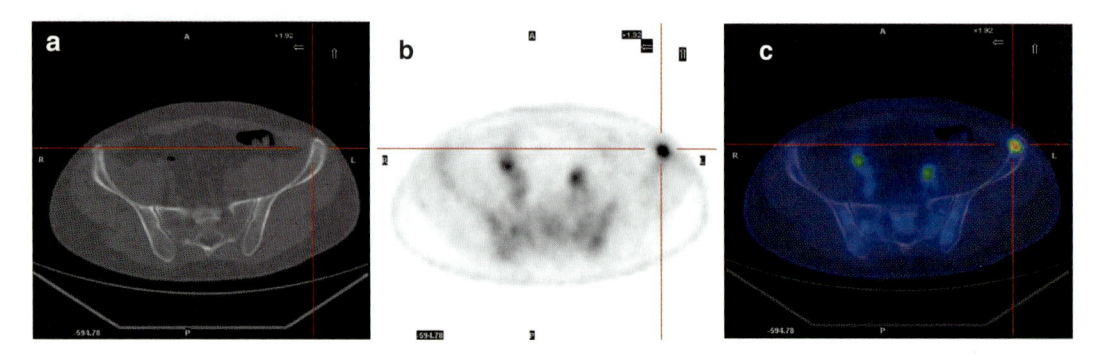

Fig. 32.5 Axial CT (**a**), PET (**b**) and PET/CT fusion (**c**) images depict a FDG-avid focus in the left iliac bone. A PET-guided bone marrow biopsy was performed at the site of tracer uptake in the left iliac bone. Based on the findings, the definitive diagnosis was non-Hodgkin's lymphoma

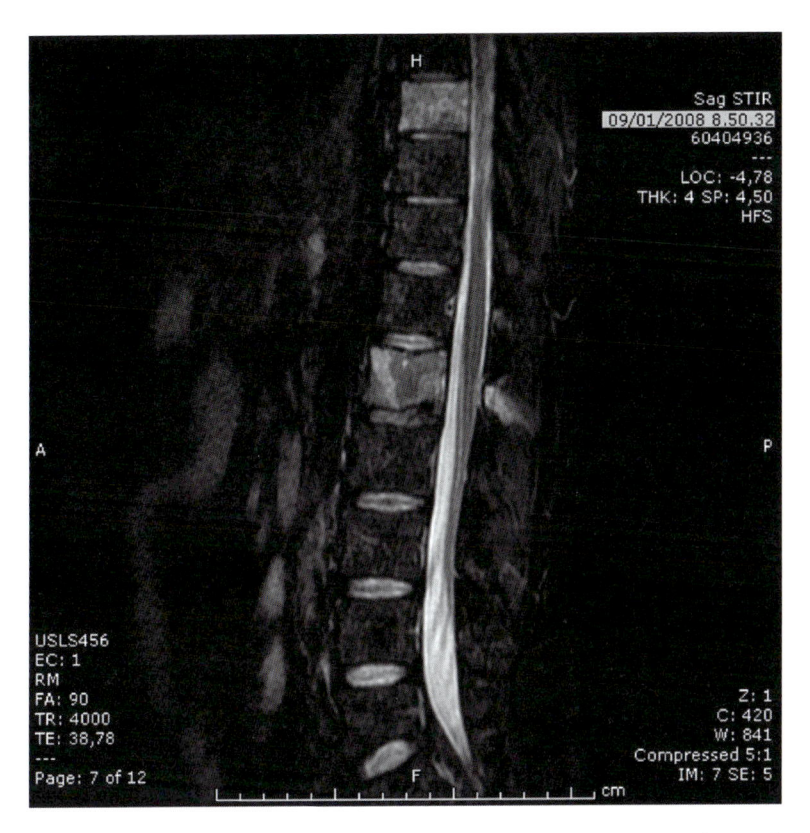

Fig. 32.6 MRI control during treatment. Sagittal T2 STIR sequence shows residual signal alteration involving the first lumbar vertebral body and a reduction of the epidural pathological tissue. Abnormal signal intensity is also seen in the ninth dorsal vertebra, with prominent vertebral body involvement

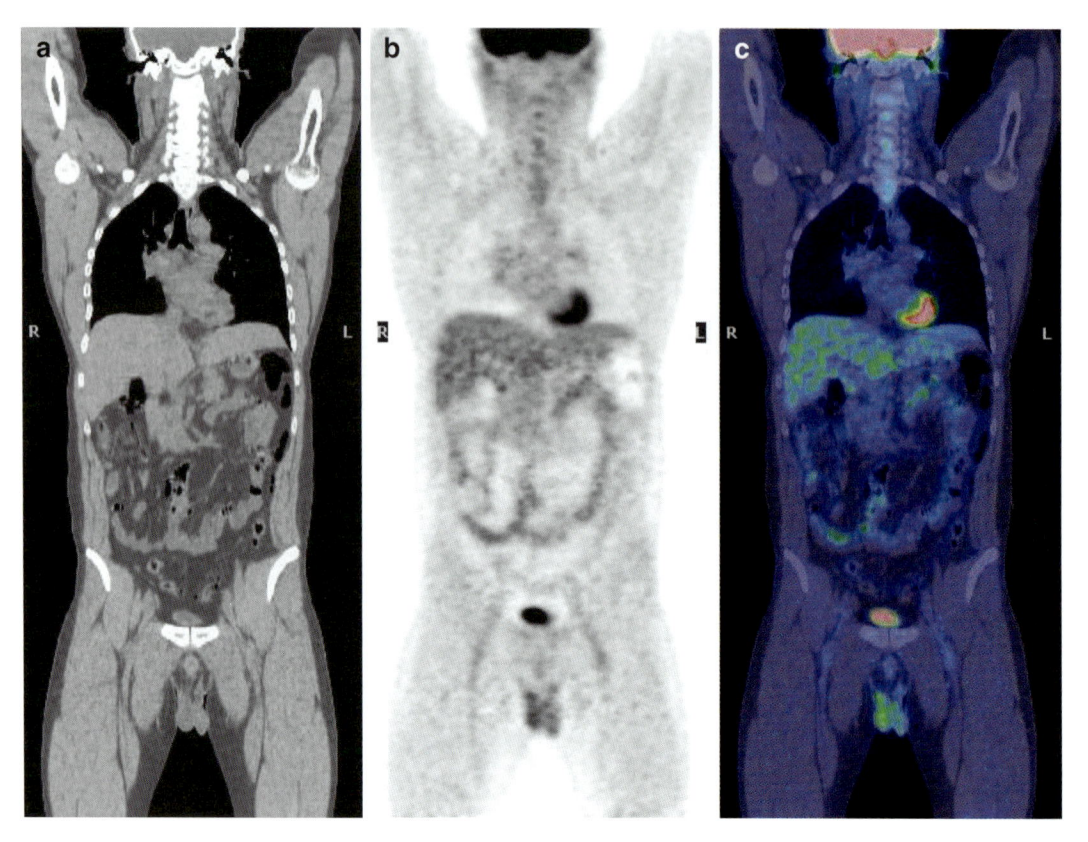

Fig. 32.7 PET control during treatment. Coronal CT (**a**), PET (**b**), and PET/CT fusion (**c**) images after six cycles of rituximab show the complete disappearance of all pathological areas of FDG uptake. The following bone marrow biopsy of the iliac bone was negative

Teaching Point
^{18}F-FDG–PET/CT can play several roles in patients with ALPS. It can confirm or rule out a diagnosis in patients with a suspected malignacy and, in case of tumor detection, allow proper staging. It also provides important information in monitoring treatment response and during follow-up. Finally, ^{18}F-FDG–PET/CT may be useful in monitoring autoimmune manifestations of symptomatic ALPS, by determining the response to therapy through the evaluation of metabolic activity in involved lymph nodes.

References

1. Clementi R, Chiocchetti A, Cappellano G et al (2006) Variations of the perforin gene in patients with autoimmunity/lymphoproliferation and defective Fas function. Blood 108:3079–3084
2. Nagata S, Golstein P (1995) The Fas death factor. Science 267:1449–1456
3. Krammer PH (2000) CD95's deadly mission in the immune system. Nature 407:789–795
4. Poppema S, Maggio E, Van den Berg A (2004) Development of lymphoma in autoimmune lymphoproliferative syndrome (ALPS) and its relationship toFas gene mutations. Leuk Lymphoma 45:423–431
5. Straus SE, Jaffe ES, Puck JM et al (2001) The development of lymphomas in families with autoimmune lymphoproliferative syndrome with germline Fas mutations and defective lymphocyte apoptosis. Blood 98:194–200

Castleman's Disease

33

Mariapaola Cucinotta and Angelina Cistaro

The first description of Castleman's disease (CD) dates back to 1954, when Benjamin Castleman and coworkers reported 13 cases of mediastinal lymphadenopathy. Two years later, they more precisely defined this uncommon benign lymphoproliferative disorder [1, 2].

There are several forms of CD, differing in their histological findings and the locations of the lesions. The histological types consist of the hyaline vascular variant (HVV), the plasma cell variant (PCV), and a mixed type. The disease can involve a single lymph node, a single chain of lymph nodes (most frequently in the mediastinum), or multiple lymph node stations. Unicentric HVV occurs in 72 % of cases, unicentric PCV in 18 %, and multicentric PCV in 10 %. The multicentric HVV is very rare, accounting for only 1 % of all CD cases [3].

The prevalence of CD is very low, especially in children, with a higher incidence in young adults. Some studies report a predominance in females, but others have found no gender differences [1, 2].

The etiology of CD is as yet unclear. Many cases, mostly those in which there is multicentric disease, are associated with a human herpesvirus (HHV)-8 and/or HIV infection and high serum levels of interleukin (IL)-6. It is thought that HHV-8, which typically infects the immunocompromised (such as transplant recipients or HIV-positive individuals), stimulates the hyper-production of IL-6 by B lymphocytes, which subsequently proliferate and differentiate into activated and generally polyclonal plasma cells [4, 5].

The high levels of IL-6 may also be responsible, at least in part, for the symptomatology of the multicentric variant, including peripheral lymphadenopathy, hepatosplenomegaly, weight loss, anemia, asthenia, night sweats, fever, skin rash, lung disorder, and kidney dysfunction [1, 6]. Patients with this form of CD usually require systemic treatment, and the disease course, especially that of PCV, is often accompanied by severe complications or evolution into a malignant neoplasm [1, 4, 7].

The unicentric form, by contrast, is generally asymptomatic, except for the associated mass effect. These patients have a good prognosis and are successfully treated by surgery [1, 2, 7].

On imaging exams, CD has several typical characteristics. Contrast-enhanced CT shows an early marked or moderate enhancement (higher in HVV than in PCV) that persists

M. Cucinotta, MD
Nuclear Medicine Unit,
Department of Radiological Sciences,
Policlinico Gaetano Martino Hospital,
University of Messina, Via Consolare Valeria 1,
Messina 98125, Italy
e-mail: mariapaola.cucinotta@gmail.com

A. Cistaro, MD (✉)
Department of Nuclear Medicine,
Positron Emission Tomography Center
IRMET S.p.A., Euromedic Inc.,
Via Onorato Vigliani 89, Turin 10100, Italy

Institute of Cognitive Sciences and Technologies,
National Research Council, Rome, Italy
e-mail: a.cistaro@irmet.com

during delayed phases. On MRI, CD lesions are iso- or hyperintense relative to skeletal muscle on T_1-weighted images and markedly hyperintense on T_2-weighted images [1, 2, 8].

Several studies have shown that PET with ^{18}F-FDG is effective in the detection of metabolically active lesions and in the assessment of disease extent, as it reveals pathological sites not seen on CT scan because of their small dimensions [5, 7, 9–11]. ^{18}F-FDG PET is also a valid tool for guiding biopsy [11] and is even better than CT in discriminating disease persistence/recurrence from post-therapeutic changes and in monitoring treatment response. As such, it is a fundamental tool in the staging and management of CD patients (Figs. 33.1 and 33.2) [5, 7, 9–11].

While CD is a benign disease, pathological lymph nodes may take up substantial amounts of ^{18}F-FDG, resulting in a high SUV. Consequently, the value of PET/CT in the differential diagnosis between CD and malignancies such as lymphoma remains to be determined in further studies [8].

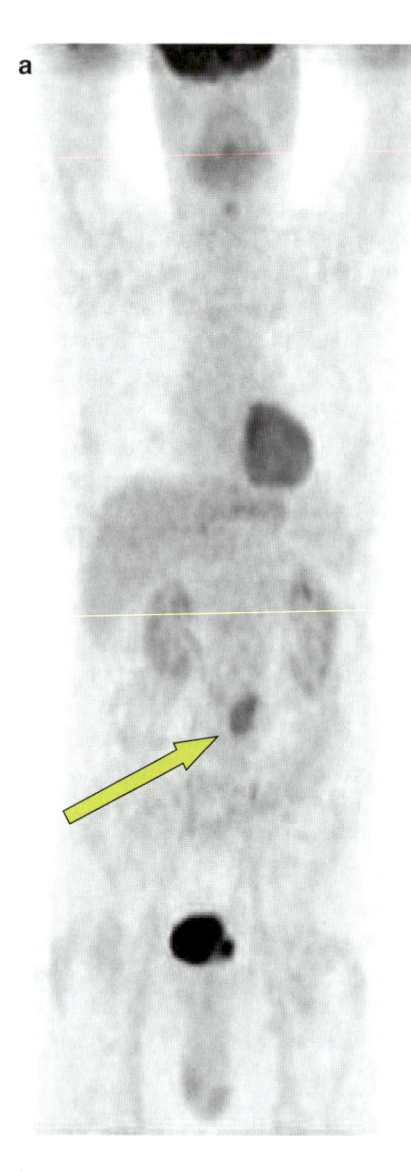

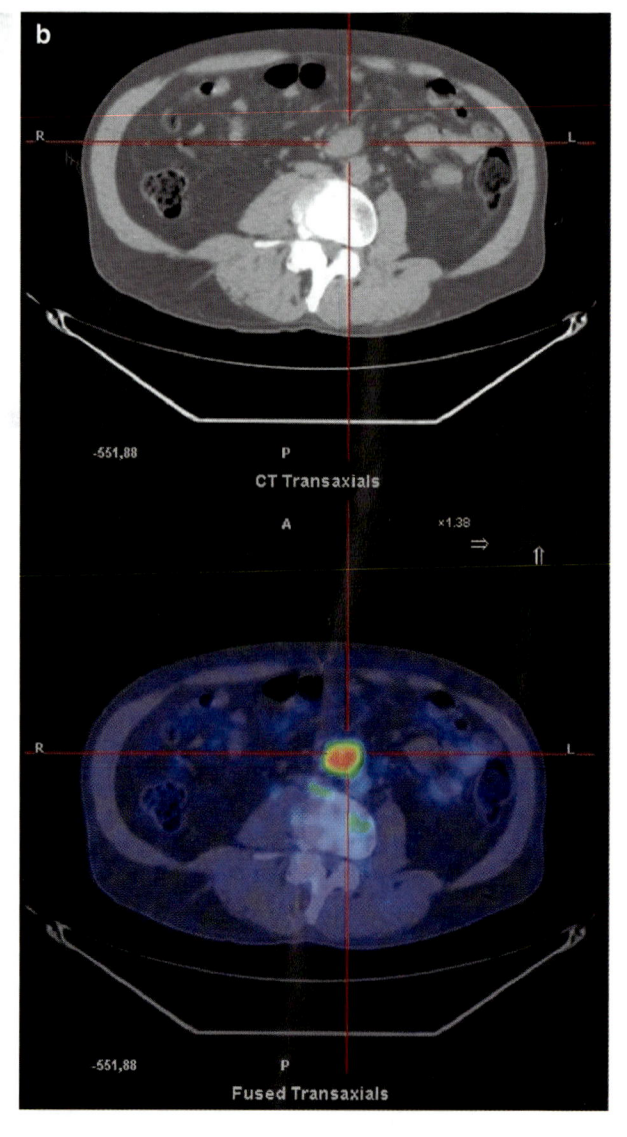

Fig. 33.1 A 19-year-old man with fever, anemia, asthenia. A mesenterial lymph node and several small iliac lymph nodes were identified on ultrasonographic examination and contrast-enhanced CT scan. (**a**, **b**) The PET study showed an ^{18}F-FDG-avid mesenterial mass (*yellow arrow* in **a**) corresponding to the large lymph node depicted on contrast-enhanced CT. Histopathological analysis showed Castleman's disease, hyaline-vascular subtype

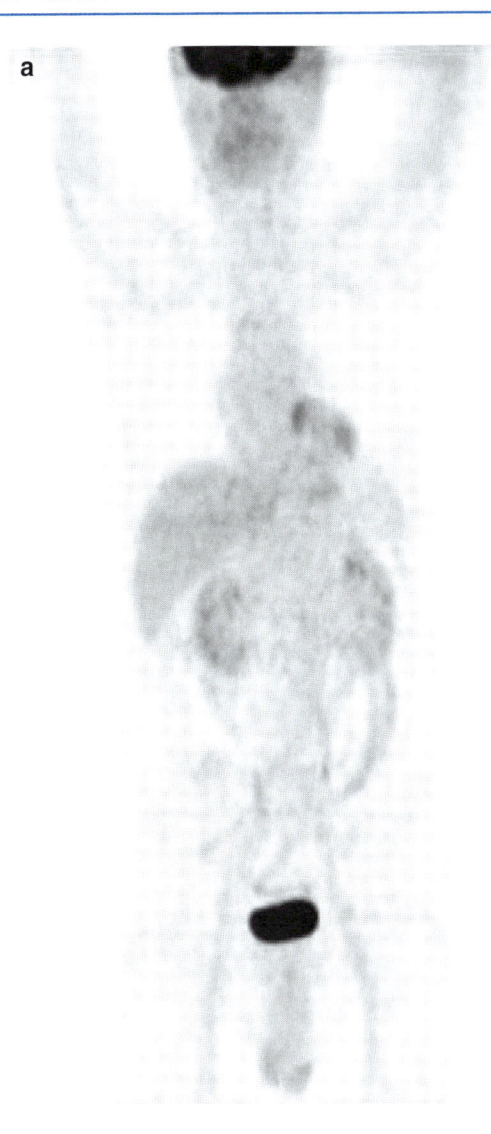

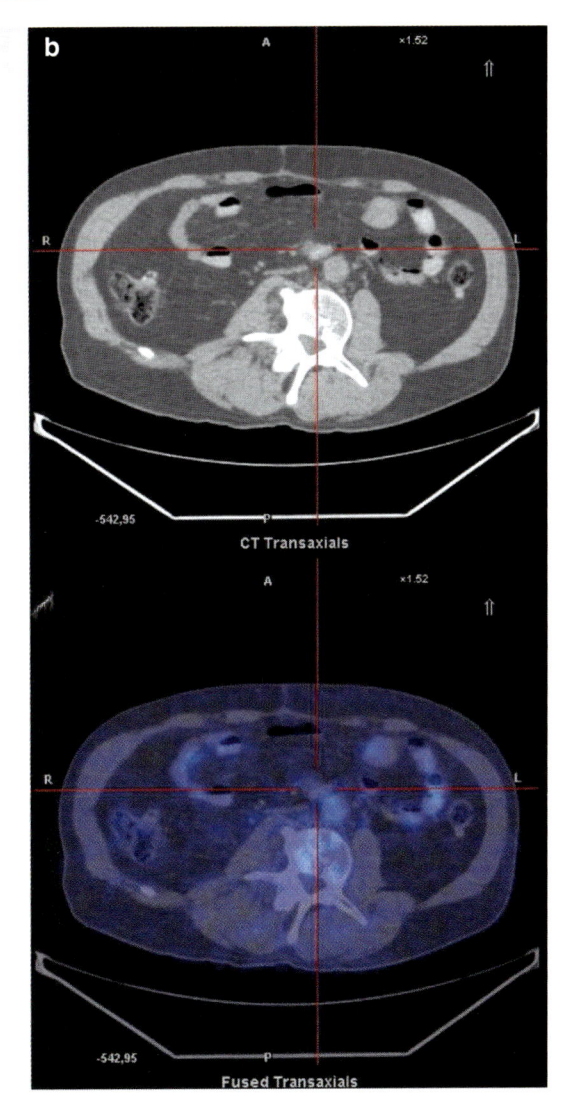

Fig. 33.2 PET study after chemotherapy. Maximum intensity projection (**a**), CT and PET/CT fusion images (**b**). Although the lymph nodes are still visible on the morphological exam, its metabolic activity on PET is not significant, suggesting a complete disease response in accordance with the clinical signs

Teaching Point

Castleman's disease is a rare lymphatic polyclonal disorder characterized by unicentric or multicentric lymph node hyperplasia and non-specific symptoms and signs, including fever, asthenia, weight loss, an enlarged liver, and abnormally high blood levels of numerous antibodies. Given the high glucose metabolic activity seen in CD, ^{18}F-FDG PET is an appropriate imaging modality to stage or restage the disease and to evaluate the response to treatment.

References

1. Farruggia P, Trizzino A, Scibetta N et al (2011) Castleman's disease in childhood: report of three cases and review of the literature. Ital J Pediatr 37:50
2. Lin CY, Huang TC (2011) Cervical posterior triangle Castleman's disease in a child – case report & literature review. Chang Gung Med J 34:435–439
3. Park JB, Hwang JH, Kim H et al (2007) Castleman disease presenting with jaundice: a case with the multicentric hyaline vascular variant. Korean J Intern Med 22:113–117
4. Van Aalderen MC, Brinkman K, Van Den Berk GE et al (2010) Vinblastine, rituximab and HART, treatment of an HIV-positive patient with multicentric Castleman's disease. Neth J Med 68:87–90
5. Toita N, Kawamura N, Hatano N et al (2009) A 5-year-old boy with unicentric Castleman disease affecting the mesentery: utility of serum IL-6 level and (18)F-FDG PET for diagnosis. J Pediatr Hematol Oncol 31:693–695
6. Arlet JB, Hermine O, Darnige L et al (2010) Iron-deficiency anemia in Castleman disease: implication of the interleukin 6/hepcidin pathway. Pediatrics 126:1608–1612
7. Enomoto K, Nakamichi I, Hamada K et al (2007) Unicentric and multicentric Castleman's disease. Br J Radiol 80:24–26
8. Liu QY, Chen MC, Chen XH et al (2011) Imaging characteristics of abdominal tumor in association with paraneoplastic pemphigus. Eur J Dermatol 21:83–88
9. Akosman C, Selcuk NA, Ordu C, Ercan S, Ekici ID, Oyan B (2011) Unicentric mixed variant Castleman disease associated with Hashimoto disease: the role of PET/CT in staging and evaluating response to the treatment. Cancer Imaging 11:52–55
10. Bertagna F, Biasiotto G, Rodella R et al (2010) ^{18}F-Fluorodeoxyglucose positron emission tomography/computed tomography findings in a patient with human immunodeficiency virus-associated Castleman's disease and Kaposi sarcoma, disorders associated with human herpes virus 8 infection. Jpn J Radiol 28:231–234
11. Barker R, Kazmi F, Stebbing J et al (2009) FDG-PET/CT imaging in the management of HIV-associated multicentric Castleman's disease. Eur J Nucl Med Mol Imaging 36:648–652

Fever of Unknown Origin

Alireza Mojtahedi, Daniele Penna, and Angelina Cistaro

34.1 Introduction

Fever of unknown origin (FUO) was recognized in the 1960s, when it was defined as a condition of increased body temperature exceeding 38.3 °C measured on several occasions and for a period of more than 3 weeks in an immunocompetent patient with no known illness [1]. More recently, FUO has been classified into three groups according to the type of patient: (1) "classical," in the case of non-immunocompromised patients; (2) "nosocomial," in neutropenic patents; and (3) "patients with HIV" [2]. The four main causes of FUO are infections, malignancies, autoimmune noninfectious diseases, and miscellaneous [3].

Molecular imaging can play an important role in diagnosing FUO, given that in these patients molecular changes usually occur earlier than morphological structural changes [4]. This determines the advantage of functional imaging with PET/CT over CT or MRI [5]. However, while the scintigraphic labeling of white blood cells has a high sensitivity and specificity to identify an inflammatory process, infection accounts for approximately one-fourth of cases of FUO, followed by neoplasm and noninfectious inflammatory diseases [4, 6]. ^{18}F-FDG–PET/CT can be used to image the inflammatory process due to the fact that inflammation causes overexpression of the GLUT-1 and GLUT-2 transporters in activated leukocytes [4, 7, 8]. Other activated inflammatory cells can also accumulate the radiotracer, as evidenced in many studies showing that, during the inflammatory processes, glucose is taken up in large amounts by granulocytes (mainly neutrophils) and monocytes/macrophages [9–11].

Multislice CT technology (MSCT) usually contributes to the final diagnosis of FUO in 40 % patients [3, 12]. PET alone is superior to CT in the detection of an inflammatory process in patients with FUO [13]. It is also more sensitive than WBC scintigraphy in the diagnosis of chronic infection [14–16]. Moreover, the combination of ^{18}F-FDG–PET and CT allows simultaneous molecular and morphological imaging [17].

^{18}F-FDG–PET/CT is therefore a potentially useful tool in the management of inflammatory disease; for example, several authors have reported its use in the diagnosis and management of abdominal and pelvic abscesses, vascular inflammations, tuberculosis, and infections of bone, soft tissue, and prostheses [11, 18].

A. Mojtahedi, MD
Nuclear Medicine Department,
Memorial Sloan-Kettering Cancer Center,
1275 York Avenue, New York City, NY 10065, USA
e-mail: ojtahea@mskcc.org

D. Penna
Department of Nuclear Medicine, Positron Emission Tomography Center IRMET S.p.A., Euromedic Inc.,
Via Onorato Vigliani 89, Turin 10100, Italy
e-mail: d.penna@irmet.com

A. Cistaro, MD (✉)
Department of Nuclear Medicine, Positron Emission Tomography Center IRMET S.p.A., Euromedic Inc.,
Via Onorato Vigliani 89, Turin 10100, Italy

Institute of Cognitive Sciences and Technologies,
National Research Council, Rome, Italy
e-mail: a.cistaro@irmet.com

Furthermore, in FUO associated with a paraneoplastic syndrome, some studies have shown that PET/CT allowed in these patients the diagnosis of malignant diseases, in particular lymphomas [19].

Clinical Case

A 6-year-old patient was seen for FUO and pain at the level of the left temporomandibular joint associated with the appearance of bilateral cervical lymph nodes (size 10–28 mm). The patient was hospitalized and the initial investigations led to the provisional diagnosis of EBV infection. A CT scan of the brain and abdomen showed no abnormal findings. Chest CT highlighted only a tissue mass of 50 mm in the anterior mediastinal, thought to represent thymic hyperplasia. A bilateral bone marrow biopsy was also performed but the specimens were not assessable. An ultrasound of the testicles showed a mild right hydrocele. In the absence of a diagnosis, an ^{18}F-FDG–PET/CT study was carried out to examine the metabolism of the adenopathies and mediastinal tissue, in view of a possible biopsy.

PET/CT (Fig. 34.1) showed abnormal radiotracer uptake in the anterior mediastinal tissue and by some of the mediastinal lymph nodes. A diffuse labeling of the skeleton with radiotracer was also observed on the PET images but the significance

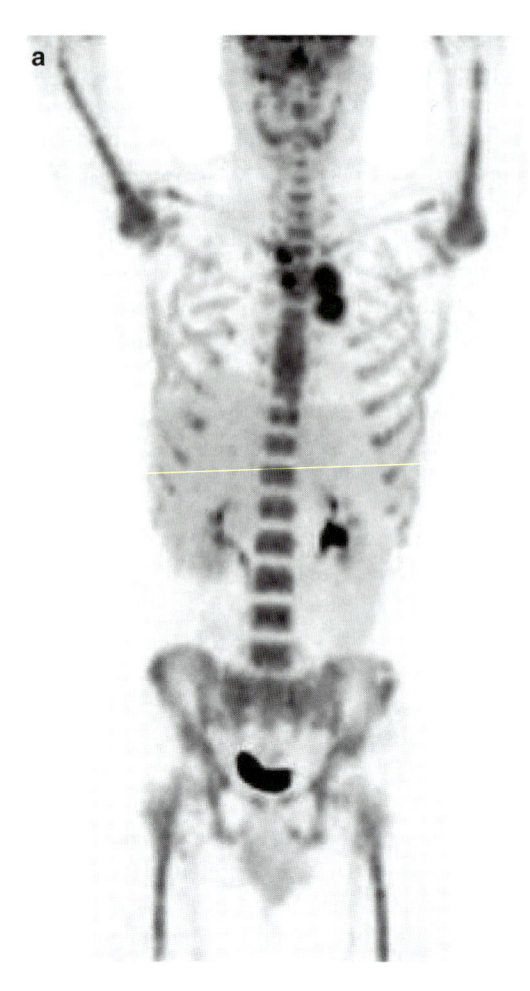

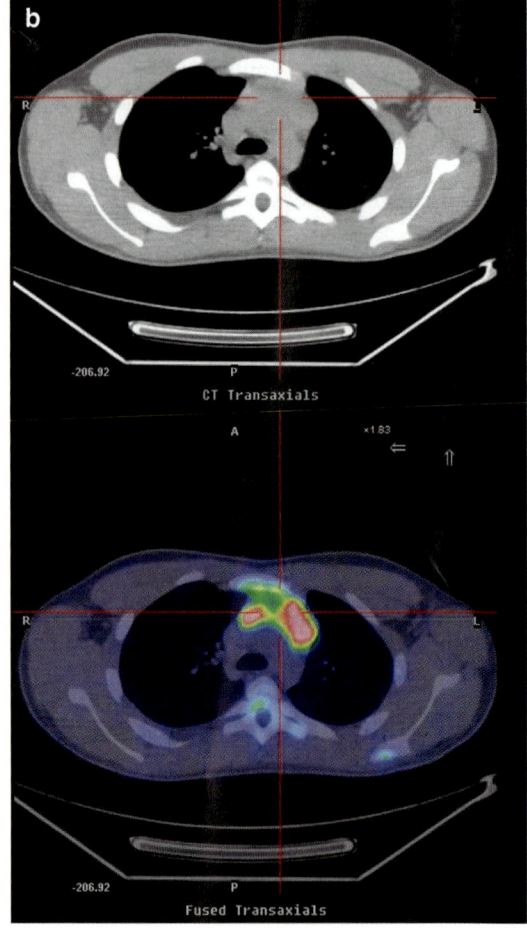

Fig. 34.1 Maximum intensity projection (**a**) shows abnormal ^{18}F-FDG mediastinal uptake. Note the absence of pathological uptake in the bilateral cervical lymph nodes detected clinically, and the absence of FDG accumulation in the testicles that corresponded to the ultrasound findings and the diffuse radiotracer uptake of the skeleton probably of functional meaning. (**b**) CT and PET/CT fusion transaxial images display intense FDG accumulation in the anterior mediastinum

was unclear. On the basis of the PET functional information, an ultrasound-guided chest biopsy was performed, which led to a histological diagnosis of T-cell lymphoblastic lymphoma. After chemotherapy, a repeat PET/CT examination with the same scanner and acquisition protocol showed the total disappearance of the anomalous uptake and confirmed the complete response to treatment.

Teaching Point

^{18}F-FDG–PET/CT evaluates molecular and functional changes and is therefore a valuable tool not only in the determination of the various possible causes of FUO but also in the detection of otherwise occult tumors or atypical infection.

References

1. Petersdorf RG, Beeson PB (1961) Fever of unexplained origin: report on 100 cases. Medicine (Baltimore) 40:1–30
2. Durack DT, Street AC (1991) Fever of unknow origin-reexamined and redefined. Curr Clin Top Infect Dis 11:35–51
3. Meller J, Sahlmann CO, Gürocak O, Liersch T, Meller B (2009) FDG-PET in patients with fever of unknown origin: the importance of diagnosing large vessel vasculitis. Q J Nucl Med Mol Imaging 53(1):51–63. Review
4. Bleeker-Rovers CP, Corstens FH et al (2004) Fever of unknown origin: prospective comparison of diagnostic value of (18)F-FDG PET and (111)In-granulocyte scintigraphy. Eur J Nucl Med Mol Imaging 31: 622–626
5. Buysschaert I, Vanderschueren S, Blockmans D et al (2004) Contribution of (18)fluoro-deoxyglucose positron emission tomography to the work-up of patients with fever of unknown origin. Eur J Intern Med 15: 151–156
6. Bleeker-Rovers CP, van der Meer JW, Oyen WJ (2009) Fever of unknown origin. Semin Nucl Med 39:81–87
7. Bleeker-Rovers CP, Vos FJ, Corstens FH (2008) Imaging of infectious diseases using [18F] fluorodeoxyglucose PET. Q J Nucl Med Mol Imaging 52:17–29
8. Blockmans D, Knockaert D, Maes A et al (2001) Clinical value of [(18)F]fluoro-deoxyglucose positron emission tomography for patients with fever of unknown origin. Clin Infect Dis 15:191–196
9. Kubota R, Yamada S, Kubota K, Ishiwata K, Tamahashi N, Ido T (1992) Intratumoral distribution of fluorine-18-fluorodeoxyglucose in vivo: high accumulation in macrophages and granulation tissues studied by microautoradiography. J Nucl Med 33(11):1972–1980
10. Jacobs DB, Lee TP, Jung CY, Mookerjee BK (1989) Mechanism of mitogen-induced stimulation of glucose transport in human peripheral blood mononuclear cells. Evidence of an intracellular reserve pool of glucose carriers and their recruitment. J Clin Invest 83(2):437–443
11. Mahfouz T, Miceli MH, Saghafifar F, Stroud S, Jones-Jackson L, Walker R, Grazziutti ML, Purnell G, Fassas A, Tricot G, Barlogie B, Anaissie E (2005) 18F-fluorodeoxyglucose positron emission tomography contributes to the diagnosis and management of infections in patients with multiple myeloma: a study of 165 infectious episodes. J Clin Oncol 23(31): 7857–7863
12. Knockaert DC, Vanderschueren S, Blockmans D (2003) Fever of unknown origin in adults: 40 years on. J Intern Med 253:263–275
13. Keidar Z, Gurman-Balbir A, Gaitini D et al (2008) Fever of unknown origin: the role of 18F-FDG PET/CT. J Nucl Med 49:1980–1985
14. Kjaer A, Lebech AM, Eigtved A et al (2004) Fever of unknown origin: prospective comparison of diagnostic value of 18F-FDG PET and 111In-granulocyte scintigraphy. Eur J Nucl Med Mol Imaging 31: 1342–1343
15. Lorenzen J, Buchert R, Bohuslavizki KH (2001) Value of FDG PET in patients with fever of unknown origin. Nucl Med Commun 22:779–783
16. Meller J, Ivancevic V, Conrad M (1998) Clinical value of immunoscintigraphy in patients with fever of unknown origin. J Nucl Med 39:1248–1253
17. Ergül N, Cermik TF (2011) FDG-PET or PET/CT in fever of unknown origin: the diagnostic role of underlying primary disease. Int J Mol Imaging 2011:318051
18. Arnow PM, Flaherty JP (1997) Fever of unknow origin. Lancet 350:350–580
19. Rosenbaum J, Basu S, Beckerman S, Werner T, Torigian DA, Alavi A (2011) Evaluation of diagnostic performance of 18F-FDG-PET compared to CT in detecting potential causes of fever of unknown origin in an academic centre. Hell J Nucl Med 14(3): 255–259, PubMed PMID: 22087445

Congenital Hyperinsulinism

35

Vittoria Rufini and Milena Pizzoferro

35.1 Introduction

Congenital hyperinsulinism (CHI) is a primary defect of the pancreatic β-cells leading to inappropriate insulin secretion. It is the most common cause of persistent hypoglycemia in infancy, with an estimated incidence of 1/50,000 live births [1, 2]. Hypoglycemia must be rapidly and intensively treated to prevent severe and irreversible brain damage. At histopathology, two typical forms of CHI are defined that are clinically indistinguishable but differ in their molecular basis and therapeutic approaches [3]. The focal form is defined as an adenomatous hyperplasia of the β-cells within the pancreatic islets; it is limited to a small area (<15 mm). This form is curable by a partial pancreatectomy restricted to the small focal endocrine lesion. The diffuse form is characterized by the presence of abnormal β-cells throughout the pancreas. It is medically treated; surgery (subtotal or near-total pancreatectomy) is required only when medical therapy is unsuccessful and carries a high risk of iatrogenic diabetes.

V. Rufini, PhD (✉)
Unit of Nuclear Medicine,
Department of Radiological Sciences,
Agostino Gemelli Hospital,
Università Cattolica del Sacro Cuore,
Largo A. Gemelli 8, Rome 00168, Italy
e-mail: v.rufini@rm.unicatt.it

M. Pizzoferro, MD
Unit of Nuclear Medicine, Department of Radiology,
Bambino Gesù Children's Hospital,
Piazza Sant'Onofrio 4, Rome 00165, Italy
e-mail: milena.pizzoferro@opbg.net

Case 1: Focal Form

A 2-year-old girl diagnosed with CHI was referred for ^{18}F-DOPA–PET/CT (4 MBq ^{18}F-DOPA/kg, administered 45 min prior to the abdominal scan) to distinguish between focal and diffuse HI. She had suffered the first episode of hypoglycemia at 3 months of age. The high plasma insulin concentration suggested a diagnosis of congenital HI. Medical treatment with diazoxide (7 mg/kg/day) had achieved a suboptimal metabolic response, with widespread hypertrichosis as a side effect.

The ^{18}F-DOPA–PET/CT study showed increased uptake in the processus uncinatus of the pancreatic head. The SUV_{max} in the head of the pancreas was 4.5, compared to 3.2 and 3.1 in the body and tail of the pancreas, respectively. The SUV ratio (SUVr, calculated between the SUV_{max} of the head of the pancreas and the mean pancreatic SUV_{max}) was 1.25, which according to Ribeiro and colleagues is suggestive of a focal lesion [4]. A sequentially coregistered contrast-enhanced CT was also performed to obtain a vascular map [5] (Fig. 35.1).

A partial resection of the head of the pancreas was performed, the focal lesion was removed (confirmed by histology), and the patient was cured without postoperative complications. The child is currently 6 years old with normal glucose levels without medical treatment. The iatrogenic hypertrichosis has disappeared as well.

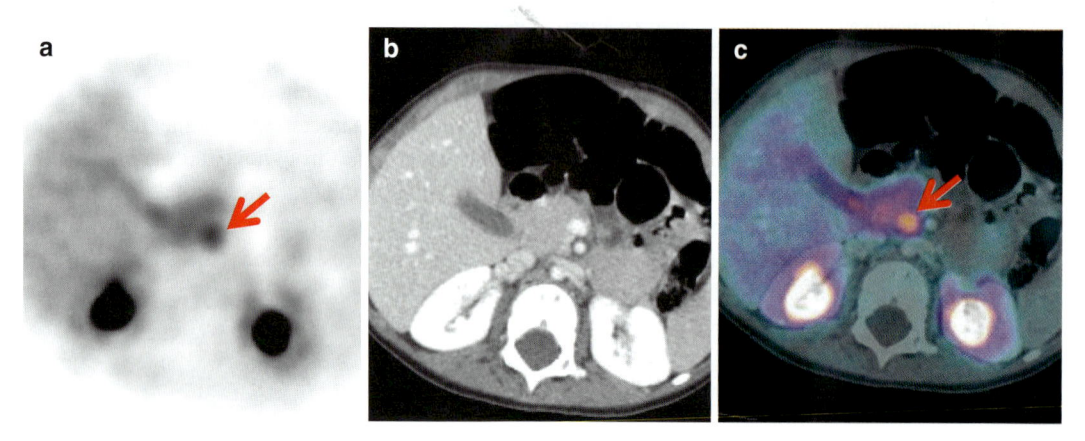

Fig. 35.1 Axial (**a**) PET, (**b**) CT, and (**c**) PET/CT images. A focal uptake is evident in the uncinatus process of the head of the pancreas (*red arrow* in **a** and **c**)

Case 2: Diffuse Form

A 2-year-old boy with severe perinatal hypoglycemia (first episode 2 days after his birth) was referred for an ^{18}F-DOPA–PET/CT study. His clinical characteristics suggested a diagnosis of hyperinsulinemic hypoglycemia. The patient was responsive to diazoxide (7 mg/kg/day) but he had a mild cognitive delay secondary to recurrent episodes of hypoglycemia in the neonatal period.

PET/CT demonstrated the homogeneous uptake of ^{18}F-DOPA, suggesting a diffuse form of congenital HI. The SUV_{max} values in the pancreas were 1.5 in the head, 1.4 in the body, and 1.4 in the tail (SUVr of each pancreatic region <1.2) (Fig. 35.2). The patient is currently under medical therapy with good control of his glucose levels.

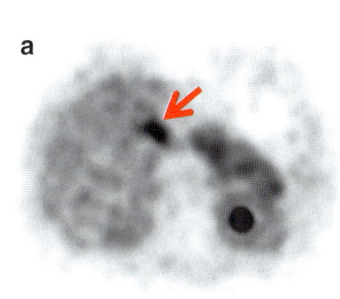

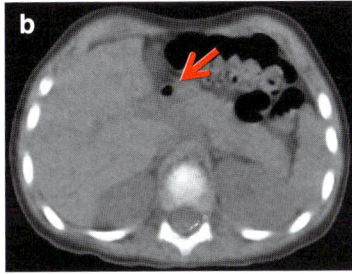

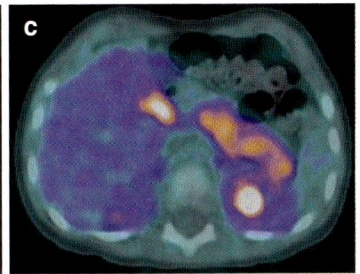

Fig. 35.2 Axial (**a**) PET, (**b**) CT, and (**c**) PET/CT images show homogeneous pancreatic uptake of ^{18}F-DOPA, suggesting a diffuse form of congenital hyperinsulinism. The *arrow* (in **a** and **b**) indicates physiologic activity in the biliary duct

Teaching Points

PET/CT with ^{18}F-DOPA is a simple and effective tool to differentiate between focal and diffuse forms of HI with high accuracy. This information cannot be obtained by other noninvasive diagnostic procedures [6]. When a focal area of intense ^{18}F-DOPA uptake is detected in the pancreatic region, a sequentially coregistered contrast-enhanced CT is useful to guide the surgeon in limited resection of the focal lesion by means of the vascular map. The SUV ratio completes the visual analysis and allows discrimination between focal and diffuse disease forms [4, 7].

References

1. De Lonlay P, Giurgea I, Touati G, Saudubray JM (2004) Neonatal hypoglycaemia: aetiologies. Semin Neonatol 9:49–58
2. Arnoux JB, Verkarre V, Saint-Martin C, Montravers F, Brassier A, Valayannopoulos V, Brunelle F, Fournet JC, Robert JJ, Aigrain Y, Bellanné-Chantelot C, de Lonlay P (2011) Congenital hyperinsulinism: current trends in diagnosis and therapy. Orphanet J Rare Dis 6:63
3. Rahier J, Guiot Y, Sempoux C (2000) Persistent hyperinsulinaemic hypoglycaemia of infancy: a heterogeneous syndrome unrelated to nesidioblastosis. Arch Dis Child Fetal Neonatal Ed 82:F108–F112
4. Ribeiro MJ, Boddaert N, Bellanne-Chantelot C, Bourgois S, Valayannopoulos V, Delzescaux T, Jaubert F, Nihoul-Fekete C, Brunelle F, De Lonlay P (2007) The added value of [^{18}F]fluoro-L-DOPA PET in the diagnosis of hyperinsulinism of infancy: a retrospective study involving 49 children. Eur J Nucl Med Mol Imaging 34:2120–2128
5. Barthlen W, Blankenstein O, Mau H, Koch M, Höhne C, Mohnike W, Eberhard T, Fuechtner F, Lorenz-Depiereux B, Mohnike K (2008) Evaluation of [^{18}F]fluoro-L-DOPA positron emission tomography-computed tomography for surgery in focal congenital hyperinsulinism. J Clin Endocrinol Metab 93:869–875
6. Treglia G, Mirk P, Giordano A, Rufini V (2012) Diagnostic performance of fluorine-18-dihydroxyphenylalanine positron emission tomography in diagnosing and localizing the focal form of congenital hyperinsulinism: a meta-analysis. Pediatr Radiol 42(11):1372–1379
7. Otonkoski T, Näntö-Salonen K, Seppänen M, Veijola R, Huopio H, Hussain K, Tapanainen P, Eskola O, Parkkola R, Ekström K, Guiot Y, Rahier J, Laakso M, Rintala R, Nuutila P, Minn H (2006) Noninvasive diagnosis of focal hyperinsulinism of infancy with [^{18}F]-DOPA positron emission tomography. Diabetes 55:13–18

Myocardial Perfusion Imaging with ^{82}Rb Cardiac PET/CT

Emmanuel Deshayes, Stefano Di Bernardo, and John O. Prior

36.1 Introduction

Rubidium-82 (^{82}Rb) has been widely used in North America as a PET radiotracer in myocardial perfusion (MP) imaging in adults since the FDA approved its clinical use in 1989, and it is gaining increasing acceptance in Europe. This potassium analogue has kinetic characteristics similar to those of the well-known myocardial perfusion agent ^{201}Tl. It has a very short half-life (76 s) but it can be produced by eluting a strontium-82 (^{82}Sr)/^{82}Rb generator, without the need for an on-site cyclotron. In addition to relative MP imaging, it allows quantitation of absolute myocardial blood flow (MBF) at rest and under stress, as well as determination of myocardial flow reserve, defined as the ratio of stress to resting MBF.

There is a paucity of data regarding the usefulness of ^{82}Rb cardiac PET in the pediatric population, and there are as yet no published guidelines for the use of cardiac PET/CT in this population. In fact, ^{82}Rb is not included in the 2010 North American Consensus Guidelines on Pediatric Radiopharmaceutical Administered Doses [1] nor in the European Association of Nuclear Medicine (EANM) pediatric dosage chart [2]. Among the few published studies on the use of ^{82}Rb cardiac PET in children, Chhatriwalla et al. described a series of 22 pediatric patients who underwent ^{82}Rb cardiac PET, with a correlation to available coronary angiography in 15 cases [3]. The authors reported a sensitivity and specificity of 100 and 82 %, with positive and negative predictive values of 67 and 100 %. It is worth noting that this small series took over 7 years to collect in a major US hospital.

36.2 Cardiac PET in the Pediatric Population

^{82}RB cardiac PET/CT should be performed with the presence of pediatric cardiologists during the entire procedure. Sedation or anesthesia is not necessarily needed, even for infants, who can be immobilized by dedicated restraints as in general nuclear medicine. In smaller children or infants, dedicated ECG electrodes should be adapted to the body size. The vasodilator adenosine can be used as a stress-inducing pharmacological agent at the same dosage per body weight as in adults (140 µg/kg/min), usually in a 4–6-min slow infusion (Fig. 36.1). Its short biological half-life (<30 s) is advantageous. Patients should be fasted and free from xanthine derivatives for 24 h. Decompensated asthma and

---

E. Deshayes, MD • J.O. Prior, PhD (✉)
Department of Nuclear Medicine,
Lausanne University Hospital, Rue du Bugnon 46,
Lausanne CH-1011, Switzerland
e-mail: emmanuel.deshayes@gmail.com;
john.prior@chuv.ch

S. Di Bernardo, MD
Pediatric Catheterization Laboratory,
Department of Pediatrics, Lausanne University
Hospital, Rue du Bugnon 46, Lausanne
CH-1011, Switzerland
e-mail: stefano.di-bernardo@chuv.ch

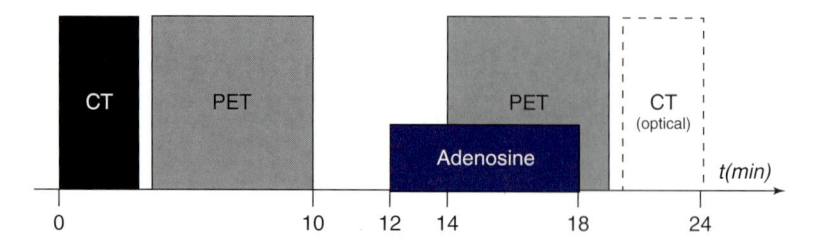

Fig. 36.1 Example of PET/CT protocol with ^{82}Rb with attenuation correction CT. PET was carried out with the patient at rest and during adenosine-induced pharmacological stress, with typical timing indications. The post-stress CT can be omitted in modern systems able to realign the rest attenuation correction CT with the stress PET

significant wheezing are contraindications to the use of adenosine.

As there are no published guidelines regarding optimal ^{82}Rb activity in a pediatric population, in most settings activity has been based on the adult recommended activity, scaled according to body weight and depending on the PET acquisition mode: 20–30 MBq/kg for 2-D and 10 MBq/kg for 3-D, with the latter preferred for use in children. In adults, the effective dose for ^{82}Rb was recently recalculated and is now lower than previously estimated, i.e., 1.1 μSv/MBq or 1.5 mSv for a resting + stress study in a 70-kg adult examined using the latest generation 3-D PET/CT scanner [4]. A dedicated dosimetry study should be carried out in the pediatric population in order to more precisely estimate the received radiation dose, but it is certainly ≤2-fold lower than that incurred with MP imaging using the corresponding technetium tracers.

36.3 ^{82}Rb Cardiac PET Imaging Protocol

As shown in Fig. 36.1, a very low-dose CT (120 kV, 10 mA) is performed first, for attenuation correction mapping. Then, ^{82}Rb is administered intravenously in a slow bolus over 30 s with the patient at rest. PET acquisition is started simultaneously in list mode for 6–8 min while the ECG gating signal is recorded. After the generator recovery period (10 min), pharmacological stress is started with adenosine (0.84 mg/kg for 6 min) infusion using a dual-channel infusion port (adenosine + ^{82}Rb) under 12-channel ECG monitoring. ^{82}Rb is injected intravenously 2 min after the beginning of adenosine infusion and stress images are acquired again in list mode with ECG gating signals for 6–8 min. A final, very low-dose CT (120 kV, 10 mA) for attenuation correction mapping may be performed, but in most cases the initial rest CT can be used for attenuation correction in modern systems able to realign PET and CT images if significant movements occurred between the two datasets.

PET images are generally reconstructed using ordered subset expectation maximization algorithms (OSEM, 2 iterations, 24 subsets). From the list mode, two datasets are extracted: (1) a series starting 2 min after injection and synchronized with the ECG (8 bins) and (2) a dynamic series (22 frames: 12×8, 5×12, 1×30 s, 1×1 and 2×2 min).

For the analysis, semiquantitative image interpretation is performed using a 17-, 20- or 25-segment model. The summed stress score (SSS) and summed resting score (SRS) can be determined, together with the summed difference score (SDS = SSS − SRS). Both the left ventricular ejection fraction (LVEF) at rest and during stress can also be derived. Finally, flow quantification measurements based on a one-tissue compartment model can be used to estimate the absolute values of myocardial blood flow at rest and during stress as well as the myocardial flow reserve.

36.4 Advantages of PET

Compared to MP imaging by SPECT, ^{82}Rb cardiac PET/CT provides several advantages: (a) shorter acquisition times, (b) better spatial resolution,

(c) built-in attenuation correction, (d) lower radiation exposure, and (e) absolute quantitation of MBF, as well as the myocardial flow reserve.

36.5 Clinical Indications

As there are as yet no guidelines for the clinical use of ^{82}Rb MP imaging PET/CT in the pediatric population, potentially useful indications could be as follows: hypertrophic and dilated cardiomyopathies, myocarditis, Kawasaki's disease, and congenital abnormalities, including single ventricle, Fallot's tetralogy, anomalous left coronary artery, unique coronary artery, and transposition of the great vessels [5]. Moreover, particularly relevant to the use of MBF quantitation are research topics such as the development of early endothelial dysfunction in early stages of type 1 diabetes in older children and adolescents [6].

Clinical Case

We report the case of a female infant born with complex congenital anomalies in association with tricuspid valve atresia, pulmonary valve atresia, and a fistula between the left anterior descending (LAD) coronary artery and the right ventricle. At 10 days of life, she underwent a Rashkind procedure and a Blalock–Taussig shunt. One week later, coil occlusion of the fistula between the LAD and right ventricle was performed (Fig. 36.2). At 3 weeks of life, she suffered episodes of ischemic events, with ST depression and cardiac enzyme elevation. The pediatric cardiologist therefore requested an MP imaging study to evaluate perfusion.

Semiquantitative analysis of the cardiac PET/CT showed a clear perfusion defect in the antero-apico-septal territory at rest, which interestingly regressed under adenosine stress (Fig. 36.3). LVEF was estimated to be 54 % at stress and 56 % at rest; these were probably overestimates due to the small size of the patient's heart.

MBF at rest was fairly high, estimated at 2.5 mL/min/g (resting heart rate of 135 min^{-1} with systolic and diastolic blood pressures of 65/35 mmHg, resulting in a rate–pressure product of 8,780 mmHg/min). MBF was 3.7 mL/min/g during adenosine-induced pharmacological stress. This resulted in a myocardial flow reserve of 1.5 (Fig. 36.4).

Following the PET/CT MP imaging study, the pediatric cardiologist and critical care pediatricians added glyceryl trinitrate and systemic vasodilator to the infant's treatment. Clinical improvement ensued, with disappearance of the ST depression, and the patient was weaned off mechanical ventilation.

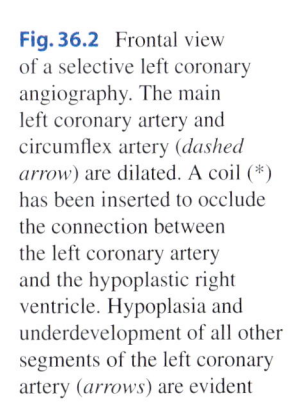

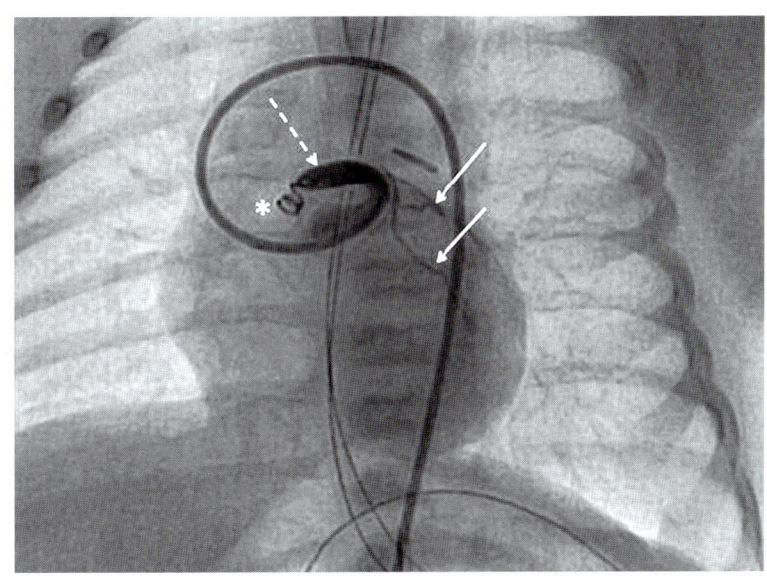

Fig. 36.2 Frontal view of a selective left coronary angiography. The main left coronary artery and circumflex artery (*dashed arrow*) are dilated. A coil (*) has been inserted to occlude the connection between the left coronary artery and the hypoplastic right ventricle. Hypoplasia and underdevelopment of all other segments of the left coronary artery (*arrows*) are evident

Clinical Case (continued)

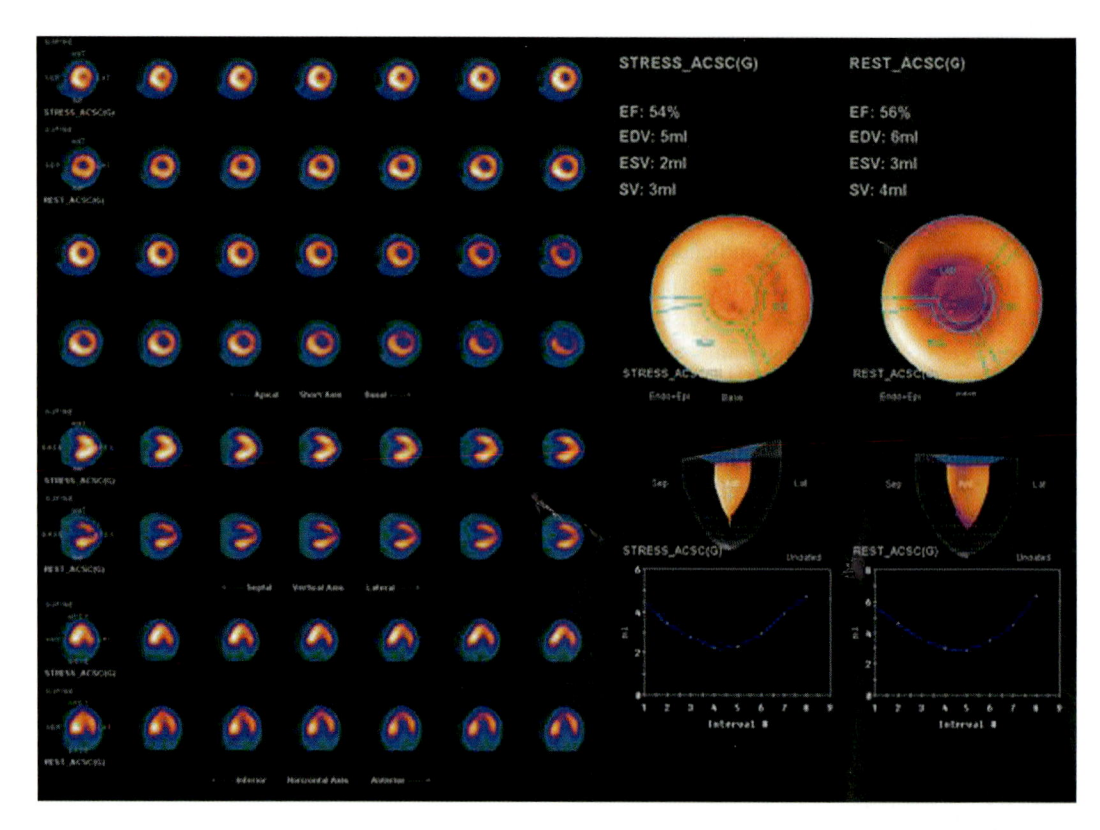

Fig. 36.3 Semiquantitative analysis of ^{82}Rb PET/CT with the patient under stress (summed stress score 1) and at rest (summed rest score 7) shows a clear perfusion defect at rest in the apical-antero-septal territories, which regressed under adenosine stress. The left ventricular ejection fraction was estimated to be 54 % at stress and 56 % at rest; both are probably overestimates due to the small size of the patient's heart

Clinical Case (continued)

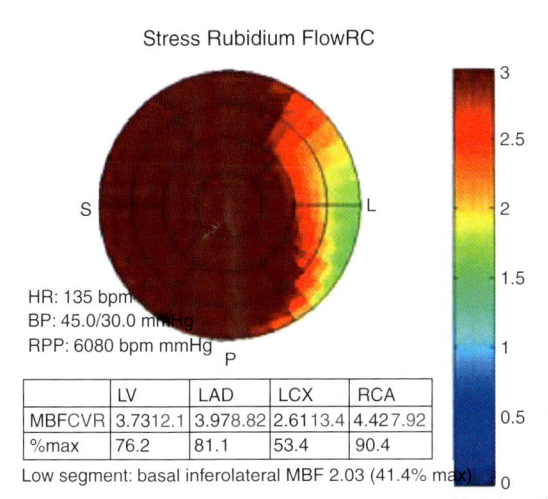

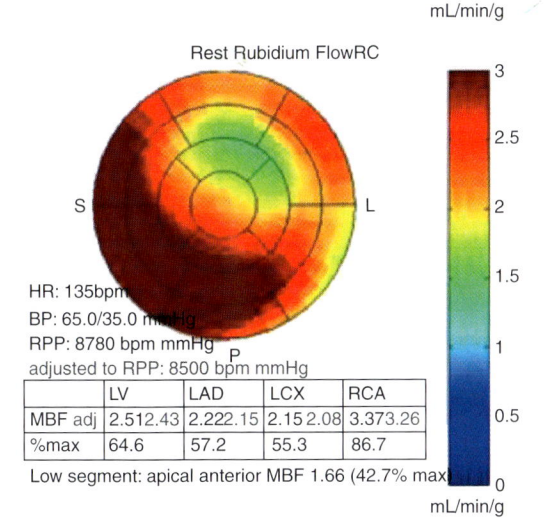

Stress Rubidium FlowRC

HR: 135 bpm
BP: 45.0/30.0 mmHg
RPP: 6080 bpm mmHg

	LV	LAD	LCX	RCA
MBFCVR	3.73 12.1	3.97 8.82	2.61 13.4	4.42 7.92
%max	76.2	81.1	53.4	90.4

Low segment: basal inferolateral MBF 2.03 (41.4% max)
mL/min/g

Stress Rubidium/Rest Rubidium

∇RPP: 0.69

	LV	LAD	LCX	RCA
∇MBF adj	1.54 1.59	1.83 1.89	1.24 1.28	1.33 1.37
%max	71.4	85.0	57.4	61.5

Low segment: basal anterolateral ∇MBF 0.92 (42% max)

Rest Rubidium FlowRC

HR: 135bpm
BP: 65.0/35.0 mmHg
RPP: 8780 bpm mmHg
adjusted to RPP: 8500 bpm mmHg

	LV	LAD	LCX	RCA
MBF adj	2.51 2.43	2.22 2.15	2.15 2.08	3.37 3.26
%max	64.6	57.2	55.3	86.7

Low segment: apical anterior MBF 1.66 (42.7% max)
mL/min/g

Fig. 36.4 Quantitative analysis shows a fairly high myocardial blood flow at rest over both the left ventricle (MBF = 2.5 mL/min/g), with decreased flow in the apical-anterior, and the latero-basal territories. Flow improved, increasing to 3.7 mL/min/g, during adenosine-induced pharmacological stress, albeit with decreased MBF in the latero-basal territory. The myocardial flow reserve was 1.5 over the whole left ventricle

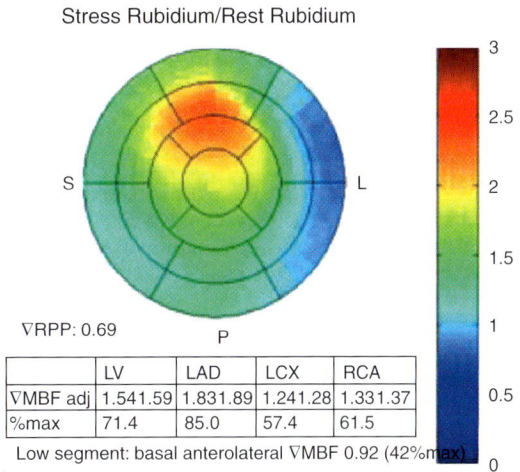

Teaching Points

^{82}RB MP imaging is feasible in pediatric populations, ranging from newborns to adolescents, and offers definite advantages over SPECT, including shorter acquisitions, better spatial resolution, lower radiation exposure, and absolute quantitation of MBF and myocardial flow reserve. There are, however, no guidelines or recommendations concerning its clinical use in children, in whom it has been implemented only in selected cases. Its superiority over other available noninvasive imaging techniques remains to be proven in clinical studies.

References

1. Gelfand MJ, Parisi MT, Treves ST (2011) Pediatric radiopharmaceutical administered doses: North American consensus guidelines (2010). J Nucl Med 52:318–322
2. Lassmann M, Biassoni L, Monsieurs M, Franzius C, Jacobs F, for the EANM Dosimetry and Paediatrics Committees (2008) The new EANM paediatric dosage card. Eur J Nucl Med Molecular Imag 35:1748
3. Chhatriwalla AK, Prieto LR, Brunken RC, Cerqueira MD, Younoszai A, Jaber WA (2008) Preliminary data on the diagnostic accuracy of rubidium-82 cardiac PET perfusion imaging for the evaluation of ischemia in a pediatric population. Pediatr Cardiol 29:732–738
4. Senthamizhchelvan S, Bravo PE, Esaias C, Lodge MA, Merrill J, Hobbs RF, Sgouros G, Bengel FM (2010) Human biodistribution and radiation dosimetry of 82Rb. J Nucl Med 51:1592–1599
5. Movahed A, Gnanasegaran G, Buscombe J, Hall M (eds) (2008) Integrating cardiology for nuclear medicine physicians: a guide to nuclear medicine physicians, 1st edn. Springer, Berlin, London, pp 401–407
6. Prior JO, Quiñones MJ, Hernandez-Pampaloni M, Facta AD, Schindler TH, Sayre JW, Hsueh WA, Schelbert HR (2005) Coronary circulatory dysfunction in insulin resistance, impaired glucose tolerance, and type 2 diabetes mellitus. Circulation 111: 2291–2298

Index

A

Abdomen, 34, 76, 113
Abdominal distension, 114
Abdominal/pelvic abscesses, 4
Abdominal window, 148
Abscesses, 245
ABVD, 33
Acetabulum, 69
Acute lymphoblastic leukemia (ALL), 21, 35, 61, 202
Acute myeloid leukemia, 62, 213
Adenoma, 147
Adenosine+^{82}Rb, 254
Adrenal gland(s), 7, 44, 113
  cancers, 147–149
  carcinoma, 148, 149
Adrenal medulla, 147
Adrenocortical, 147
Aggressive, 169
ALCLs, 35
ALK$^+$, 35
ALL. *See* Acute lymphoblastic leukemia (ALL)
Allelic, 141
ALPS. *See* Autoimmune lymphoproliferative syndrome (ALPS)
Amino acid analogs, 158
Amino acid transporter systems, 158
Amphotericin B, 215
Amygdala, 173
Anaplastic astrocytoma, 157, 173, 175
Anaplastic large B cell lymphoma, 32
Anaplastic large cell lymphoma (ALCL), 33, 35, 50
Anaplastic oligoastrocytoma, 172
Anesthesia, 8
Aneurysmal bone cyst, 67
Ann arbor staging system, 32, 33
Anteriorly, 21
Anterior mediastinum, 19
Aortic arch, 19
Apo-1, 233
Appendicitis, 18, 201–202
Appendicitis inflammatory response (AIR), 201
Arms, 225
Aspergillosis, 4, 213
Aspergillus fumigatus, 213
Ataxic, 168
Attenuation correction, 255

Autoimmune lymphoproliferative syndrome (ALPS), 20, 233–238
Axial bone, 70
Axial fluid attenuated inversion recovery (FLAIR), 159
Axial mediastinal, 71

B

Basal ganglia, 3, 17
B-cell lymphoblastic lymphoma, 35
Benign fibro-osseous lesions, 40
Benzodiazepines, 8
Bevacizumab, 161
Biliary atresia, 170
Biogenic amines, 103
Biomarkers, 158
Bladder, 13
Blade, 125
Blastomas, 4
Bleomycin, etoposide, doxorubicin, cyclophosphamide, vincristine, procarbazine, prednisone (BEACOPP), 33
Blood–brain barrier, 158, 161
Bone involvement, 57
Bone marrow, 17, 57, 116
Bone metastases(is), 114, 124
Bowel, 34
Brain, 76
Brainstem symptoms, 189
Brain tumors, 31, 157
Brain window CT, 167
Breast, 141, 142
Brown adipose tissue, 7
Brown fat, 10
Brown fat activation, 51
Buccal cavity muscles, 7
Bulb, 178
Burkitt's lymphoma (BL), 32–34

C

Carcinoid(s), 99, 104, 106
Carcinoid syndrome, 104
Carcinoma, 137, 147
Cardiac enzyme elevation, 255
Cardiac muscle, 17

Cardiovascular, 39
Cartilaginous disks, 205
Catecholamine metabolites, 114
CD3, 35
CD4, 35
CD5, 35
CD10+, 35
CD15, 31, 32
CD20, 31, 32, 34, 36
CD20–, 35
CD30, 31, 32, 35
CD45, 35
CD79+, 35
CD95, 233
CD1a, 35
CD79a, 31, 32, 36
Celiac lymph nodes, 55
Celiac region, 54
Cell-mediated immunity, 213
Cells, 3
β-Cells, 249
Central nervous system (CNS), 34, 61, 157, 189
Cerebellar medullobastoma, 178
Cerebellum, 175
Cerebral activity, 182
Cerebral cortex, 17
Cerebral tumors, 4
Cervical vertebra, 48
^{11}C-flumazenil, 185
Chemotherapy, 5
Chest, 113
CHI. *See* Congenital hyperinsulinism (CHI)
Cho/Cr ratio, 170
Chondroblastoma, 67
Chondromyxoid fibroma, 67
Chondrosarcoma, 67
^{11}C-hydroxyephedrine (^{11}C-HED), 109
^{11}C-hydroxytryptophan (^{11}C-HTP), 109
Classical Hodgkin's lymphoma (cHL), 31
^{11}C-methionine, 158
α-^{11}C-methyl-l-tryptophan, 185
CNS. *See* Central nervous system (CNS)
Colon, rectum, 104
Congenital biliary atresia, 24
Congenital hyperinsulinism (CHI), 249–251
Consciousness, 170, 189
Conventional closed-mouth acquisition, 7
Coronary angiography, 253
Cortical bone, 70
Cranial nerve, III branch of, 177
Craniopharyngioma, 157
^{11}C-WAY, 185
Cystic, 175
Cystosarcoma phylloides, 141
Cytotoxic T cells, 233

D
Delayed acquisition, 176
Dendritic cells, 4

Denys–Drash syndrome, 54
Dermoid cyst, 151
Diabetic patients, 5
Diametaphyseal junction, 40
Diaphragm, 7, 33
Diaphysis, 17
Diffuse large B-cell lymphoma (DLBCL), 33, 35–36
Diplopia, 168, 175
Diseases (mycobacterial, fungal, and bacterial), 64
Dose distribution, 84
D7S522, 141
D22S264, 141
Dysembryoplastic neuroepithelial tumor (DNET), 166

E
Electroencephalography (EEG), 187
Enchondroma, 67
Endothelial cytotoxicity of shiga-toxin, 189
Eosinophilic granuloma, 67, 212
Ependymoma grade II, 174
Ependymomas, 157
Epilepsy, 181–185
Epileptogenic temporal lobe, 183
Epiphrenic area, 7
Epiphyseal growth cartilage, 22
Epiphysis, 17
Epithelial membrane antigen (EMA), 35
Epstein–Barr virus (EBV), 31, 54, 56, 246
Erector muscle of spine, 70
Event-free survival (EFS), 35, 67
Ewing family of tumors (ESFT), 68
Ewing's sarcoma (EWS), 8, 67, 68, 72, 103
EWS-FLI-1, 68
Excretory system, 122
Extraocular muscles, 7, 9
Extrapulmonary metastases, 75
Extratemporal, 184–185
Eyes, 223

F
Facial muscles, 7
Fas, 233
Fas–FasL, 233
FasL, 233
18F-FDG–PET/CT, 88–90, 131–134
^{18}F-DOPA, 121
Feet, 225, 227
Femora, 118
Femur, 40, 67, 79, 125
Ferrioxamine E (FOXE), 215
Fever of unknown origin (FUO), 245–247
^{18}F-fluorodeoxyglucose (^{18}F-FDG), 109
^{18}F-fluorodopamine (^{18}F-FDA), 109
Fibroadenoma, 141
Fibroblasts, 4, 217
Fibro-epithelial tumors, 141
Fibrosarcoma, 67
Fibrous dysplasia, 67

Index 261

Fibula, 78
Fine-needle aspiration, 137
First lumbar vertebral, 234
Foramen, 70

G
^{68}Ga, 215
GABAergic system, 185
^{67}Ga-citrate, 213
Gadolinium, 157, 174, 175
^{68}Ga-DOTATOC, 121–123
Ganglioglioma, 159, 161, 171
Ganglioneuroma, 113
Gastric disease, 56
Gastroenteropancreatic (GEP) carcinoid tumors, 104
Germinoma, 176
Glial cells, 4
Glial tumor, 168, 170
Gliomas, 157
Gliomatosis cerebri, 159
Glucose transporter (GLUT), 3
GLUT-13, 3
Gluteus, 69
GLUT-1 transporters, 3, 245
GLUT-2 transporters, 245
Gonads, 143
Granulocyte(s), 17, 245
Granulomatous reactions, 228
Gray matter, 190

H
Headache, 168, 177
Head–neck region, 48
Hemangioma, 67
Hemiparesis, 189
Hemolytic anemia, 189
Hemolytic-uremic syndrome (HUS), 189–194
Hemorrhage, 169
Hemosiderin deposits, 168
Heparinized, 13
Hepatoblastoma, 5
Hexokinase, 3
Hilar, 33
HIV, 245
HIV infection, 34
Hodgkin's lymphoma (HL), 22, 31–33, 142, 210, 218
Human herpesvirus-8 (HHV-8), 241
Humerus, 22
HUS. *See* Hemolytic-uremic syndrome (HUS)
Hyaline vascular variant (HVV), 241
Hydrocele, 246
Hyperinsulinism, 251
Hyperplasia of thymus, 51

I
IBD. *See* Inflammatory bowel disease (IBD)
Ictal, 181

Ileocecal area, 34
Iliac, 124
Iliac bone, 69, 70, 125
^{123}I-MIBG, 121
Immature teratomas, 151
Immunocompetent tissues, 17
Immunodeficiency-related BL, 34
Infected joint prostheses, 4
Inferior frontal gyrus, 159
Inflammatory acne, 26
Inflammatory bowel disease (IBD), 199–200
Inflammatory infiltrate, 31
Inflammatory pathologies, 18
Inguinal regions, 225
Insular, 137
Intercostal muscles, 7
Interictal, 181
Interleukin-2 (IL-2), 119
Interleukin-6 (IL-6), 241
Intervertebral disc, 206
Intestinal inflammation, 200
Intra-axial tumors, 157
Intralesional bleeding, 176
Invasive fungal infections (IFIs), 213
Isotretinoin, 119

J
Jaw, 177

K
Kidney(s), 3, 7, 143
Kidney dysfunction, 241
Kingella kingae, 205
Kinsbourne syndrome, 114

L
Large bowel, 24
Large cell non-Hodgkin's lymphoma, 26
Lateral pterygoid muscles, 9
Laterocervical lymphadenopathy, 233
Laterocervical regions, 10
Laterocervical regions of neck, 7
LBL of B-cell origin (B-LBL), 35
Left anterior descending (LAD), 255
Left brachiocephalic vein, 17, 21
Left cavernous sinus, 177
Left common carotid artery, 21
Left frontal white matter, 160
Left laterocervical region, 225
Left lung hilus, 108
Left parietal cortex, 160
Left posterior, 11
Legs, 79, 226, 228
Lesions, 170
Lethal liver disease, 24
Leukemia, 31, 113
Leukocytes, 3, 245

Li–Fraumeni syndrome, 67
Liver, 3, 76
 carcinoids, 104
 lesions, 44
 transplantation, 24, 170
L3-L5 vertebral, 118
LSA2-L2-like, 35
Lumbar region, 205
Lung(s), 57
 metastases, 72
 nodules, 72
Lymphadenopathy, 17
Lymphatic polyclonal disorder, 243
Lymph node(s), 137, 223
Lymphoblastic lymphoma (LBL), 32, 33, 247
Lymphocyte, 233
Lymphocyte-depleted, 31
Lymphocyte predominant (LP), 32
Lymphocyte-rich, 31
Lymphocytes macrophages, 4
Lymphoepithelial tissues, 17
Lymphoid structure, 33
Lymphoma(s), 4, 31, 147

M
Macrophages, 217
Malignant peripheral nerve sheath tumors (MPNST), 229
Malignant teratoma, 153
Maxillary sinusitis, 27
Maximal intensity projection (MIP), 4, 24
Mechloretamine, vincristine, procarbazine and prednisone (MOPP), 32
Medial and lateral rectus, 9
Mediastinal, 14, 15, 17, 34, 81, 246
Mediastinum, 7, 14, 34, 225
Medulloblastoma, 157
MEN types IIA, 104
MEN types IIB, 104
Mesenchymal stem, 67
Mesenteric lymph node, 45
Metaiodobenzylguanidine (MIBG), 114
Metaphyseal portions, 67
Metaphysis, 40
Metastasectomy, 72
Metastases(is), 72, 147
Metastatic disease, 72
Microangiopathy, 189
Mixed cellularity, 31
Monocytes/macrophages, 245
Mouth, 9
Multifocal Langerhans cell histiocytosis, 212
Multiple endocrine neoplasia (MEN), 103
Muscles, 5, 76
MYC, 34
MYCN, 113
Mycobacteriosis, 217–218
Mycobacterium avium intracellulare complex (MAC), 217
Myelolipoma, 147
Myocardial blood flow (MBF), 253
Myositis, 53

N
NAA/Cr ratio, 170
Nasal cavity, 226
Nasopharyngeal carcinoma (NPC), 131
Nasopharyngeal tonsils, 17
Nasopharynx, 17, 23
NB. *See* Neuroblastoma (NB)
Neck, 113, 119
Necrotic, 175
Neocortical, 184
NETs. *See* Neuroendocrine tumors (NETs)
Neuroblastoma (NB), 103, 113, 118, 147
Neuroblastoma stage IV, 124
Neuroectodermal cells, 113
Neuroendocrine tumors (NETs), 103, 109
Neurofibromatosis 1 (NF-1), 103, 229
Neurofibromatosis (NF), 229–231
Neurogenic tumors, 231
Neuronal, 189
Neutropenic, 245
Neutrophil granulocytes, 217
Neutrophils, 245
NF-1. *See* Neurofibromatosis 1 (NF-1)
NK cells, 233
Nodular lymphocyte predominant Hodgkin's lymphoma (NLPHL), 31, 32
Nodular sclerosis, 31
Non-Hodgkin's lymphoma (NHL), 19, 31
Nonossifying fibroma, 40, 67
NPM-ALK translocation, 35
NPV, 77

O
Octreotide, 107
O-(2-[^{18}F]fluoroethyl)-l-tyrosine, 158
Old, 168
Open-mouth acquisition, 7
Oral cavity, 5
Orbicular muscles, 9
Oropharynx, 17
Osteoarthritis, 48
Osteoblastoma, 67
Osteochondroma, 67
Osteogenic sarcoma (OS), 67
Osteoma, 67
Osteosarcoma, 7, 67
Osteosarcoma of humerus, 74
Otalgia, 168
Oval foramina, 177
Ovarian follicle, 18, 47
Ovarian teratoma, 151
Ovaries, 17

P
Paget's disease, 67
Palatine tonsils, 23
Pancreasectomy, 249
Pancreatic β-cells, 249
Paragangliomas, 103–104

Para-hippocampus, 173
Paraneoplastic syndrome, 246
Paravertebral regions, 11
Paravertebral thoracic regions, 7
Parotid glands, 226
Partial complex, 183
Partial seizures, 182
Patella, 227
Peduncle, 178
Pelvis, 18, 47, 70, 109
Pericolic lymph node, 25
Peri-orbital, 34
Peri-skeletal soft tissue, 81
Peritoneal, 152
PET/MRI fusion image, 159
Pheochromocytoma(s), 103–104, 109, 147
Photopenic, 171
Phylloid tumor, 141, 142
Phylloid tumor of breast, 141–142
Pilocytic astrocytomas, 157
Piriform muscles, 69
Plasma cell variant (PCV), 241
Pleural, 34
Plexiform neurofibroma (PNF), 229, 230
Pons, 169, 178
Poorly differentiated thyroid carcinoma, 137–140
Portal node, 33
Posterior right, 11
Posttransplantation, 34
Posttransplantation lymphoproliferative diseases (PTLD), 4, 18
Posttransplantation lymphoproliferative disorders (PTLD), 35, 54, 56
PPV, 77
Primary tumor, 5
Primitive neuroectodermal tunor (PNET), 25
Protein synthesis, 158
Proximal humerus, 50, 67
Proximal right tibia, 49
Proximal tibia, 67
Proximal ureter, 122
Pseudoprogression, 158
Pseudoresponse, 158, 161
PTLD. *See* Posttransplantation lymphoproliferative diseases; Posttransplantation lymphoproliferative disorders
Pulmonary, 39
    aspergillosis, 213
    hilar region, 224, 225
    valve atresia, 255

R
Radioimmunotherapy, 138
Radionecrosis, 174
Radiotherapy, 5
Radiotherapy planning, 157
Reed–Sternberg (RS) cells, 31, 32
Renal pelvis, 122
Rhabdomyosarcoma (RMS), 87
Right bowel, 25

Right cerebral hemisphere, 159
Right femur, 49
Right knee, 225, 227
Right laterocervical lymph nodes, 63
Right scapula, 50
Right tibia, 41
Rothmund–Thomson syndrome, 67
Rubidium-82 (^{82}Rb), 253, 254

S
Sacral/sacrum, 70
Salivary glands, 223
Sarcoidosis, 64
Sarcomas, 4, 5
Scalp, 76
Scenium™, normalization, 193
Sedation, 8
Seizures, 183
Serotonin, 104
Simple bone cyst, 67
Sinusitis, 27
Skeletal muscle(s), 8, 223
Skull, 116, 166
Soft-tissue infections, 4
Soft-tissue sarcomas (STS), 87
Solid neoplasm, 157
Spectroscopy, 170
Spine, 117
Spleen/splenic, 17, 33, 42, 45, 152
Spoiled gradient recalled (SPGR) sequence MRI, 175
Spondylodiscitis, 4, 205–206
Squamous carcinoma, 7
Standard uptake value (SUV), 250
Staphylococcus aureus, 205
Statistical parametric mapping (SPM), 190
Sternum, 50
Sternum beyond spine, 22
Stomach, 54, 55
Strabismus, 168
Striatum, 159
Strontium-82 (^{82}Sr), 253
Subdiaphragmatic region, 57
Sub-glissonian, 152
Superior frontal gyrus lesion, 170
Superior mediastinum, 21
Supraclavicular regions, 10
Supradiaphragmatic lymph nodes, 41, 42
Supradiaphragmatic region, 57
Supratentorial tumors, 157
Surgery, 5

T
Tachykinin, 104
Tacrolimus, 24
^{99m}Tc-antimicrobial, 214
T-cell lymphoblastic lymphoma, 35, 177
T-cell lymphoproliferative, 56
^{99m}Tc-fluconazole, 214
^{99m}Tc-interleukin-8, 214

^{99m}Tc-1, 214
TdT, 34
TdT+, 35
Temozolomide, 172, 173
Temporal lobe, 183
Temporal pole, 183
Temporomandibular joint, 246
Terminal ileum, 25
Testes, 17
T2/FLAIR MRI, 161
Thrombocytopenia, 189
Thrombotic vasculitis, 189
Thymic, 34
Thymus, 17, 19–21, 33
Thyroid, 39
Tibia(s), 40
TP53, 141
Transverse colon, 24
Treatment planning, 158
Triacetylfusarinine (TAFC), 215
Tricuspid, 255
Trochlear area, 225
Tuberculosis, 4, 217, 245
Tumor-like disorders, 67
Tumor necrosis factor receptor (TNFR), 233
T1-weighted, 159

U
Ulcerative colitis (UC), 199
Urinary bladder, 122

V
Vascular, 170
  endothelial growth factor, 161
  inflammations, 245
Vasculitis, 4
Vasoactive peptides, 104
Vertebra, 58
VHL. *See* von Hippel–Lindau (VHL) disease
Visual disturbances, 189
Vomiting, 177
von Hippel–Lindau (VHL) disease, 103, 104

W
Waldeyer's ring, 17, 33
Warburg effect, 4
WBC scintigraphy, 245
Werner syndrome, 67
Wilms tumor (WT), 54, 143–145

Printing and Binding: Stürtz GmbH, Würzburg